Psychiatry in Primary Care

Fourth Edition

Patricia R. Casey
Richard Byng

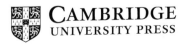

CAMBRIDGE
UNIVERSITY PRESS

CAMBRIDGE UNIVERSITY PRESS
Cambridge, New York, Melbourne, Madrid, Cape Town,
Singapore, São Paulo, Delhi, Tokyo, Mexico City

Cambridge University Press
The Edinburgh Building, Cambridge CB2 8RU, UK

Published in the United States of America by Cambridge University Press, New York

www.cambridge.org
Information on this title: www.cambridge.org/9780521759823

Fourth edition © Cambridge University Press 2011

First edition published by Wrightson Biomedical Publishing 1990
Second edition published by Wrightson Biomedical Publishing 1997
Third edition published by Wrightson Biomedical Publishing 2005
Fourth edition published by Cambridge University Press 2011

Printed in the United Kingdom at the University Press, Cambridge

A catalogue record for this publication is available from the British Library

Library of Congress Cataloguing in Publication data
Casey, Patricia R., 1952– author.
Psychiatry in primary care / Patricia R. Casey and Richard Byng. – Fourth Edition.
  p. ; cm.
Includes bibliographical references and index.
ISBN 978-0-521-75982-3 (pbk.)
1. Psychiatry. 2. Primary care (Medicine) I. Byng, Richard, author.
II. Casey, Patricia R. Guide to psychiatry in primary care. revision of (work). III. Title.
[DNLM: 1. Mental Disorders. 2. Primary Health Care. WM 140]
RC454.4.C374 2011
616.89–dc22   2010051570

ISBN 978-0-521-75982-3 Paperback

To my sons – James and Gavan McGuiggan

– Patricia Casey

To my wife Melanie and children, Joe, Felix and Calypso

– Richard Byng

Contents

Section 5 The wider mental health system

Preface to the fourth edition

The book aims to support family doctors and other primary care practitioners in providing care to the very many people with mental health problems at some time in their lives. As a psychiatrist and general practitioner, we have written this book together in order to find the best of both perspectives. We are determined both to lay bare the complexities and also to identify relatively straightforward solutions to the problems practitioners face. Primary care clinicians do not need to choose between the medical or social models of illness; it is possible to embrace both with skill and flexibility, in the consultation and from a public health perspective. This book is a synthesis of evidence, experience and a modern patient-orientated and evidence-informed approach to primary care psychiatry.

In the consultation, family practitioners need to be able to make diagnoses as a part of an overall formulation, ensuring the needs of the individual, rather than simply a label, and define the content of care provided. NICE and other agencies have produced guidance on the diagnosis and management of mental illness by GPs. These guidelines make it sound easy by promoting a 'detect and treat' model of care. But many GPs doubt the relevance of this simplified approach to the complexities of primary mental health care. Instead they need a framework for integrating psychiatric diagnoses and evidence-based treatment with an approach which values the strengths of individuals, their preferences for treatment and the often complex social context of their lives.

Furthermore, strong psycho-social currents are at work in the consulting room. The stigma of mental illness and a healthy desire to be independent may prevent some from engaging with care. Conversely, the security afforded by a diagnosis might lead to dependence on the doctor and over-treatment. Negotiating these dilemmas requires knowledge and skills. This book aims to support the reflective practitioner.

It will also provide important information on the epidemiology of common and rarer conditions, the likely co-morbidities and the latest evidence on treatment. This is useful as a resource when facing uncertainties in the consulting room. This information, alongside the chapters on health services, in the final section of the book, provides ammunition for those wishing to engage in quality improvement and redesigning services.

While our book is aimed largely at general practitioners, we are confident that other mental health professionals, such as psychiatrists in training and public health specialists with an interest in mental health, will also find this book useful. Placing the patient in the context of their social network, be it family, friends or local community, it provides a perspective that is often lacking in the mainstream text books of psychiatry. We hope that the case vignettes we have provided, based on real patients, will bridge the gap between theory and practice and bring to life the complexities of treating mental health problems whether in a general practice setting or an outpatient clinic.

Foreword

It is a pleasure to provide the foreword for the most recent edition of this well-respected textbook. On this occasion Patricia Casey has joined forces with Richard Byng to provide an integrated set of perspectives drawn from their clinical and academic backgrounds across psychiatry and primary care. Aided by judicious collaborations with a range of colleagues from related disciplines, the result is a text even richer and more valuable than we found in previous editions.

Psychiatric problems are common in primary care, with about one-third of consultations having a mental health component to them. There have been considerable advances in both the assessment and management of such problems during the past three decades, and these are well represented in the breadth and scope of this excellent book. This volume will be of great benefit to doctors and other health professionals working in primary care, particularly those in training and early in their professional careers. For those of us who are longer in the tooth and feel set in our ways, it also brings fresh evidence and new insights.

The book is well organized and easy to follow, with chapters embedded within several clearly defined sections. Each chapter begins with specific learning objectives, which enable readers to orientate themselves to the key elements within it, and ends with a focused summary of essential points. The texts include a very helpful combination of formal psychiatric diagnostic information, research evidence and detailed worked case examples. References include reading relevant to family and patients, useful websites and contact points with relevant third-sector organizations.

The first section begins with a clear exposition of the scale of psychiatric problems in primary care, combining epidemiological perspectives with valuable insights into the context within which primary care is delivered, including the centrality and scope of the consultation. It moves on to an effective exposition of current psychiatric classifications and how they may be applied in primary care.

The next section provides a clear and helpful exposition of the diagnosis and management of the mental disorders found most commonly in primary care. It includes important and updated chapters on adjustment problems (including grief reactions) and personality disorders, both of which are less well understood within primary care than anxiety, depression or substance misuse – and both of which draw on the particular research and clinical expertise of Patricia Casey. The role and limitations of pharmacological approaches are carefully considered, and practitioners are encouraged to think beyond the reflex movement towards the prescription pad. The particular contribution of primary care to the management of physical health problems in schizophrenia is highlighted. The assessment and management of suicidal ideation is sensitively addressed, and there is a strong chapter on psychosomatic problems as they present in primary care, including evidence-based proposals drawn from Richard Byng's experience of creating effective management structures.

Psychiatric disorders through the life cycle are addressed by several contributors. The section on children focuses helpfully on common behavioural disorders, and provides practical tips for their management, while the adolescent chapter includes essential information on the early detection of psychosis. Dementia and depression are common in older patients, and their differentiation and management are effectively described.

The next section, on evidence-based psychological interventions, explains the principles and application of cognitive behaviour therapy, problem-solving therapy, solution-focused therapy and counselling. This is followed by chapters on family therapy and interventions for sexual problems. These chapters are helpful reading for primary care practitioners in providing insights into how these therapeutic approaches operate, even if they are felt to be beyond our own set of skills or aptitudes. Some aspects, such as the use of genograms as part of problem formulation, may well prove beneficial for many clinicians within their routine practice. An invaluable new resource is the inclusion of a set of audiotapes providing practising clinicians with 'how-to-do-it' introductions to the three main psychological therapies discussed in the text.

In the final section the focus becomes broader, looking at the wider systems within which primary care practitioners operate and how these can be brought to bear for the benefit of practitioners and – importantly – their patients. New models of care, both existing and envisaged, are described in ways that encourage innovative thinking. This is particularly pertinent for practitioners in the UK, during the current period of major turbulence and upheaval in the organization and delivery of our health services.

Christopher Dowrick
Professor of Primary Medical Care
University of Liverpool, UK

Authors and guest contributors

Authors

Patricia R. Casey
Professor of Psychiatry,
University College, Dublin; and
Consultant Psychiatrist, Mater
Misericordiae University Hospital, Dublin,
Ireland

Richard Byng
Clinical Senior Lecturer,
Primary Care Group, Institute of Health
Services Research, Peninsula College of
Medicine and Dentistry, University of
Plymouth, UK

Guest contributors

Gerard J. Butcher
CBT Therapist, Dublin, Ireland

M. Elena Garralda
Professor of Child and Adolescent
Psychiatry, Academic Unit of Child and
Adolescent Psychiatry, Imperial College
London, St Mary's Campus,
London, UK

Daniel Hacking
Specialist Registrar in Psychiatry,
St Charles Hospital, London, UK

Mary Kerrisk
Assistant Director of Nursing,
South Lee Adult Mental Health Services,
Cork, Ireland

Maja Lelandais
Community Development Worker,

BME Mental Health and Wellbeing, Health
Promotion Devon, NHS Devon, South
Molton, Devon, UK

Breda McLeavey
Principal Psychologist and Clinical
Neuropsychologist,
Manager HSE South Lee Psychology
Services, Cork University Hospital, Cork,
Ireland

Chukumeka Maxwell
Senior Community Development Worker,
BME Mental Health and Wellbeing,
Health Promotion Devon, NHS Devon,
and Torbay Care Trust Universal Services
Directorate Provider Service, Culm
Valley Integrated Centre for Health,
Cullompton, UK

James de Pury
Project Manager for IAPT,
South West Development Centre,
Bridgwater, Somerset, UK

Neill Richardson
IAPT Clinical Lead – Plymouth Options,
NHS Plymouth, UK

Raghuram Shivram
Consultant Child and Adolescent
Psychiatrist, Leicestershire Child and
Adolescent Mental Health Services, UK

Nigel Smith
Family and Systemic Psychotherapist,
Plymouth Psychotherapy Department,
NHS Plymouth, UK

Aaron K. Vallance
Clinical Research Fellow, Academic Unit of Child and Adolescent Psychiatry, Imperial College London, St Mary's Campus, London, UK

Panos Vostanis,
Professor of Child and Adolescent Psychiatry, University of Leicester, Greenwood Institute of Child Health, Leicester, UK

James Warner
Consultant/Reader in Old Age Psychiatry, St Charles Hospital, London, UK

Graeme Webster
Cognitive Behavioural Psychotherapist, Plymouth Options, NHS Plymouth, UK

Cornelis de Wet,
Consultant Psychiatrist, Dorset Healthcare University NHS Foundation Trust, UK

Acknowledgements

I am indebted to the many GP's who read the previous editions of this book and who offered insightful advise for this one. I am grateful to the contributors who so willing rose to the challenge of contributing to the book and the accompanying DVD, some at very short notice. My husband and sons showed immense patience at my many hours of absence as I worked on this edition. Finally with the immense enthusiasm and commitment of my co-author Richard Byng this project would never have come to fruition.

– Patricia Casey

I am grateful to all the people with mental health problems I have had contact with in my clinical work; suffering or coping in admirable ways, I have learnt so much from them. I am also indepted to colleagues from around the UK and beyond, particularly the band of practitioners linked to the Royal College of GPs mental health forum and other networks, with whom so many challenging and creative encounters have emerged. And of course thanks to Patricia Casey for both generously allowing me to add a generalist stance to the book, while also quietly keeping me on the right track.

– Richard Byng

Chapter

Scope and extent of mental health problems in primary care

Learning objectives

Knowledge of the prevalence of psychiatric morbidity in the general population
Knowledge of the prevalence of psychiatric morbidity in primary care, detected and undetected

Primary care clinicians provide the majority of care and treatment for adults with mental illness, particularly those suffering from depression and anxiety ('common mental health problems'), but also those with 'severe mental illness'. This chapter outlines the extent of mental health problems and psychiatric disorders in the community as a whole and in the primary care setting. Each chapter in Sections 2 and 3 of the book provides more detailed information about the epidemiology of individual conditions.

Patients' lives and illnesses are complicated and interlinked and while each is unique, there is value in understanding the extent of different mental health problems. Hence the need for excellent epidemiological studies, based on psychiatric definitions and linked to measures of deprivation and social adversity. GPs do not need to choose between the medical or social models of illness; it is possible to embrace both with skill and flexibility, in the consultation and from a public health perspective. Studies of pathways to care, from the community, to the consulting room, and from recognition to onward referral are important, both to help us plan and also to evaluate health systems. Understanding the prevalence of different conditions in the social context will support GP commissioners to design more effective care.

'Common mental illness' is generally a euphemism for non-psychotic diagnoses. The 'worried well' can actually be 'worried sick'. As well as depression, anxiety and adjustment disorder, it includes other neuroses such as post-traumatic stress disorder (PTSD), obsessive-compulsive disorder (OCD) and specific phobias. Scales such as the GHQ provide an estimate of the severity and extent of common mental health problems in the individual and community. Often patients have associated drug and alcohol dependence, and chronic physical conditions which also affect their mental health. Patients' personalities add further complexity both because of the symptoms presented, and the way in which patients engage with their doctors. Personality disorder is rarely diagnosed in primary care, and though not strictly an illness, recognition can be useful when planning treatment since it may impact on the doctor–patient relationship. In comparison severe mental illness is relatively uncommon, yet the role of primary care can be critical for early diagnosis as well as ongoing mental and physical care.

Psychiatric epidemiology has mostly been concerned with studies of prevalence rather than incidence as even common mental health problems are often long-term or recurrent.

Prevalence studies might look at lifetime prevalence (proportion affected over a lifetime), annual prevalence or point prevalence (morbidity at a point in time). Measures include specific diagnoses (either estimated or based on diagnostic interviews) and general measures of morbidity (e.g. GHQ), and also of associated social problems. Mortality is also important, particularly related to suicide and to the excess death rate from physical illness seen in people with severe mental illness.

Psychiatric illness in the community

Total psychiatric morbidity in the community can only be ascertained by screening whole communities or by studying representative samples from them. Despite some efforts in the early part of the twentieth century the first such study was conducted in 1956, when a community sample in Sweden was interviewed to determine the distribution of both personality disorder and psychiatric disorder using predetermined criteria. Of that population, 8.5% had evidence of definite psychiatric disorder and a further 45% possible or probable psychiatric disorder. Personality disorder and the neuroses predominated. After a lull, the early 1960s ushered in a number of epidemiological studies, mainly from the United States. These found that between 45% and 81% of the population had psychological problems, suggesting that psychological dysfunction was the norm! These early attempts, whilst well-meaning in their intentions, were criticized for the broadness of their concepts of psychological dysfunction and for their failure to use diagnostic labels. They do, however, provide a foretaste of the ongoing debates relating to defining psychiatric morbidity simply in terms of symptom numbers with relatively arbitrary cut-offs rather than being grounded in a number of dimensions that include personality, social context and symptom patterns.

Goldberg and his colleagues developed the General Health Questionnaire (GHQ) in the 1970s, which adopted cut-off scores to define the threshold for psychiatric disturbance. The GHQ does not provide a definitive diagnosis but gives an indication of those likely to be ill at a single point in time. Of those interviewed, 11% had scores in the range suggestive of illness and these were mainly women (Goldberg et al. 1976). Slightly higher figures have been found by others using this schedule.

A further development in the detection of psychiatric illness was the use of the structured interview, which both standardized the interview, thereby improving reliability, and provided a diagnosis. This was the approach adopted in the famous study by Robins et al. (1984). Known as the Epidemiological Catchment Area (ECA) study it measured psychiatric disturbance at five sites scattered throughout the USA according to DSM-III criteria (see Chapter 4). A 1-year prevalence ranging from 13.7 to 15.2% and a lifetime prevalence from 23 to 25.2% was found, with major depression, substance abuse and phobias predominating.

The National Co-Morbidity Survey (NCS) (Kessler et al. 1994) was conducted among 8, 000 adults throughout the USA and the diagnostic schedules were administered by trained lay interviewers. An extraordinarily high lifetime rate of almost 50% for any psychiatric disorder was found and the rate for 1 year was 30%. Major depression, alcohol dependence, social phobia and simple phobias were the most common disorders. Fewer than 40% with a lifetime disorder had received professional help, whilst fewer than 20% with a recent disorder had been on drug treatment. Major depression and anxiety were more common among women and the reverse applied to substance use disorders and antisocial personality disorder. However, these data were re-analysed using criteria that incorporated information on the impact of symptoms on functioning and relationships and using this more stringent methodology the 1-year rate for any disorder dropped to 18.5%, of which 16% were rated as mild and the rest moderate, serious and severe (Narrow *et al.* 2002). These findings led to criticism that many of these so-called disorders might in fact be normal reactions to life events which generally resolve spontaneously with time.

One of the early studies in Britain set out to investigate psychiatric illness in the community (Casey and Tyrer 1986), in which the investigators attempted to measure the prevalence of all psychiatric disorders including personality disorder and social functioning: 8% met the criteria for psychiatric disorder and depressive illness predominated; 13% of those interviewed also had personality disorder independent of illness and the emotionally unstable (borderline) type was the most common.

A much larger study, the National Psychiatric Morbidity Surveys (Jenkins *et al.* 1997), selected 13 000 adults aged between 16 and 65 for interview. Over 10 000 were assessed using structured interviews for the presence of neurotic disorders as well as alcohol and drug dependence by lay interviewers. Psychiatrists evaluated the presence of psychotic disorders. Overall 16% of subjects scored above the cut-off for any neurotic disorder. Men had a 1-week period prevalence of 12.3% and women of 19.5%. Those who were married and those in social class 1 had the lowest rates and urban dwellers the highest. All disorders were significantly more common in women with the exception of panic disorder, which was equally prevalent in both. Surprisingly generalized anxiety was more common than depressive episode (3.1% vs. 2.1%), followed by obsessive-compulsive disorder (1.2%) and phobias (1.1%). For psychotic disorders the 1-year prevalence was 0.4%, being equally common in both sexes, and for alcohol and drug dependence the prevalence was 4.7% and 2.2% respectively, with a large male preponderance in each.

Although the overall prevalence of disorder was similar in both studies, after re-analysis of the NCS data the pattern of diagnoses differed from the Jenkins study (1997), pointing to the problems of generalizing from data obtained in one country to another with a very different culture.

Other countries have conducted similar surveys. For example, a study in Australia (Andrews *et al.* 2001) also using a structured interview found that 23% met the criteria for a disorder in the previous year and 14% for a current disorder but only 35% had consulted for this (Andrews *et al.* 2001).

Psychiatric illness in primary care

There are two components to epidemiological investigations in primary care – one relates to studies of psychiatric morbidity among those consulting, but not necessarily disclosing this or being identified as having a mental health problem. The second deals with studies of those identified by their general practitioner as having a psychiatric disorder. The latter is often referred to as conspicuous psychiatric morbidity and the difference between both components is a measure of the level of unrecognized psychiatric morbidity in primary care.

Studies of both of these elements were pioneered by Goldberg and Blackwell (1970), who assessed 553 consecutive attendees at a general practitioner's surgery using the GHQ to measure the extent to which psychological factors contributed to the consultation. Some degree of psychiatric disturbance was found in 24.4%, but only 7.8% had entirely psychiatric illness. Over a quarter had mild or subclinical disturbances. A similar study (Goldberg *et al.* 1976) showed that 33% of consecutive attendees at a surgery had scores on the GHQ suggestive of psychiatric disturbance and that 12% of attendees were not so identified by their doctor. And while the GHQ is not a diagnostic instrument, these studies point to the magnitude of the problem of psychological distress and morbidity in the primary care setting over and above that in the community.

More recent studies have continued to identify even higher prevalence rates for mental illness in primary care. For instance a multi-practice study involving 86 practices in Belgium (Ansseau *et al.* 2002) found an overall prevalence for all disorders of 42.5%, with mood disorders predominating (31%) while anxiety and somatoform disorders were next in frequency (19 and 18% respectively) followed by alcohol abuse/dependence (10.1%). These figures represent evaluation of the total population of consulters and must be set against the actual proportion (5.4%) who stated their reason for consultation as due to mental health problems. A study from Denmark (Toft *et al.* 2005) found an even higher prevalence, with 50% of those attending with a new complaint meeting ICD-10 criteria for a mental disorder and one-third having more than one disorder. As in other studies mental disorders were higher in women and for specific diagnoses 35.9% had somatoform disorders, 13.5% mood disorders, 16.4% anxiety disorders and 2.2% alcohol abuse. Rates increased with increasing age. These increasing rates of mental health problems, seen dramatically in repeated surveys of teenage girls using the GHQ, may be due to increased morbidity but it is also possible that the general and specific diagnostic instruments are performing differently as individuals become more used to and willing to disclose emotions (Sweeting *et al.* 2009).

Detected psychiatric morbidity in primary care

While much focus has been directed at those whose illnesses are not detected, it is important to consider the profile and diagnostic status of those who are identified with mental illness, also termed conspicuous psychiatric morbidity. This can include both illness which is recognized and that which is actually discussed or treated. Studies in this area date back half a century when, using case note identification, in a single practice, Kessel (1960) found that 9% of the sample had psychiatric illness and a further 5% had personality abnormalities independent of illness. Both were more common in women than men and consisted of anxiety states and hypochondriacal and depressive reactions. Only 10% were referred to the specialist services. A number of multi-practice studies were then conducted; Shepherd *et al.* (1966) is the most quoted. A random sample of case notes was selected from 12 London practices and the GP identified the reason for consultation in the subsequent year. In addition, each patient was classified into one of the major diagnostic categories. Overall the neuroses predominated (8.8%) and formal psychiatric illness was identified in 10.2%, but when psychosocial and 'psychiatric associated' conditions were included the total with psychiatric morbidity was 13.9%. With the exception of personality disorder, all disorders were higher in women than men. Although the broad diagnostic categories of illness were identified, no attempt at a more specific classification was made. This last study showed a staggering nine-fold inter-practice variation in reported morbidity.

Others have identified a psychiatric component in 40% of the consulting population (Skuse and Williams 1984) and correcting for the fact that only a subsample was seen, a prevalence of 26% for depression and of 8% for other diagnoses was estimated. Casey and colleagues (1984; 1990) investigated the diagnostic breakdown of those with conspicuous morbidity, in an inner-city and in a rural practice. Assessments were made clinically and using structured interviews. This study was unusual in that it was the first of its kind to assess personality independent of illness. Using the general practitioner to screen for psychiatric disorder a prevalence of 5% was found; 33% of these also had personality disorders. Depressive illness predominated, followed by anxiety states and adjustment reactions. A large-scale study of the prevalence of psychiatric illness in primary care under the aegis of the World Health Organization was carried out among 15 international centres (Sartorius *et al.* 1993). Almost 26 000 subjects were screened using a structured interview schedule and 243 per 1000 of the sample were diagnosed with at least one of depressive illness, anxiety or alcohol-related disorders. A recent study (Rait *et al.* 2009) using the Health Improvement Network (THIN) electronic scheme found that between 1996 and 2006 the incidence of recorded depressive illness fell from 22.5 to 14 per 1000 person years at risk (PAYR) while the incidence of depressive symptoms rose three-fold. Combining both the incidence was stable over time. This may reflect not so much a reduction in the incidence of diagnosed depression as a change in diagnostic habits, possibly born of a desire to use non-stigmatizing terminology by avoiding the depression diagnosis. It may also represent a recognition that not all depressive symptoms amount to a depressive disorder. This study shows also that the incidence of diagnosed depression is lower than that identified in epidemiological studies using structured interviews, raising questions about the validity of this diagnosis when made using the latter technique.

In the USA equivalent studies are difficult to assess because of the differing health care delivery systems. One such study in a very large practice in California (Olfson *et al.* 1997) found that the overall prevalence for any disorder was 19.8% and that anxiety disorders were the most common at 11.6%, followed by affective disorder (8%). Substance abuse was the diagnosis in 6.3%. A study in New Zealand (MaGPIe 2003) identified those with psychiatric disorder using various screening instruments but it also examined the proportion who were identified by the general practitioners as having a psychiatric disorder. GPs thought that 54% of female and 46% of male patients had experienced some level of psychological problem in the past year while the structured diagnostic instruments identified one-third with a diagnosable psychiatric condition in the previous 12 months, with depression, anxiety and alcohol abuse predominating. All disorders were more common in the younger age group. Contrary to studies showing that GPs fail to identify those with psychiatric disorder, this study found that over 50% were correctly identified as having a psychiatric disorder by their family doctor but only one in ten were believed to have a condition that was moderate or severe.

Screening for psychiatric disorders in primary care

The high prevalence of psychiatric disorders identified in primary care has led to recommendations that patients in primary care be routinely screened for mental disorders and this has intuitive appeal. A number of studies have now been conducted to evaluate the impact of screening on the detection, management or outcome of psychiatric disorder, especially depression by general practitioners. Surprisingly a meta-analysis (Gilbody *et al.* 2005) published in the Cochrane Library found that screening made no difference to these outcome measures and led the authors to conclude that the routine use of a screening questionnaire is not supported by the available best evidence. They subsequently reiterated this view but with the caveat that there may be benefits from screening high-risk groups, such as those with a prior history, those with alcohol dependence or those with certain physical illnesses such as diabetes (Gilbody *et al.* 2006). Given the wide range of recognition rates, it is also feasible that patients registered with GPs who are poor recognizers may benefit from screening. While there is a paucity of such studies, one recent investigation of a group of high-risk patients seen in general practice, chosen because they were frequent consulters or had unexplained somatic symptoms or mental health problems (Baas *et al.* 2009), found no benefit from screening for major depression because of the poor uptake of treatment.

This chapter has shown the high level of psychiatric morbidity, both in the community and in those attending general practitioners and other family physicians. The varying rates of morbidity in the community, based on different ways of measuring, hint at an underlying philosophical conflict within both professional and patient groups about whether or not mental health problems should be labelled and specified as disorders or treated as 'cares of life'. The difference between recognized illness (or conspicuous morbidity) and actual morbidity in those attending primary care highlights the importance of primary care both in supporting individuals and in managing the system as a whole. The next chapter discusses this central role of primary care.

Summary

- The prevalence of psychiatric illness varies in different populations, being highest in community samples and lowest when hospital populations are examined.
- The broader the concept of illness, the higher the prevalence, and screening schedules arrive at higher prevalence rates than diagnostic instruments.
- Psychiatric disorder predominates in women, both in the general population and in general practice patients.
- Rates of up to 50% for psychiatric morbidity have been identified in some studies.
- The principal diagnosis in both populations consists of affective disorders, anxiety disorders and somatoform disorders.
- Evidence for the benefits of screening is lacking.

References

Andrews, G., Henderson, S., and Hall, W. (2001). Prevalence, co-morbidity, disability and service utilisation. *Overview of the Australian National Mental Health Survey*, **178**, 145–153.

Ansseau, M., Dierick, M., Buntinkx, F., *et al.* (2002). High prevalence of mental disorders in primary care. *Journal of Affective Disorders*, **78**(1), 49–55.

Baas, K. D., Wittkampf, K. A., van Weert, H., *et al.* (2009). Screening for depression in high risk groups: prospective cohort study in general practice. *British Journal of Psychiatry*, **194**, 399–403.

Casey, P. R., and Tyrer, P. (1986). Personality, functioning and symptomatology. *Journal of Psychiatric Research*, **20**, 363–374.

Casey, P. R., and Tyrer, P. (1990). Personality disorder and psychiatric illness in general practice. *British Journal of Psychiatry*, **156**, 261–265.

Casey, P. R., Dillon, J., and Tyrer, P. (1984). The diagnostic status of patients with conspicuous psychiatric morbidity in general practice. *Psychological Medicine*, **14**, 673–682.

Gilbody, S. M., House, A. O., and Sheldon, T. A. (2005). Screening and case finding instruments for depression. *Cochrane Database Systematic Review*, **4**, CD002792.

Gilbody, S. M., Sheldon, T. A., and Wessely, S. (2006). Should we screen for depression? *British Medical Journal*, **322**, 1027–1030.

Goldberg, D., and Blackwell, B. (1970). Psychiatric illness in general practice. A detailed study using a new method of case identification. *British Medical Journal*, **2**, 439–443.

Goldberg, D., Kay, C., and Thompson, L. (1976). Psychiatric morbidity in general practice and the community. *Psychological Medicine*, **6**, 565–569.

Jenkins, R., Lewis, G., Bebbington, P., *et al.* (1997). The National Psychiatric Morbidity Surveys of Great Britain – initial findings from the Household Survey. *Psychological Medicine*, **27**, 775–789.

Kessel, N. (1960). Psychiatric morbidity in a London general practice. *British Journal of Social and Preventive Medicine*, **14**, 16–22.

Kessler, R. C., McGonagle, K. A., Zhao, S., *et al.* (1994). Lifetime and twelve-month prevalence of DSM-111-R psychiatric disorders in the United States. *Archives of General Psychiatry*, **51**, 8–19.

MaGPIe Research Group. (2003). The nature and prevalence of psychological problems in New Zealand primary healthcare: a report on Mental Health and General Practice Investigation MaGPIe). *New Zealand Medical Journal*, **116**(1171), U379.

Narrow, W. E., Rae, D. S., Robins, L. N., *et al.* (2002). Revised prevalence estimates of mental disorders in the United States: using a clinical significance criterion to reconcile two surveys' estimates. *Archives of General Psychiatry*, **59**(2), 115–123.

Olfson, M., Fireman, B., Weissman, M., Leon, A., Sheehan, D., *et al.* (1997). Mental Disorders and disability among patients in a primary care group practice. *American Journal of Psychiatry*, **154**(12), 1734–1740.

Rait, G., Walters, K., Griffin, M., *et al.* (2009). Recent trends in the incidence of recorded depression in primary care. *British Journal of Psychiatry*, **195**, 520–524.

Robins, L. N., Helzer, J. E., Weissman, M. M., *et al.* (1984). Lifetime prevalence of specific psychiatric disorders in three sites. *Archives of General Psychiatry*, **41**, 949–958.

Sartorius, N., Ustun, T. B., Costa e Silva, J. A., *et al.* (1993). An international study of psychological problems in primary care. Preliminary report from the World Health Organization Collaborative Project on 'Psychological Problems in General health care'. *Archives of General Psychiatry*, **50**(10), 819–824.

Shepherd, M., Cooper, B., Brown, A. C., *et al.* (1966). *Psychiatric Illness in General Practice.* Oxford University Press.

Skuse, D., and Williams, P. (1984). Screening for psychiatric disorder in general practice. *Psychological Medicine*, **14**, 365–377.

Sweeting, H., Young, R., and West, P. (2009). GHQ increases among Scottish 15 year olds 1987–2006. *Social Psychiatry and Psychiatric Epidemiology*, **44**, 579–578.

Toft, T., Fink, P., Oernboel, E., *et al.* (2005). Mental disorders in primary care: prevalence and co-morbidity among disorders, results from the functional illness in primary care (FIP) study. *Psychological Medicine*, **35**(8), 1175–1184.

The central position of primary care in the detection and treatment of psychiatric disorder

Learning objectives

The factors influencing the decision to consult
The factors influencing the recognition of mental health problems
Does training or screening improve recognition and treatment?

The process determining which patients decide to consult their doctors, which are labelled as ill and which are referred for specialist assessment is not just a haphazard chain of events but is governed by a set of 'filters' which have been the subject of much investigation. These serve to deter some and to include other patients at each stage of the process. Chapter 1 described the totality of psychiatric morbidity in the community (known as level 1), among all general practice consulters (level 2) and among those identified as psychiatrically unwell by their family practitioners (level 3). These different levels were described by Goldberg and Huxley (1980) as a model for explaining the prevalence rates of mental illness in different parts of the health system. The fourth and fifth levels describe the disorders seen among psychiatric outpatients and amongst inpatients. Between each stage there is a shortfall of patients so that the total number identified in the community is not the same as the total number seen in hospital settings. There are key variables which affect the rate of 'filtration' between the levels or stages of care in this model. These are described below; the chapter ends with an elaboration of the basic model of filters, by describing the central position of primary care in the pathways of patients with a variety of conditions.

The first filter – the decision to consult

The relationship between symptom frequency and the likelihood of consultation is not straightforward. Many variables affect the decision to seek medical advice. Symptom surveys have shown that more than two-thirds of people surveyed believed themselves to have a health problem yet only a small proportion consulted with this. Furthermore some seek advice for trivial symptoms whilst others with serious symptoms do not seek help. This 'illness behaviour' (Mechanic 1962) has been investigated in detail over the past 40 years.

Where depression or anxiety are the presenting symptoms epidemiological studies of depression have shown that up to 60% of those with depressive illness have sought help, even in communities which are relatively deprived. The Defeat Depression Campaign of the Royal Colleges of Psychiatrists and General Practitioners found that 60% of those surveyed said they would consult their general practitioner first. The presence of stress as measured by life events in the 3 months prior to consultation also increases the propensity to seek help. For those with physical problems the likelihood of consultation is increased by the presence of concomitant psychological symptoms.

In addition to symptom severity, the degree of subjective distress and the extent of dysfunction also impinge upon this process. There is often an incongruity between the severity of symptoms and the degree of social disruption and where the latter is high, help is more likely to be sought. It is hardly surprising that the sufferer whose usual activities are disrupted or whose subjective level of distress is high will seek help promptly. A number of other features relating to symptoms also contribute to the process: thus symptoms of insidious onset are more often tolerated without treatment than those of acute onset, and those that are generally believed to be common are unlikely to prompt a visit to the doctor. Interestingly attitudes to illness and to consultations follow clear trends within families across generations and have been shown to account for a significant proportion of the variance in predicting consultation. The importance of sociodemographic factors may not at first seem relevant but they have indeed emerged as exerting an influence on this complex process. A consistent finding is that women have more contact with their family doctors than men and that consultation increases with increasing age. Whether this is due to an excess of symptoms and illness in women or whether they are more willing to acknowledge them is as yet unresolved. Also unresolved is the influence social class may have on consultation rates. It is not surprising that the lonely seek help more frequently than those who are in close, confiding relationships – the consultation will not only provide reassurance but is also a source of human contact. This has been verified by the repeated finding that the separated, single and widowed as well as those in relationships of conflict consult more frequently than their married counterparts.

The second filter – the recognition of psychiatric illness

A proportion of those with illness are not identified when consultation with the family practitioner takes place – the hidden psychiatric morbidity. Average recognition rates are thought to be about 50% in the United Kingdom, although over time most significant enduring depression is picked up in primary care (Coyne *et al.* 1995; Boardman 1987; Kessler *et al.* 2002). A number of variables contribute to the process of recognition of psychiatric disorders in primary care; these are discussed in detail in the following sections.

More detailed analysis of real-time consultations has demonstrated that the process of recognition is very far removed from textbook descriptions of how to diagnose mental illness. GPs may recognize problems but not attempt to elicit symptoms and patients may resist engaging in emotional talk. Even when the pair explicitly discuss emotional distress there is often no mutual agreement about the possibility of a mental health problem. For those agreeing there is a mental health problem most do not go on to discuss an explicitly psychiatric diagnosis. Thus the old idea of doctor as 'detector' does not hold. Both doctors and patients are active and at times resistant to diagnosis.

Patient variables

Patients may offer only physical symptoms even though their primary pathology may be psychological for a number of reasons.

(1) The common physical symptoms of depression or anxiety such as anorexia, fatigue, etc., may be described.

(2) Patients may feel their doctors only want to hear of physical symptoms and thus avoid mention of those concerned with the emotions.

(3) Some patients have a sense of guilt or stigma about feelings such as gloom and sadness when 'there is nothing to be depressed about' or when such complaints are viewed as evidence of weakness.

(4) The patient may consult with some other physical illness and both doctor and patient feel the psychological sequelae are understandable in the circumstances.

(5) Many patients, especially those who are not psychologically minded or those from some other cultures, may not have a vocabulary for or a concept of emotional hurt.

In addition to the manner in which symptoms are presented a number of demographic variables are associated with the non-identification of those with psychiatric disorder and vice versa. Thus, the unemployed, those of low socio-economic status and those who are separated, widowed or divorced are more likely to be correctly identified than their counterparts. This is probably related to stereotyped views of those who constitute the psychiatric population in this setting which either heighten or diminish the doctor's vigilance for detecting these disorders.

GP variables

It is important to examine two aspects of the process of general practitioner diagnosis. The first of these is referred to as 'bias' and is defined as the doctor's tendency to make or to avoid making a psychiatric diagnosis, whilst the second is 'accuracy' and refers to the correctness of diagnosis in terms of either severity or labelling. Since different factors influence each, they will be considered separately.

Bias towards making psychiatric diagnosis is determined by emphasis and interest in this area. It is reflected in interview style by questions with a psychiatric focus, by emphatic and psychotherapeutic comments and by an awareness of psychological factors in illness. The doctor will make enquiries about home and work and will identify the verbal and non-verbal cues that emotional problems exist. The style of questioning will commence with open questions and later proceed to closed and more focused enquiry.

A doctor with a high bias towards diagnosing psychiatric illness may incorrectly label patients as being psychologically disturbed where in fact no such disturbance exists. The appropriateness of the psychological tag is described as accuracy and is governed both by the personality attributes of the doctor and by the style of interview he conducts. Thus self-assured doctors, those who are extrovert and who are aware of their own feelings are more accurate than their counterparts. Involvement in academic activity also facilitates accuracy. In relation to interview style, dealing with over-talkativeness, clarifying symptoms, making eye contact and not reading notes during interview all contribute to the accuracy with which psychiatric disturbance is diagnosed. In addition, asking questions that follow from what a patient has just said rather than from theory increases the number of verbal distress cues, thus improving the likelihood of detection.

Systematic improvement of recognition

Recognition of depression and other mental health problems in primary care by general practitioners is therefore considered by many to be sub-optimal and in need of a remedy (Hickie et al. 2001; Paykel and Priest 1992; Coyne et al. 1995). Although screening interventions have not usually improved outcomes (Katon 1995; University of York 2002) and earlier recognition is not always associated with reduction in depression (Katon 1995; Dowrick and Buchan 1995), policy makers, professional and patient groups have generally advocated training doctors to increase rates of recognition (Rix *et al.* 1999). Significant efforts have been made to improve recognition but these have not been successful in improving outcomes. For example, in the Hampshire Depression Study, motivated practices engaged in a quality improvement intervention but recognition rates and outcomes did not improve (Thompson *et al.* 2000). In a smaller study in Newcastle, the two practices achieved improved recognition rates (Scott *et al.* 2002), and in a larger London-based study modest improvements in recognition, but not in care or outcomes, were achieved in the intervention practices (Bashir *et al.* 2000). The failure to improve outcomes, despite some success in addressing recognition, has led to reduced emphasis on recognition training programmes. The Quality and Outcome Framework (QOF) indicators for depression reward the use of objective scales as a part of the diagnostic process, aiming to avoid over- and under-diagnosis, but have introduced case finding for those with long-term conditions at high risk of depression.

Behind the average recognition rates, however, lies significant heterogeneity, with rates of less than 1% and higher than 80% being reported for some practitioners (Boardman 1987). The Exeter Depression Study took two practices and audited recognition rates before and after an educational intervention (Evans *et al.* 2002). While on average there was no significant improvement in recognition rates, the detail of the results demonstrates that in one practice recognition rates were already high and did not change but that in the practice where recognition rates were low an improvement from 44% to 79% in recognition index was achieved. Improvements appear greater for practitioners achieving lower baseline recognition rates and this is supported in a similar Newcastle-based study. As yet there is only the indirect evidence above that training the less good 'detectors' can make a difference, but it this may be the most strategic approach

The third filter – referral to the psychiatric services

Only between 5 and 10% of those patients identified as having mental health problems by their general practitioners are referred to the specialist services. This may well increase with the development of more accessible psychological therapy services. The new IAPT (Improving Access to Psychological Therapy) teams in England represent an additional step between low- and high-intensity therapy. Direct access to the psychiatric services has been rare in Britain and Ireland and a number of obstacles have to be overcome before the patient reaches the psychiatrist – these form the components of the third filter. However, the development of direct access to the new IAPT services has been shown to increase uptake in some areas, specifically those with a high proportion of ethnic minorities.

The reasons for referral are various. A common feature is failure to respond to treatment from the primary care team. Further reasons include requests for a specialist opinion on diagnosis or management. Up to a quarter are referred because they seek this themselves or because others request it on their behalf, particularly when behavioural disturbance becomes problematic.

Patient variables

Men are more likely to be referred than women, probably a reflection of the perceived impact of psychiatric illness upon the traditional breadwinner. Younger patients pass this filter more easily than older patients possibly because illness in the young is believed to be more socially restricting than in those who are retired. Those belonging to high socio-economic groups are over-represented among psychiatric clinic attendees partly because they seek referral them-selves. The role of marital status is uncertain in this filter.

Illness variables

Those who are referred are generally more seriously ill than those who are not. In particular GPs tend to refer all those who are psychotic and those who are suicidal. Those who have behavioural disturbances pass this third filter easily as a result of the social disruption they often generate. Some patients with depression have been referred for counselling, while a small number of treatment-resistant cases are referred to community mental health teams. Many such cases are not seen by psychiatrists and in some areas community mental health teams have strict criteria excluding all but the most depressed. In other areas a model of liaison and link working encourage patients to be seen by specialists in primary care settings.

GP variables

In general older doctors have higher referral rates than their younger colleagues, as do those in urban areas, the latter presumably due to ease of access for the patients to the services. A similar high referral rate has been noted among single-handed practitioners. Competencies in detec-tion are not clearly linked to referral rates; some high referrers have made little attempt to provide treatment and some low referrers also recognize less mental illness.

Service variables

The Goldberg and Huxley model (Goldberg and Huxley 1980) has been a useful tool for understanding the flow of patients towards specialist care. However, it does not adequately account for the active role of the patient nor, as discussed above, for the less than dichoto-mous nature of the recognition process. Furthermore the functions of both primary and secondary care have changed with the development of specialized community teams (see Chapter 21) and the development of shared care. In addition there are two new but potentially conflicting imperatives: to reduce stigma and increase effective early intervention.

Pathways in Primary Care Mental Health, shown below in Figure 2.1, is complementary to the Level and Filter model of Goldberg and Huxley and depicts both flow and function (Byng, personal communication).

Five of the many potential patterns are illustrated which demonstrate the varied roles of primary care mental health.

A. The classic 'common mental health problem' pathway, with appropriate recognition and treatment. Possibly better or failing to attend for other reasons.

B. Significant and recurrent mental health problems, e.g. comorbid depression, PTSD and personality disorder. Detected in primary care, referred promptly to a specialist worker based in primary care. Not taken on, but advice on management given. This is followed by intermittent access to primary care during crises.

C. Classic pathway for an individual with stress reaction following a significant life event. The GP is able to reassure with minimal intervention.

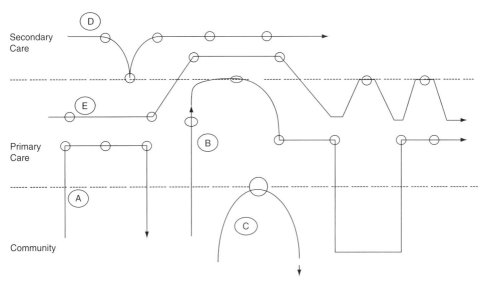

Figure 2.1. Pathways in Primary Care Mental Health

D. Patient with chronic psychosis, under specialist services and occasional GP contact for physical care.

E. Patient with less severe chronic mental health problems, initially referred and taken on by specialists but discharged to shared care with practice-based mental health workers.

Summary

- Women and those who are isolated and unsupported are more likely to consult. Several variables relating to the illness govern this decision also. Up to two-thirds of those with psychological problems consult their doctors. These variables constitute the first filter.

- The second filter identifies those factors which assist the GP in identifying the psychological component to the consultation. A number of social and demographic variables increase the GP's vigilance for detection, as do attributes of the doctor himself.

- Fewer than 10% of those with psychological disturbance are referred to the psychiatric services. Men and young patients pass this third filter more easily than women or the elderly. In particular the extent of social dysfunction caused by psychiatric illness is an important determinant of referral.

- Increasing complexity of community-based mental health services and more varied mental health functions in primary care indicate a need for a more complex model.

References

Bashir, K., Blizard, B., Bosanquet, A., Bosanquet, N., Mann, A., and Jenkins R. (2000). The evaluation of a mental health facilitator in general practice: effects on recognition, management, and outcome of mental illness. *British Journal of General Practice*, **50**(457), 626–629.

Boardman, A. P. (1987). The General Health Questionnaire and the detection of emotional disorder by General Practitioners.

A replicated study. *British Journal of Psychiatry*, **151**, 373–381.

Coyne, J. C., Schwenk, T. L., and Fechner-Bates, S. (1995). Nondetection of depression by primary care physicians reconsidered. *General Hospital Psychiatry*, **17**(1), 3–12.

Dowrick, C., and Buchan, I. (1995). Twelve month outcome of depression in general practice: does detection or disclosure make a difference? *BMJ* (Clinical Research Ed), **311** (7015), 1274.

Evans, P. H., Lloyd, K. R., Powell, R. A., *et al.* (2002). The Exeter Depression Audit Package: pilot study findings. *Primary Care Psychiatry*, **8**(2), 47–54.

Goldberg, D., and Huxley, P. (1980). *Mental Illness in the Community. The Pathway to Psychiatric Care*. London: Tavistock.

Hickie, I. B., Davenport, T. A., Scott, E. M., *et al.* (2001). Unmet need for recognition of common mental disorders in Australian general practice. *Medical Journal of Australia*, **175** Suppl, S18–S24.

Katon, W. (1995). Will improving detection of depression in primary care lead to improved depressive outcomes? [comment]. *General Hospital Psychiatry*, **17**(1), 1–2.

Kessler, D., Bennewith, O., Lewis, G., and Sharp, D. (2002). Detection of depression and anxiety in primary care: follow up study.

BMJ (Clinical Research Ed), **325**(7371), 1016–1017.

Mechanic, D. (1962). The concept of illness behaviour. *Journal of Chronic Diseases*, 189–194.

Paykel, E. S., and Priest, R. G. (1992). Recognition and management of depression in general practice: consensus statement. *BMJ* (Clinical Research Ed), **305**(6863), 1198–1202.

Rix, S., Paykel, E. S., Lelliott, P., *et al.* (1999) Impact of a national campaign on GP education: an evaluation of the Defeat Depression Campaign. *British Journal of General Practice*, **49**(439), 99–102.

Scott, J., Thorne, A., and Horn P. (2002) Quality improvement report: effect of a multifaceted approach to detecting and managing depression in primary care. *British Medical Journal*, **325**(7370), 951–954.

Thompson, C., Kinmonth, A. L., Stevens, L., *et al.* (2000) Effects of a clinical-practice guideline and practice-based education on detection and outcome of depression in primary care: Hampshire Depression Project randomised controlled trial. [See comments]. *Lancet*, **355** (9199), 185–191.

University of York. (2002). Improving the recognition and management of depression in primary care. *Effective Health Care*, **7**(5).

Chapter 3

The consultation in primary care

Learning objectives

Components of a 'good' consultation
History taking in primary care
Safety netting and reviewing care
Letter writing

Primary care and general practitioners (GPs), in particular, are responsible for delivering mental health care for the majority of those in contact with the health services. Most consultations in primary care involve dealing with the emotional response to physical illness and a significant minority involves diagnosable psychiatric illness. Mental health problems are often dichotomized into common mental health problems and severe mental illness; and the GP consultation has sometimes been seen as a mechanism for ensuring adequate detection, treatment and sometimes onward referral. However, this model negates the critical contributions of patient and GP to a dialogue which can, we believe, in itself, contribute to better mental health. This chapter provides a framework (see Table 3.1) for structuring consultations for mental health problems which takes into account the complexities of comorbidity, individuals' lives and beliefs, and organization of services. It also provides a summary of the key elements of psychiatric history-taking which can be incorporated into a series of general practice consultations.

Recognition and engagement

Achieving recognition by a mutual agreement about diagnosis and understanding about the patient's emotional distress appears to involve a number of important stages. Talk about emotional issues is often imbedded within consultations about physical health. Both patient and practitioner may dance around the possibility of entering an in-depth discussion about the emotional; perhaps due to stigma or for fear of upsetting an existing comfortable relationship. On the whole though, we believe that continuity of care, a prized element of general practice, is likely to help the process of engagement with the emotional.

Listening to narrative and subtly encouraging talk about psychosocial issues may also be an important prerequisite to achieving mutual acknowledgement about emotional distress. Once achieved, the conversation will need to address the patient's ideas and beliefs about the cause of their own distress and whether they see the problem as being part of 'the cares of life' – a social model – a biochemical phenomenon or genetic predisposition. This

Table 3.1. Important components of consultations for mental health problems

- Listen to narrative

- Engage in a conversation encompassing psychological or emotional distress

- Elicit ideas and beliefs about well-being and mental illness

- Reach a mutually agreed formulation or diagnosis in medical and/or social terms

- Make a risk assessment

- Be positive while acknowledging difficulties

- Provide information about a range of management options – medication, talking therapy and social or health promoting strategies

- Elicit concerns and expectations about treatments

- Reach a shared decision about management plan

- Reinforce the contribution of the patient – reinforcing strengths and promoting self care

- Arrange review and follow-up

- Look after your own emotions

understanding will help a practitioner to gain trust and explain mental illness and its treatment in terms accepted and understood by the patient; by understanding their life world, problems can be understood in terms of the social so that recent losses, abandonment or abuse, and general life pressures can become part of the agreed formulation.

Medical practitioners do have an important role in making a diagnosis, but it does not always need to be pivotal (see Chapter 4). A diagnosis can be helpful for some patients: as a way of feeling understood, to feel less isolated, to explain their symptoms and distress, or to obtain sick notes. In some conditions it helps define the optimal treatment. There will be differences of opinion, with the practitioners wishing to normalize or de-medicalize a condition while patients want something done, perhaps in the form of medication; or alternatively, with the patient reluctant to enter the medical realm and accept a psychiatric diagnosis. Being open about these differences of opinion is part of a concordant consultation.

A risk assessment is required to ensure that significant risks of self-harm or suicide are managed; it is also worth considering the possibilities of harm to others, and in primary care this is most likely related to the patients' ability to care for dependants, particularly children. Other chapters in this book will provide detailed accounts of how specific conditions can be diagnosed accurately, whereas this chapter focuses on how, in the context of primary care, comorbidity and past history affect the process of engagement with the psychosocial. This may well take several consultations, as well as relying on the trust derived from months or years of contacts.

Formulation and diagnosis in general practice

A good overall 'formulation' of the problem will incorporate information from the past, and bring together an understanding of social context, psychological assessment and the

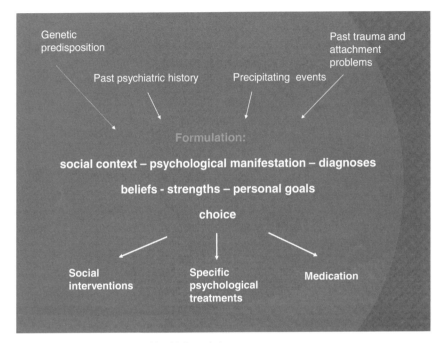

Figure 3.1. Primary care mental health formulation

psychiatric diagnoses. But in addition it should consider an individual's strengths and personal goals. This primary care mental health formulation (drawn from the best traditions of general practice and psychiatry) should take the form of an iterative conversation resulting in a shared understanding and mutual trust. This sets the scene for the difficult, but shared task of deciding on a management plan. Figure 3.1 depicts these elements.

Treatment decisions

Management options for mental health problems can broadly be divided into three groups: (1) medication, (2) psychotherapy so as to change thinking patterns and (3) lifestyle interventions. All of these may involve some elements of self-care and sharing responsibility with the patient.

The 'stepped care' model for depression and other disorders provides a useful framework for rationing intensity (and cost) of treatment against need (NICE 2009). For instance the NICE guidance for depression has usefully uncoupled the diagnosis from the imperative to provide medication with the concept of *watchful waiting*. The term is a misnomer, however, and rarely involves doing nothing; it might include the use of basic counselling and cognitive behavioural approaches, normalization of distress in response to life events, reattribution of somatic symptoms for those with medically unexplained symptoms, and the provision of health-promoting advice about exercise, substance misuse, sleep and sensible work patterns if appropriate. These may require skilful psychological manoeuvres by generalist clinicians embedded within short consultations.

For those being considered for more involved and costly treatment, an explanation about the treatment required, possibly with the help of written information sheets, or sign-posting to websites, combined with a dialogue about patients' concerns and expectations is an essential foundation for shared decisions about treatment. More patients are likely to receive effective treatments if choice of modality is based on their beliefs and setting, according to convenience, rather than on interventions based on the limited evidence base of fitting specific treatments to specific conditions. The Stepped Care approach to the delivery of psychosocial interventions then allows a number of options for each level of need, in order, for example, to save longer-term and specialist therapies (steps three and four) for those not responding to antidepressants or brief treatment.

Safety netting and reviewing care

Proactive review of care has been shown to improve outcomes for people with mental health problems (von Korff and Goldberg 2001). Safety netting at the end of a consultation and ensuring that care is reviewed are relevant to the range of presentations within primary care and are established as a key component of the consultation (Neighbour 2005). For those thought likely to have self-limiting conditions, a critical component of 'normalization' or signposting to care, away from specialist care settings, is to ensure that if problems worsen patients feel empowered to return for review. For those with common mental health problems, such as single episodes of depression, there is increasing, although not conclusive, evidence that follow-up in primary care should be more proactive, using procedures such as medication adherence education and telephone reviews. As a minimum patients should be advised to return at a set time.

For those under specialist care, there is less need for primary care to have systems for review, although the GP contract rewards contact between such patients and general practitioners as a way of ensuring physical health needs are met. For others, out of contact with specialist services but with chronic psychosis and bipolar affective disorder, this review may become a critical mechanism for ensuring safe ongoing care, particularly if it can be combined with timely, proportionate specialist advice. Brief assessments of risk, mental state, psychosocial needs, combined with a recovery and crisis oriented care plan, will need to be further developed in primary care.

Those patients with complex long-term non-psychotic mental health problems might also benefit from a primary-care-based review, going beyond renewed repeat prescriptions of antidepressants. This review function could be integrated with systems of chronic disease management for physical health problems such as diabetes and asthma; this will help break down the mind–body divide. Many older patients with dementia and chronic depression will also fall into this category. This proactive care would incorporate a range of the options described above, including an emphasis on self-care, timely support from specialist mental health workers, signposting to community resources, referral for brief episodes of therapy, involvement of carers and family and the development of crisis and recovery plans, known as Wellness Recovery Action Planning.

Psychiatric history-taking in primary care

The consultation should be conducted in a relaxed manner, creating an atmosphere of having time to listen. This will elicit more information than if the doctor appears to be in haste (Goldberg *et al.* 1993). The practitioner may have information from previous knowledge of the patient and will therefore be able to concentrate, in most cases, on current symptomatology and precipitating stresses.

The question of taking notes is problematic where a lot of information is being given. Ideally they should not be taken whilst the patient is with the doctor. However, this may be impractical and unobtrusive writing may be acceptable in certain circumstances. The 'open' sitting position can be used – this refers to sitting with the hands resting on the lap and feet on the ground. Folded arms or a hunched position creates an impression of tension or defensiveness. Interruptions from the telephone make a psychiatric interview difficult and if possible telephone calls should not be taken.

It is best to begin the interview with open questions followed later by closed questions in order to clarify the presenting complaints. The doctor can begin the interview with an open question such as 'How can I help you Mrs X?' or 'Tell me about your problem?' Later in the interview clarification of symptoms will require closed questions, e.g. 'Do you wake up early?' There is evidence to suggest that clarification of symptoms is an important factor in determining accuracy of diagnosis. A single question, 'How is your appetite?', is preferable to 'How is your appetite and your concentration?' Avoid leading questions, e.g. 'I suppose you don't drink too heavily?' or vague questions, e.g. 'Do you ever have odd experiences?' The latter are often used by inexperienced doctors when trying to elucidate psychotic symptoms.

In order to encourage the patient during the interview, techniques such as nodding, saying 'I see' and 'I understand' are useful. Expressions of empathy, both verbal and non-verbal, are particularly helpful when emotional information as distinct from factual information is being given. Summarizing is a useful means of ensuring the patient has been understood. The interviewer who is verbally active during the session (known as floor-holding) and who interposes questions while the patient is speaking freely rarely elicits extra information. It is, however, important for the interview to be controlled if it is not to ramble and be nothing more than a social exchange. The doctor can gently guide the patient through the interview and where necessary return the patient to the area under discussion.

Some patients are vague and circumstantial and the skill of the doctor in such interviews is of paramount importance if they are to be of clinical use. Controlling the responses is crucial and statements such as 'We will return to that later' or 'Perhaps we could concentrate on your panics for the moment' are useful when the patient is moving on too quickly or deviating from the questions asked.

Further difficulties arise when a patient avoids or refuses to answer questions. Reluctance may represent a painful area for the patient and if so can be returned to at a later interview. In general, however, the reluctance of patients to answer questions is related to a lack of understanding about what the doctor is trying to achieve. Reassurance can be given that the interest is not prurient but that the aim is to understand the present difficulties and the context in which they have arisen.

The GP must be finely attuned to the sensibilities of the patient who may resent or be embarrassed by questions of a personal nature. In particular questions about sexual abuse, sexual orientation and activity, previous abortions or criminal involvement and those dealing with religious matters should be handled with delicacy. In general it is difficult not to enquire directly about criminal activity. This latter is not as irrelevant as many believe since it gives the therapist an insight into the patient's value system and into a potential area of support from which the patient may derive benefit. Questions relating to sexual abuse in childhood should rarely be broached at the first interview; often it is not necessary to elicit detail about abuse; just acknowledging it can be important in itself.

Some doctors are reluctant to enquire about suicide but failing to do so is potentially negligent. The subject can be broached by initially enquiring of the patient whether he sees hope for the future followed by 'Do you ever get so depressed you wish you were dead?' If the patient answers positively the doctor may then ask 'Do you ever think of harming yourself?' followed by questions about any such plans and finally questions and assessment as to true intent.

The format of the history

There is a standard format for psychiatric history-taking to which psychiatrists adhere. However, the general practitioner because of his unique position in having a personal and long-term knowledge of the patient will not necessarily need to cover all areas. For new problems the history can be taken over several consultations. Moreover, pressure of time will make it impossible to obtain all the information described below but in most instances this will not be necessary anyway since the GP will have prior knowledge of the patient and his background. The following areas are considered when taking a psychiatric history.

History of presenting complaint – This is a description in the patient's own words of the symptoms and problems which bring him to the doctor.

Family history – The family history includes information about siblings and parents, especially information on any psychiatric history, including alcohol abuse and details of any psychiatric disturbance in more distant relatives, e.g. grandparents.

Personal history – The personal history incorporates information on the patient's childhood and upbringing. Details of neurotic traits in childhood such as bed-wetting and nightmares are sometimes a clue to the development of future psychiatric difficulties. This should also include details of the patient's schooling and any difficulties with peers, teachers or education, generally followed by an employment history and finally a history of psychosexual relationships. For the married person this will include details of their relationship with their spouse at present and for those who are not married or cohabiting information on any current relationships. Those who claim not to have had any boyfriends/girlfriends should be questioned about reasons for this, especially shyness of the opposite sex, lack of interest or over-protectiveness by their family. The GP's knowledge of the patient's family and the degree of support which they give to the patient should be included here. This is vital information frequently not available to the psychiatrist who has little contact with the patient's immediate family and social circumstances. This is of more than theoretical interest since the adequacy of support is one of the factors determining the outcome of many psychiatric illnesses.

Past medical and psychiatric history – This includes disorders treated by the general practitioner, by counsellors or by psychiatrists. The diagnosis made during previous episodes of disorder should be noted along with response to treatment, if this information is available. This is particularly true where certain approaches to therapy, e.g. behaviour therapy, have failed or where certain pharmacological treatments have been successful or failed, e.g. ECT or certain groups of antidepressants.

Drug history – The drug history should include information on current prescribed as well as non-prescribed medication and in particular enquiries should be made about any tendency to use tranquillizers prescribed by others. This may sometimes be associated with dependence on these drugs which the patient will not admit to unless specifically questioned. Where referral to a psychiatrist is being considered the duration of medication should be noted as this will have a special bearing on the decision to prescribe or to change antidepressants.

Pre-morbid personality – The personality of the patient must be assessed and the GP is in a special position to do this in view of his knowledge of the patient over a long period of time and of the patient's response to previous stresses. The importance of distinguishing between long-term personality traits and current symptoms is emphasized in Chapter 9. Information about the person's alcohol consumption (if this is not the presenting complaint) should be given here also.

Mental state

The information obtained in the history is then followed by an assessment of the *mental state*, which is the psychological equivalent of the physical examination and is considered under the following headings:

- Speech – pressure, slowing, 'word salad'. Abnormalities of speech, making it seem incomprehensible, or changing from topic to topic, may be found in those with schizophrenia or hypomania/mania, while slowing of speech is a feature of severe depression. Speech may also appear pressured in those with anxiety.

- Behaviour – compulsive behaviour, such as repeated checking or washing, is found in OCD or when obsessional symptoms occur as part of depressive illness; Anxiety evident in tremors, sweating and so on can be part of any psychiatric condition; Agitation such as pacing and restlessness can occur in most conditions but is more common in severe illnesses such as depression and psychotic disorders. Akathisia or a compulsion to keep moving, psychomotor retardation, mannerisms or stereotypies also occur in many disorders.

- Mood – elation is seen in those with hypomania/mania. Tearfulness is a feature of most psychiatric conditions and of normal emotional responsiveness also. Emotional lability or changing from sadness to joy is a feature of hypomania/mania. Emotional incontinence, defined as sudden uncontrollable outbursts of crying or laughing often associated with exaggerated facial expressions, is seen in many post-stroke victims and in other central neurological conditions also such as MS. Mood is said to be reactive when it changes according to circumstances, such as crying when a sad topic is raised or smiling when a happier matter is discussed. Mood is non-reactive when it does not change with the immediate circumstances and this is particularly a feature of depressive illness.

- Perception – hallucinations, defined as perception without a stimulus, are typically seen in psychotic disorders. They can occur in any sensory modality. Visual hallucinations are a feature of organic conditions such as delirium tremens or dementia. Tactile hallucinations occur in those misusing substances, especially cocaine. Illusions or visual misinterpretations can occur in those without any psychiatric disorder, such as the bereaved when a person is mistaken for the deceased.

- Disorders of thought – (a) Thought content:– delusions or false fixed beliefs out of keeping with the person's cultural or social background are found in a variety of psychotic disorders and also in organic states. The content is varied and may be of persecution, reference, hypochondriasis, nihilism, guilt, grandiosity and so on. Over-valued ideas are less fixed than delusions and are found in many psychiatric disorders and not just psychoses.

Obsessional ruminations are recurrent, intrusive senseless thoughts that are recognized as the individual's own. They may be resisted, leading to anxiety. Typically they include counting, or pondering on a theme repeatedly, e.g. the meaning of life. They occur most frequently in OCD and in depression but can also be found in schizophrenia, where they can be difficult to distinguish from delusions. The focus of ruminations is occasionally on suicide or on harming others. These differ from suicidal or homicidal thoughts since they are unwelcome and resisted.

Depersonalization, or the feeling of being cut off or 'outside' oneself, and derealization, feeling that objects are distant from one, occur in states of extreme anxiety, in depression and in rare instances as a primary disorder. These can also occur in the absence of any psychiatric disorder such as when a person is exhausted, hungry or intoxicated.

(b) Thought form – also known as formal thought disorder: this is seen in schizophrenia. It represents a disorder of the conceptual or abstract thinking and manifests itself as a lack of connection between thoughts. Flight of ideas or the occurrence of rapid shifts from one thought to the next is seen in mania.

- Concentration – distractibility is found in hypomania/mania and other acute psychoses. Concentration may be impaired in those with severe depression.

- Orientation – disorientation in time, place or person is found in acute and organic conditions. In severe depression it resembles dementia (called depressive pseudodementia) but resolves with treatment of the underlying depressive disorder.

- Insight/motivation – acceptance that treatment is needed; knowledge about the particular condition and motivation to change (especially for substance misusers) are important especially in relation to treatment adherence.

Further and more detailed information on psychopathological symptoms is available from other sources (Casey and Kelly 2007).

An attempt must next be made to *formulate a diagnosis* (see above and Chapter 4 for the multiaxial diagnostic system).

Letter writing

Letter writing as a key means of communication between doctors has received little attention. This is often the only mode of communication used and optimizing its usefulness is therefore important. The ultra-brief referral '?Depressed?' is to be deplored, as is the tendency of the specialist to reply in a five-page letter. Somewhere between these two extremes lies a mutually acceptable compromise.

A number of key items required by psychiatrists in *referral letters* have been identified (Pullen and Yellowlees 1985). These include family history, reasons for referral, past and current psychiatric history and medication prescribed so far. The knowledge that the family doctor has of the patient's personality and usual methods of coping is of great import, especially when considering the likely outcome, and should be included.

In return general practitioners have expectations of the type of letter they should *receive from psychiatrists* (Yellowlees and Pullen 1984). They should if possible not be longer than one page and should include the essential points: diagnosis and wider formulation, mental state exam, agreed management plan, prognosis and contingencies. Some doctors utilize sub-headings in their letters but this can be too rigid and is not favoured by most. A criticism of psychiatrists' letters is that they fail to mention prognosis, even after several consultations have taken place, and anticipated duration of treatment is seldom indicated.

Letter-writing does not stop with the initial letter following the patient's first appointment, but should continue whilst the patient is under the specialist mental health team's care. Unfortunately, many GPs fail to receive any correspondence once other members of multidisciplinary teams take over routine care, apart from Care Programme Approach documents, which are bulky and incomprehensible to most GPs. Whilst it is important to update the family doctor on progress there is no necessity to correspond following each and every visit, especially for those with protracted illnesses, unless there is a change in the patient's condition or alterations are being made to treatment. A further problem arises with those who default from treatment, and whilst most psychiatrists convey this information to the general practitioner when it involves new referrals, there is evidence that family doctors are not informed when those coming for follow-up fail to attend (Killaspy *et al.* 1999). This is particularly relevant since this group are likely to be the most seriously ill.

Communication during and following inpatient stays is also important. Knowing that someone has been admitted and whether sectioned is important. Communication when patients start to go on trials of leave at home is important, and a well-structured and immediate communication on discharge is important. It should include information about diagnosis and formulation, progress on the ward, management plans and review plans, and detail about mental state on discharge is probably more important than on admission. A further omission is that general practitioners are seldom informed of what details have been given to relatives about the disorder. This is pertinent in relation to psychotic and organic states. Some doctors may wish to receive an interim letter after initial inpatient assessments have been made but this may be an unrealistic request in all but the most well-staffed units. A large proportion of psychiatric case notes have been shown to contain pejorative remarks which could be expressed in a more acceptable manner and there is a danger that these would be conveyed also in letters, particularly those which are lengthy. This could be minimized by an ongoing hospital audit of letter writing (Shah and Pullen 1995).

From 2004 onwards, patients were to be routinely sent copies of all correspondence between clinicians working in the NHS. Pilot schemes suggest that patients value this but that doctors frequently omit information that it is considered may distress the patient (Murray *et al.* 2002). There were also concerns about security, especially for those patients who frequently change address. This has only been implemented fully in a few locations although a number of psychiatrists and GPs have embraced it voluntarily.

The increasing use of computers might have been expected to produce a significant rise in this method of corresponding between psychiatrists and general practitioners. This, however, does not seem to have occurred, possibly because of fears about confidentiality, but more likely as a result of the general decline in interactions between psychiatrists and GPs.

Summary

- The purpose of the interview is to arrive at a formulation.
- This should take account of the context of the symptoms, the person's past history, their strengths and vulnerabilities.
- The formulation sets the scene for an agreed management plan.

- The components of a skilled interview include listening, raising questions about emotional issues, discussing expectations of treatment and so on.
- The interview technique is important. Frequent interruptions by the doctor and the use of closed questions are best avoided. Clarification of symptoms and problems may make closed questions necessary at the end of the interview.
- The skilled interviewer takes control of the interview without appearing intrusive. Failure to achieve control will cause the patient to wander from the essential problems and a diagnosis may not be formulated.
- Psychiatrists frequently send excessively long letters to general practitioners but these should be no longer than one page and should include details of causation, treatment and its duration and prognosis. Information given to relatives should be mentioned also.

References

Casey, P., and Kelly, B. (2007). *Fish's Clinical Psychopathology. Signs and Symptoms in Psychiatry, 3rd edn.* London: Gaskell.

Goldberg, D. P., Jenkins, L., Millar, T., and Faragher, E. B. (1993). The ability of trainee general practitioners to identify psychological distress among their patients. *Psychological Medicine*, **23**, 185–193.

Killaspy, H., Banerjee, S., King, M., and Lloyd, M. (1999). Non-attendance at psychiatric out-patient clinics: communication and implications for primary care. *British Journal of General Practice*, **49** (448), 880–883.

Murray, G. K., Nandhra, H., Hymas, N., and Hunt, N. (2002). Doctors omit information from clinic letters when they know patients will be sent copies. *British Medical Journal*, **325** (rapid responses).

National Institute for Clinical Excellence. (2009) Depression: treatment and management of depression in adults, including adults with a chronic physical problem.

Neighbour, R. (2005). *The Inner Consultation: Developing an Effective and Intuitive Consulting Style.* Oxford: Radcliffe.

Pullen, I. M., and Yellowlees, A. J. (1985). Is communication improving between general practitioners and psychiatrists? *British Medical Journal*, **290**, 31–33.

Shah, P. J., and Pullen, I. (1995). The impact of a hospital audit on psychiatrists' letters to general practitioners. *Psychiatric Bulletin*, **19**, 544–547.

Von Korff, M., and Goldberg, D. (2001). Improving outcomes in depression. *British Medical Journal*, **323**, 948–949.

Yellowlees, A. J., and Pullen, I. M. (1984). Communication between psychiatrists and general practitioners. What sort of letters should psychiatrists write? *Health Bulletin*, **42**, 285–289.

How psychiatric disorders are described and classified

Learning objectives

The different classification systems currently used in psychiatry
The drawbacks and benefits of these in general practice psychiatry
The major categories of psychiatric disorder

Medicine as a whole is built upon the classification of different diseases and there are some doctors who find detailed sub-classification a useful tool. Mental health is a particularly active arena for the debates between 'lumpers' and 'splitters'. Because much of the classification in psychiatry is based on descriptive psychopathology, the study of symptoms, rather than studies of the brain, the scope for debate is wider still. Examples include: is 'depression with anxiety' an affective or neurotic condition? Can psychological trauma induce the hallucinations seen in schizophrenia?

In primary care these debates can sometimes appear as intellectual irrelevances. Our view is that diagnostic classification is an important activity for doctors in primary care. We do, however, have a number of caveats:

(1) Detailed sub-classification, beyond the point at which management changes significantly, is largely irrelevant to the general practitioner, whose work is treatment-oriented.

(2) When uncertainty exists differential diagnoses should be actively stressed as possibilities.

(3) The classification system is a construct created by doctors and psychologists to aid in decisions about treatment and is only one representation of mental illness as lived by individuals.

(4) Many individuals do not fit easily into this (necessarily) imperfect system. They may appear to fit no categories or several and changes may occur over time. These issues are illustrated in the following case vignette.

Case 1

C, a 57-year-old woman, presented to her general practitioner with significant depression and anxiety with panic attacks related to fear of meeting an ex-neighbour who had bullied her. Initially the presentation was of depression with poor sleep and rumination relating to the original episode of bullying and a subsequent encounter with the individual in some local shops. It became apparent that the fear of meeting this individual meant that C no longer left home if not accompanied by her son, and had resigned herself to not returning to work or engaging in anything other than a minimal number of social activities. While both depressive and anxiety symptoms, in particular the panic, had abated, she had restricted her life to her house and continued to attend her GP. Over the years she developed an increasingly low mood, and intense feelings of failure. CBT was not available and there was limited motivation to engage in therapy. Counselling was attempted, but did not result in any significant clinical change. A number of antidepressants had only short-lasting success or no success.

C then had a breakdown in the relationship with her mother with significant arguments over relatively minor issues. This altercation lasted for about a year, but then her mother died. C was able to deal with the funeral, and was able to get out a little more, but the depression intensified and rumination relating to the period of conflict increased and was associated with significant worsening depression, although at no time did C consider taking her own life. Again there was no motivation to engage in CBT, but eventually she attended bereavement counselling and gradually came to terms with her mother's death, by focusing on positive periods in their relationship.

Comment

This vignette illustrates the interplay between depressive and anxiety-related problems; and also the shift in diagnosis over time in response to events and social context. Initially she had sufficient symptoms to warrant diagnoses of depression and panic disorder; as the symptoms following the acute stressor subsided the criteria for adjustment disorder would have been reached. Later depression returned, with anxiety only obvious when challenged by her GP to go out of the house. Diagnosis is a useful component of an overall formulation, and can point towards evidence-based treatments, but is subsidiary to the social, psychological and biological components of the whole formulation, as this case illustrates.

Individual patients therefore should always be treated as such, and not as disorders. As discussed in Chapter 3, their social situation and their views on mental illness should also be considered both when making an 'objective' diagnosis, and also when negotiating a shared view on describing it. The act of making a diagnosis lies at the heart of the tension between 'labelling' as disorders, or 'normalizing', mental health problems. When there is significant disagreement between the doctor and patient, as to the appropriate diagnosis or descriptive label, the doctor may find it necessary to express his honest views on this while respecting the different perspective of the patient. Typically a patient may view herself as 'stressed out' while the GP may believe that she is experiencing a depressive episode.

Having stressed these limitations we believe that diagnosis, particularly when associated with evidence on treatment and prognosis, remains an important tool, not only to formulate management plans but also to help the patient understand their symptoms (see Chapter 3).

The psychiatric classification systems

In the United States psychiatric disorders are classified according to the system outlined in the Diagnostic and Statistical Manual, 4th edition (DSM-IV) (American Psychiatric Association 1994) whilst the European approach is embodied in the International Classification of Diseases, 10th edition (ICD-10). There are some differences between these, centring largely on the specific categories which have been included. The principles underlying both are broadly similar although the multiaxial system of providing an evaluation of various dimensions of the patients' current status is much better developed in the DSM. Unlike the DSM, the current ICD-10 for use in clinical practice does not use operational definitions.

Since primary care has special requirements and most psychological problems are seen in that setting, there is also a version of ICD-10 for use there (ICD-10-PC). ICD-10-PC consists of a brief description of the disorder and the diagnostic features and differential diagnoses. Definitions for 25 conditions are provided and a shorter version of six disorders for use by other primary care workers is also incorporated. Management guidelines incorporate information for the patient as well as details of medical, social and psychological interventions. Finally, assistance on when to refer for specialist treatment is provided. DSM-IV also has a primary care version (DSM-IV-PC) that is similar to ICD-10-PC, focusing on the most common disorders seen in primary care (anxiety, depression, substance abuse, etc.).

However, these classifications although developed for use in primary care do not assist the general practitioner in classifying the more nebulous social, behavioural and sub-syndromal problems that dominate their mental health consultations. To overcome this deficit the World Organization of Family Doctors has developed its own classification – The International Classification of Primary Care (ICPC). It incorporates the reason for the consultation and the symptoms dominating the consultation. Thus it is possible to provide a symptom as well as a syndrome classification.

Several studies have now examined the utility of these purpose-designed classifications, especially ICD-10-PC, in diagnosing disorders in general practice, on the accuracy of diagnosis and on outcome (Ustun et al. 1995). Unfortunately these studies suggest that although their use does significantly increase the numbers diagnosed with depression and with unexplained physical symptoms, they make little difference to diagnostic accuracy or to outcome (Croudace et al. 2003).

Why diagnose?

Psychiatric diagnosis, seen by some as labelling, has been the butt of criticism from disciplines as diverse as philosophy and statistics, sociology and psychiatry itself. The arguments against psychiatric diagnosis are varied, but the central theme is the dehumanizing nature of labelling, the inadequacy of using single labels to describe human problems and the poor reliability of the specific diagnoses. The original diagnosis often changes from admission to admission and different psychiatrists may make different diagnoses on the same patient. The overall agreement for diagnosis between psychiatrists is poor and lies between 30% and 60%, being lowest for personality disorder and highest for the functional psychoses. Diagnosis does not predict treatment or outcome and the label gives a spurious notion of understanding. Many feel that using a label only serves to mystify rather than assist and hence confers power on doctors which they can abuse. It has been argued that psychiatric illness does not exist, as anything other than a construct, and is a convenient epithet for the eccentric, the deviant or those whom society tries to scapegoat.

It is not the purpose of this chapter to enter in detail into this controversy, which has been eloquently stated by Kendell (1975), but it is important to understand the value of diagnosis and classification. As with many controversies, there is an element of truth in some of the anti-psychiatry arguments. It is undoubtedly true that psychiatric labels have been given to those who were not ill but protesting and that these people have all too often been subjected to humiliation and degradation. On the other hand we do not hold the view that schizophrenia does not exist, and is designed only by psychiatrists to perpetuate their own interests. There is good biological evidence from genetic, imaging and biochemical studies that people with schizophrenia have distinctive biological features. However, there is not a clear one-to-one match between biological markers and symptoms. Hence the ongoing debates.

The statistical arguments pointing to the low reliability of psychiatric diagnoses and the evidence that diagnosis does not have good predictive value are therefore partly true. One approach to improving the reliability of psychiatric diagnosis is to define the criteria for making the diagnosis. Thus defined, the diagnostic term can be applied more accurately. This is referred to as an operational definition and this technique underpins DSM-IV although not ICD-10.

Providing an operational definition, however, does not prove the existence of the condition defined. The next stage, proving its validity or existence, is to examine populations of patients so defined in terms of sydromes, course, response to specific treatments and common aetiological factors. It is this task, i.e. identifying specific diseases, which makes operational definitions fundamental to further progress.

In psychiatry no less than in general medicine, it is useful to label and classify patients so that features common to them can be examined. Classification in the research setting allows us to assess the stability of diagnosis, the prognosis and response to treatments. At the individual level, diagnosis can then be used first to make a judgement about whether an individual is similar to those who have been allocated a specific diagnosis and second to make judgements about whether specific treatments are likely or not to be effective.

A further element of classification is its facility to communicate; thus, describing a person as tall or small implies a system of classification which is distinct from that describing them as male or female. In psychiatry, as in all branches of medicine, the capacity to succinctly describe a patient and to use terminology which conveys meaning is of fundamental importance. For this it is important to have a basic understanding of how psychiatric disorders are grouped and to be aware of the difficulties inherent in this process as well as recent changes in the approach to the classification and description of the common psychiatric conditions. These issues will be discussed in the context of the DSM and the ICD systems.

Multi-axial classification

The argument that single labels are inappropriate to describe a patient's difficulties will be recalled. As outlined above, the psychiatric profession responded by devising a dimensional or multi-axial system of classification. This means that several aspects of the patient can be described. In ICD-10 the axes are poorly developed and there are three:

(1) Mental state and personality disorder

(2) Psychosocial/environmental problems

(3) Impact on functioning.

DSM-IV, however, has different and more comprehensive axes:

Axis 1: refers to mental state diagnosis

Axis 2: refers to personality disorder

Axis 3: describes physical illnesses contributing to the emotional problems

Axis 4: refers to the level of social functioning at a designated point, e.g. at admission or discharge

Axis 5: refers to stressors in the previous 6 months.

In this way a clear and succinct picture of the patient, his background and problems can be presented and communicated to those charged with his management.

These systems of classification are currently being revised and DSM-V is expected to be published in 2012 and ICD-11 in 2015.

Changes

The neuroses

The term neurosis was coined in 1772 in Edinburgh by Cullen, a physician. Freud used the term psychoneurosis to describe specific disorders (anxiety, phobic, hysterical and obsessional neurosis) as well as to indicate unconscious conflicts which he believed were aetiologically important. This dual usage has continued. Some clinicians use 'neurosis' to describe those disorders which are associated with distressing symptoms but where reality testing is intact, i.e. it is used as a descriptive term. Others, however, use it aetiologically. Those of the psychodynamic school adopt the aetiological usage and believe that unconscious conflicts always underlie the traditional neurotic illnesses, but most clinicians now accept that there are other theories to explain the development of these disorders. These include cognitive, learning and biological models. Unfortunately, the word neurosis is also often used pejoratively as a way of describing difficult patients. This confusion paved the way for some clinicians to suggest that the term neurosis be abandoned, as obfuscation rather than clarification was its legacy. Inevitably this caused dismay to many but was welcomed by others.

When the American Psychiatric Association published DSM-III in 1980 the term neurosis did not appear and the cluster of disorders subsumed by this rubric were classified under affective, anxiety and other disorders. In ICD-l0 the traditional dichotomy between neurotic and psychotic has been abandoned although the former does find occasional use, as in the cluster headed 'Neurotic, stress-related and somatoform disorders'. However, categories such as 'neurotic depression' have been abandoned and the concept of neurosis can be said to be almost defunct in the current system of classification. This change in terminology may not directly affect family doctors in the immediate future, but in the longer term this will have an inevitable impact on the way psychiatric illnesses are conceptualized and on the terminology used when describing our patients.

Personality disorder

Many textbooks of psychiatry still contain a chapter entitled 'The Neuroses and Personality Disorder', suggesting that the two are linked. This has its foundation in the work of the nineteenth century psychiatrists who felt that personality predisposition was the real source of the malady and that psychiatric disturbances were reactions to stress. In the 1930s some questioned the interlinking of personality and mental state diagnosis and held that both were separate although of course in individual patients there may be an association. This separation has been the approach of the ICD and DSM classifications for many years. The clinical implication is that individual patients are no longer viewed in terms of either mental state diagnosis or personality disorder but may have one or other or both. Unfortunately many clinicians still retain a single-dimension model in which the person is believed either to have a personality disorder or to have some other condition such as schizophrenia. On the other hand there is some evidence of links, in terms of both aetiology and symptomology, between psychiatric illnesses and personality disorder. Trauma and abandonment appear to be common and powerful aetiological factors for mood disorders, obsessional traits and border-line personality disorders as well as PTSD.

Psychoses

The distinction between manic depressive and schizophrenic psychosis was made by Kraepelin and this separation has rarely been subject to dispute. The only change has been the recognition that schizophrenia may have a good prognosis in some and successful attempts have been made in the identification of factors which make for this – a view not held by Kraepelin in his original description of 'dementia praecox', which he believed always had a poor outcome. Schizophrenia and manic depressive psychosis are thus retained as distinct entities in both the European and American systems of classification.

Other conditions

Psychotic and neurotic illnesses following childbirth have been referred to as puerperal psychosis and postnatal depression respectively. In other words they were classified by aetiology. Post-traumatic stress disorder is similarly classified by aetiology. There is now evidence that the treatment and outcome of disorders following childbirth are no different from those occurring at other times. The practice of classifying by aetiology has now been abandoned and has been replaced by symptomatic classification. If a patient has symptoms of schizophrenia or of depressive illness, they are described accordingly rather than by the precipitant.

For this reason the term reactive depression is no longer used either. The latter had a number of meanings and for some it described a depressive illness which had a precipitant, for others an understandable reaction to stress and for still others was used interchangeably with neurotic depression. Thus a person who developed a depressive illness with psychotic features following a bereavement could have been described as having a psychotic depression or a reactive depression depending on local practice. Similar arguments have led to the abandonment of 'endogenous' depression, although the American system retains a similar concept in its recognition of depression with melancholic features. As with 'reactive' and 'neurotic' depression the term 'endogenous' was used variously to describe depression with a particular pattern of biological symptoms or to delineate an illness which had no precipitant.

A category of particular importance to general practice is the 'adjustment disorder'. Although included in the previous editions of ICD, this section has been expanded consid-erably in recognition of the multifaceted aspects of stress reactions, both acute and long-term, that, unlike depressive illness, are driven entirely by the presence of a stressor and resolve when the precipitating stress is removed or with the passage of time as a new level of adaptation is gradually achieved. These must be distinguished from depressive illnesses and indeed other disorders precipitated by stresses whose resolution is not contemporaneous with removal of causation. In clinical practice the distinction can often be difficult. Acute stress reactions are also included in this section and this diagnosis is made when a person has the typical symptoms of PTSD (flashbacks, hypervigilance, intrusive symptoms) occurring in response to a serous stressor. If the symptoms last longer than 6 weeks the diagnosis changes to PTSD.

Conclusion

It is recognized that general practitioners see large numbers of patients with psychiatric disorders and that many are distinct in their mode of presentation from those seen in secondary care. The classifications used by psychiatrists, ICD-10 and DSM-IV, although valid as descriptors are over-complicated for everyday use in general practice. The World Health Organization (1992) and the American Psychiatric Association have modified their classifications specifically in recognition of this.

Adhering to internationally recognized systems of classification is important as a first step in overcoming the confusion about diagnostic labels that has existed. To some the debate about classification may seem ephemeral, and while care is required to avoid unnecessary stigma, the true value of a valid and reliable system rests in the accuracy of communication about patients at the interface between psychiatrists and general practitioners, and the predictive power for prognosis and treatment.

Summary

- There has been debate about the usefulness of psychiatric diagnosis, but there are forceful arguments against abandoning it, while recognizing limitations.

- Psychiatric diagnosis has been unreliable but by specifying the criteria, known as operational definitions, this can be improved and can be a springboard from which to validate these syndromes. This approach is currently used by the DSM but not by the ICD system.

- The modern approach to diagnosis favours describing the patient along dimensions (known as a multi-axial system) and in this way captures the multifarious aspects of the patient's condition.

- Modern classifications avoid commonly used terms such as 'neurosis', 'post-natal depression' and a number of others.

- A classification for use in primary care has been developed but its value has yet to be convincingly demonstrated.

References

American Psychiatric Association. (1994). *Diagnostic and Statistical Manual*, 4th edn (DSM IV). Washington DC: American Psychiatric Association.

Croudace, T., Evans, J., Harrison, G., *et al.* (2003). Impact of the ICD-10 Primary Health Care (PHC) diagnostic and management guidelines for mental disorders on detection and outcome in primary care. *British Journal of Psychiatry*, **182**, 20–30.

Kendell, R. E. (1975). *The Role of Diagnosis in Psychiatry*. Oxford: Blackwell Scientific.

Ustun, T. B., Goldberg, D., Cooper, J., *et al.* (1995). New classification for mental disorders with management guidelines for use in primary care: ICD-10 PHC chapter five. *British Journal of General Practice*, **45**, 211–215.

World Health Organization. (1992). *Mental Disorders: glossary and guide to their classification in accordance with the Tenth revision of the International Classification of Diseases*. Geneva: World Health Organization.

Chapter

5

Adjustment to stress

Learning objectives

What is meant by stress

How stress, vulnerability and symptoms relate

Common stress reactions – normal adaptive reactions, adjustment disorder, acute stress
reactions and PTSD

Stress is the term used to describe the overall reaction of individuals as they adapt to or attempt to adapt to circumstances or events which threaten to disrupt their physical or psychological well-being. These circumstances or events are referred to as stressors. Life stressors vary and can be: acute (e.g. accidents) or chronic (e.g. long-term illness); positive (e.g. promotion) or negative (e.g. theft of a car) or catastrophic (repeated sexual abuse). There is a large body of work linking stressors or life events to mental illness (Brown and Harris 1978). The association between the event and the response is not a simple cause and effect relationship but is governed by intervening variables known as mediators (see Figure 5.1). It is these which determine the magnitude and duration of the response to a particular stressor as well as whether the reaction might be considered pathological or normal.

Some people respond to significant stressors, such as arduous working conditions or family crises, with great resourcefulness and increased performance. Others react to even minor stressors and become unable to cope with normal activities, develop increased agitation, anxiety, depression or other symptoms and show impairment in day to day functioning.

Normal adaptive reactions

Some reactions to stressors, such as sadness following bereavement or avoidance of certain locations after being mugged, are not considered pathological but normal, adaptive reactions to events. They are time-limited and resolve spontaneously. Some doctors call these 'adjustment reactions' but this term will not be used in this book as it may lead to confusion with 'adjustment disorders' (see below), which are considered abnormal.

Figure 5.1. The stress model

MEDIATORS

↓

STRESSOR → REACTION

Table 5.1. Internal and external mediators

Internal	External
Personality and defences, e.g. denial	Social supports, e.g. family, relationships, workplace
Cognitive interpretation	Role
Biological predisposition	Societal norms, e.g. stigma, beliefs
Genetic factors	Beliefs (religious, philosophical, cultural)

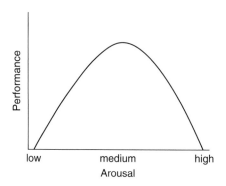

Figure 5.2. Yerkes–Dodson curve

The relationship between what is a normal adaptive reaction and an abnormal reaction is illustrated by the Yerkes–Dodson curve (Figure 5.2). This shows that as the severity of the stress reaction (arousal) increases, performance improves and plateaus but thereafter diminishes. The point at which performance diminishes represents the point of transition from normal to abnormal and this is determined by the mediators.

Mediators are the factors which determine the reaction to each stressor. Without these, each stressor would have an entirely predictable effect on the recipient. Both internal (e.g. personality) and external (e.g. family) mediators (Table 5.1) have been identified. Their importance, particularly those linked to personality, to cognitive interpretation and to social supports, lies in their relevance to treatment, prevention of recurrence and resilience enhancement.

Dealing with stress – broad principles

It is clear that no interventions other than general support are required to deal with normal adaptive reactions. Interventions to help manage abnormal stress can be problem-focused, mediator-focused or response-focused.

Problem-focused: a problem-oriented response implies avoiding or minimizing the stressor *ab initio*. This may not always be possible since events occur without warning and are often not amenable to outside control. However, it may, on occasion, be possible to avoid stress, as when a person already under pressure declines extra work. When events occur that are not predicted, intervention to reduce their impact, e.g. if they have caused a sudden increase in workload, can offset the negative effect. Cognitive techniques can be used to

Table 5.2. Defence mechanisms

Positive	Negative
Planning	Denial
Suppression of competing activities	Substance misuse
Social supports for instrumental reasons	Social supports for emotional reasons
Active coping	Disengagement

reframe and re-evaluate the significance of the stressor or to consider it within a framework of problem-solving. This involves a staged process as follows: (i) assessing the problem, (ii) setting realistic goals, (iii) planning a strategy, (iv) action to solve the problem, (v) evaluating the effects of this action, and (vi) re-adjusting the strategy on this basis. This technique is illustrated in the CD (Problem Solving) and see also Chapter 16.

Mediator-focused: mediator-based responses to stress are not often applied since they may be ill-defined. Essentially their purpose is to reduce the vulnerability of the person to the effects of stressors. Included in this group is the use of prophylactic medications such as antidepressants for known psychiatric disorders which render the person vulnerable to abnormal stress responses. Bolstering support from others is also helpful, particularly when used to provide advice on practical solutions. Many assume that all support is helpful but when used only for emotional ventilation it is of much less benefit than when used in a practical way. In addition, by using healthy coping skills the mediators may be modified and this should include knowledge of the faulty strategies which are used as well as healthy defences. These are listed in Table 5.2.

Symptom-focused: the third approach to stress responses, and perhaps the best-known to doctors, is the symptom-focused one in which either medication or some other technique, such as relaxation, is used to reduce symptoms. These approaches can be very effective with rapid symptomatic control, especially using anxiolytics to reduce symptoms of anxiety. This is usually a short-term intervention but its benefit in reducing symptoms may enable the doctor to engage in other strategies as outlined above. Once a depressive illness has supervened, the approach to management is as outlined in Chapter 7 since there is no difference in response to pharmacotherapy or in outcome between those episodes which have a precipitant and those which occur spontaneously.

The effects of stress

The effects of stressors may be to produce reactions which stimulate performance, as indicated in the Yerkes–Dodson Curve (Figure 5.2), and in these circumstances the stress is beneficial. However, when performance is impaired the result can be physical, behavioural and psychological.

Abnormal physical reactions include exacerbation or precipitation of existing illnesses such as psoriasis or migraine. There is also increasing recognition that a wide range of physical symptoms are manifestations of emotional stressors. These medically unexplained symptoms include focused problems such as tension headaches or 'globus' (lump in throat) and the non-specific symptom clusters found in chronic fatigue.

Personality disorders, particularly Cluster B (borderline and antisocial) (see Chapter 9 p. 121), are increasingly recognized as being the result of significant early stressors such as abuse or poor attachment. Relapses in schizophrenia have been linked to stressors and life events but more controversially some primarily psychotic reactions are considered by some to be the result of intensive traumatic experiences (Read *et al.* 2005). Burn-out, although not included in the modern psychiatric classifications, is frequently mentioned in books dealing with stress. It is defined as an increasingly intense pattern of psychological, physical or behavioural dysfunction in response to a continuous flow of stressors and best regarded diagnostically as a variant of either adjustment reactions or depressive illness, requiring treatment accordingly.

Stress in the current classifications

In the modern classifications (ICD-10 and DSM-IV) the only disorders listed under the 'stress reaction' heading are post-traumatic stress disorder (PTSD), acute stress reactions and adjustment disorders and it is these which will be considered in more detail in this chapter. Even though many disorders such as depressive episodes or even psychotic reactions can also be triggered by stressors they are categorized separately since the presence of a stressor is not essential to their genesis, unlike adjustment disorders, acute stress reaction and PTSD, where the diagnosis cannot be made in the absence of a stressor. Bereavement ordinarily is not classified as a psychiatric disorder but when complicated or prolonged would be subsumed under either the adjustment disorder or the depressive illness categories depending on the symptom profile. Normal adaptation to stress, as illustrated in Case 1, does not require a diagnosis.

Case 1

A 21-year-old woman, M, presented to a general practitioner with a 10-day-long episode of acute anxiety, low mood, suicidal thoughts (but no plans or intent) and significant physical symptoms including inability to sleep, tiredness, tremor and a tight feeling in her chest. She had taken time off work because of her distress. The symptoms had been triggered by the breakup of a 2-year relationship and although she recognized the link she had become increasingly worried that her psychological symptoms were a sign of madness. Her grandmother had suffered from schizophrenia and she felt very alone due to the loss of her relationship and the fact her mother was living some distance away.

Her main concern was to obtain treatment to prevent her from having a breakdown. She was particularly concerned about an exam which she was due to sit in 3 days time. The general practitioner quickly recognized that the main aim of this consultation was to provide some immediate relief, but more importantly to help M realize that her psychological and physical symptoms were a normal reaction to a traumatic event. She could see that both the physical and emotional symptoms were in response to her distress after an explanation of the physiological stress reaction. She was particularly keen to make sure she had some sleep and the pros and cons of sedatives for the short term were discussed. She agreed to take a prescription for 2 or 3 days, but that this may not be needed, as by the end of the consultation she was greatly relieved to understand that her reaction to stress was entirely normal. She was reviewed 10 days later and had managed to get to the exam and had significantly improved sleep and reduced anxiety. She was still feeling low in mood and had normal feelings about the loss, but could now see that they were likely to diminish over time. She did not go on to have a depressive disorder or abnormal loss reaction when reviewed 3 weeks later.

Comment

This case illustrates the importance of the role of the general practitioner at the interface between medical and lay worlds. This GP was able to interpret the patient's loss and emotional and physical reactions to it, and by listening to her concerns reassure her that it was a normal, and probably temporary, reaction. Because her functioning was not impaired she did not reach the threshold for regarding this as an adjustment disorder. An empathic response, a clear explanation relating to her concerns and a follow-up to ensure that the problem did not deteriorate were all appropriate. This is an excellent example of how primary care can provide a cost-effective response to mental health problems and avoid unnecessary stigma.

Adjustment disorder

Adjustment disorder (AD) is a useful category that describes an understandable but exaggerated response to stress. It is broadly similar to what used to be called 'reactive depression'. AD is not often diagnosed in clinical practice except in liaison psychiatry. Its importance is two-fold – first, it is usually self-limiting and unlike depressive illness does not require antidepressants and its management is largely psychotherapeutic. Second, it is commonly the diagnosis made in the context of deliberate self-harm and therefore carries a suicide risk in that context. Pragmatically its usefulness as a non-stigmatizing description of an exaggerated and incapacitating reaction to stress is important and can be used for those individuals whose 'normal adaptive reaction' does not resolve. The term adjustment disorder has been in the psychiatric literature since 1968 in DSM and 1976 in ICD although the concept was recognized for over a decade before it entered the modern classifications.

Three broad categories are described according to the predominant symptom cluster, i.e. AD with depression, with anxiety, with conduct disturbance or various combinations of these. They may brief (less than 1 month) or prolonged (less than 2 years). Unfortunately, there are no specific diagnostic criteria given to assist the clinician apart from stipulating that if the criteria for another condition are met then AD cannot be diagnosed. Thus, AD is regarded as a sub-syndrome that lies in the hinterland between normal reactions to stress and a clearly defined disorder such as depressive illness or generalized anxiety.

Clinical features

Adjustment disorders are closely related in time to a stressful event. These are not the traumatically significant events required for PTSD, but include job losses, relationship breakdowns and other such common events. The reactions may be depressive, anxious or behavioural in content and the latter are described mainly in teenagers. Physical symptoms such as poor sleep or headache are also common. Patients feel overwhelmed and unable to cope. These reactions occur in the absence of any pre-existing psychiatric disturbance although personal vulnerability is said to play a role, but the evidence base for this is limited due to the paucity of research into AD.

ADs occur generally within 1 month or 3 months of the original stress, depending on whether the criteria of ICD or DSM are followed. The symptoms continue until resolution, either when the stressor is removed or until a new level of adjustment is reached. Of course if the stressors themselves or their consequences continue, then the symptoms may also be prolonged, as for example when a person is bullied at work and resigns but then pursues a

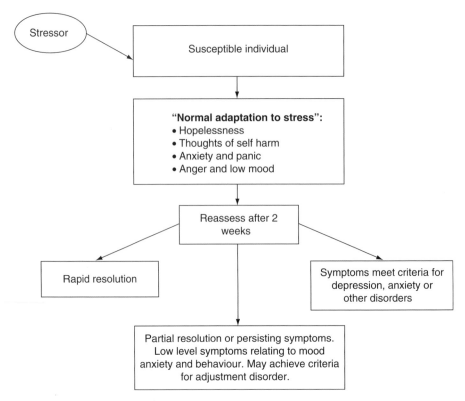

Figure 5.3. A pragmatic approach to assessment

legal case against the employer. The reminders of the incidents during the preparation of the legal case can prolong the symptoms.

A pragmatic approach is summarized in Figure 5.3.

The symptoms of AD are often conflated with depressive illness and there is little to distinguish one from the other apart from the close time relationship to a stressful event in AD and the presence of typical vegetative symptoms in depressive illness such as early-morning wakening, diurnal mood swing and psychomotor retardation. In essence a reaction is considered an AD if it is in excess of what would be normally expected and the symptoms are believed to be driven by the external stressors rather than having their own momentum. Thus ADs have the likelihood of spontaneous resolution when the stressor is removed. It is clear that a great deal of judgement is required when considering a diagnosis of AD that takes into account individual vulnerability, the meaning of the event for the person and cultural norms for the expressions of distress along with the stressor and the subsequent symptoms (Casey 2009).

Epidemiology

Among adolescents the stressors are related mainly to school and parental problems, while they are more diverse in adults. Demographically, women outnumber men by a ratio of 2:1. The diagnosis is made largely in the under-30 age group and over 50% are single, separated or divorced.

There is little information on the prevalence of ADs in the community at large. Among general practice attendees recent studies are lacking but older data suggest a prevalence of between 17 and 25% of those consulting with emotional problems (Blacker and Clare 1988; Casey *et al.*, 1984).

Differential diagnosis

1. The first consideration is whether the reaction is in fact abnormal at all. Emotion is always a feature in response to events, be they positive or negative. With the emphasis on the detection and treatment of depression and anxiety and the availability of effective treatments, it is tempting to regard any emotional responses as pathological and to 'do something' such as prescribing psychotropic medication. This concern has recently been articulated by one of the founding fathers of the current criteria for major depression in DSM-IV (Spitzer 2007). Many of these responses to stress can be considered normal adaptive reactions.

2. The second differential is from depressive illness, which also frequently has a precipitant. Appetite, sleep and concentration disturbance may be present in both. Anxiety is also common to each. One of the problems is that the threshold for reaching the criteria for major depression is now so low that almost anybody who is distressed for longer than 2 weeks would be so diagnosed, with the likely consequence of being prescribed an antidepressant. Since AD is a diagnosis based on the longitudinal pattern of being provoked by a stressor and resolving spontaneously, a course that cannot be known at the time of making the evaluation, the cross-sectional diagnosis of major depression trumps that of AD.

   If the stress is long-standing, arriving at a definitive diagnosis is more difficult. It may be that the ongoing stressors are prolonging the symptoms or that the person has now tipped into a depressive illness. Sometimes the pragmatic decision is to give a trial of antidepressants coupled with psychotherapy and then re-evaluate the person's symptoms and functioning.

   If the dominant symptoms are those of anxiety and tension then generalized anxiety must be ruled out.

3. It should always be borne in mind that those who seem to have AD may in fact be in the early stage of an evolving disorder and so follow-up is important so as to evaluate any deterioration in symptoms, especially if there appears to be a disjunction between the presence of the stressor and symptom severity.

4. When the person has been exposed to an overwhelming stressor such as a major traffic accident it is tempting to diagnose PTSD. Yet this diagnosis should only be made when the characteristic symptoms are present, since PTSD is not the inevitable consequence of a major event and other conditions such as AD can also be among the sequelae.

Treatment and prognosis

By definition the minimum of pharmacological treatment is required since this condition is not conceptualized as an illness but rather as a reaction which is self-limiting. Pharmacotherapy has little role to play except in the acute phase if symptoms such as anxiety or insomnia are overwhelming. Antidepressants are not indicated and there is no evidence to suggest that they reduce depressive symptoms.

The psychological interventions should begin with an explanation of the basis for the symptoms along with reassurance that these are understandable in the circumstances and linked to patients concerns. Frequently patients will ask whether they are likely to 'break down' and again this fear should be dispelled so as to limit the pressure to prescribe. Relaxation techniques may be encouraged to reduce anxiety symptoms.

Once the problem causing the reaction has been revealed, patients will often talk openly about what has happened. Frequently the doctor will find himself unable to 'do' anything to effect change in the patient's circumstances. The value of listening, 'just being there', should not be underestimated since many who consult with such reactions will be isolated socially or unsupported and have few personal resources. Acting as a confidant and a support may at times be life-saving. The value of formal counselling, problem-solving or CBT is uncertain due to the paucity of studies in this area. Because most symptoms resolve quickly it may be more appropriate to use 'micro-therapy' (Chapter 20) within the primary care consultation, taking a reflective counselling stance while incorporating a problem-solving or cognitive behaviour approach to discussions. Resolution without formal therapy has the advantage of allowing the patient to believe more in their own internal resources.

A definitive offer of follow-up is critical, as an 'insurance policy' for the patient so as to provide an opportunity to explore other diagnoses if there is no resolution and to reassess suicide risk.

Referral for psychological therapy or other social interventions may well be appropriate if the problems or symptoms do not resolve and a range of therapies may be employed, including problem-solving or solution-focused interventions, relationship therapy, cognitive therapy or longer-term psychodynamic interventions. The specifics of these will depend on the nature and background to the problem as well as the mediators determining the vulnerability of the individual.

An example of AD is described below, which evolved slowly but resolved rapidly.

Case 2

Mr. X was a 55-year-old man admitted to the psychiatric unit having been rescued when he attempted to jump from a bridge into the river. He had left a suicide note in his car. He reported increasingly low mood since his relationship broke up 6 months earlier. Shortly thereafter he was made redundant, although he had since got another job. His salary was now much less than previously. This had resulted in mounting debt. When he moved out of his partner's house he rented a one-bedroom bedsit that was cold, damp and poorly furnished but was all he could afford. He ceased meeting his friends and siblings because he was embarrassed about his situation. His evenings were spent in the pub where he drank, usually on his own, and had food, because his accommodation was so poor. He returned home only to sleep. He continued to go to work and was satisfied that he was doing it well. Seeing no solution to his debts or accommodation problems he decided to end his life.

During his stay in hospital he was not given any medication apart from hypnotics for the first two nights. He was reported to be eating well, attending all activities and engaging in conversation with staff and fellow-patients. His mood was euthymic and he reported relief that his life had been saved. He also felt happy to be away from his situation and to be receiving help for the same. He received visits from close friends and from his siblings, who were disappointed that he had not confided his predicament to them. Offers of accommodation were made and he accepted this. Meanwhile he was referred to a free financial advice service for help in addressing his debts and to the local council for help with housing. He began to discuss his problems in more detail with the team social worker and was discharged 2 weeks post-admission. Throughout the period of follow-up he remained symptom-free and continued the process of resolving his debt and accommodation problems. He was discharged to his GP 6 months post-admission and did not require medication.

Comment

This gentleman's history showed that the onset of symptoms was closely related in time to the breakup of his relationship and was maintained and eventually worsened by a number of factors, which included financial difficulties and housing problems. In addition he was socially isolated and so had no support from those who might have been able to help him, either emotionally or practically. Although his mood was low he continued to work. His use of alcohol may have contributed to his low mood. His increasing hopelessness and sense of helplessness led to him making a serious suicide attempt. Once he was in an environment that removed him from his adverse circumstances and offered practical assistance and emotional support his symptoms resolved rapidly with the minimum of pharmacotherapy. This case study indicates that AD can persist while adverse social circumstances continue and also that it can in some instances be associated with near-miss suicide. This history illustrates the overlap between AD and depressive episode since this man might easily have been prescribed antidepressants when in fact his symptoms were driven exclusively by his circumstances.

Outcome

The favourable prognosis for those with AD is demonstrated by studies showing that in comparison with depressive illness hospitalization times are shorter and readmission rates are lower after an index episode (Jones *et al.* 2001). Sometimes the diagnosis changes to alcohol misuse or personality disorder but this is unsurprising since alcohol can cause depressive symptoms, the cause of which may not be evident due to failure of disclosure. Those with personality disorder are particularly prone to experience AD in response to stressful events and this subgroup may have a poorer prognosis than the generality of those developing AD since their problem-solving skills are often limited and they may have limited social supports to mitigate the effects of adverse events.

Acute stress reactions

Acute stress reactions are those disturbances which develop in response to exceptional physical or mental stress. The symptoms are present in the early hours and days following such a stressor and consist of the same symptoms as those seen in PTSD.

Initially there may be a dazed feeling and withdrawal from the surrounding situation. Physical symptoms of anxiety are particularly common, as are flashbacks, numbing and nightmares. They usually appear within minutes of the impact of the stressful event and may resolve within hours or days but can last up to 4 weeks after the traumatic incident.

If they persist for longer than 1 month the diagnosis changes to PTSD. Usually, however, there is a gap of months between the resolution of the acute stress reaction and the onset of PTSD. Acute stress reaction is a risk factor for the later development of PTSD. PTSD can also develop without any acute prodrome when an individual appears to have coped, apparently unscathed, with a major stressful incident.

It has become commonplace to recommend counselling following intensive trauma, but there is evidence that debriefing in the early days after such an event may induce PTSD, while psycho-education is of little benefit (Wessely *et al.* 2008) although it is unclear whether it is harmful. It is better practice to allow patients to talk, if they wish, rather than being prescriptive.

Post-traumatic stress disorder

Post-traumatic stress disorder (PTSD) is distinct from most others in psychiatry in that a stressor is required without which the condition would not have developed. The current classifications specify that the stressor be such that 'the event is of an exceptionally threatening or catastrophic nature, which is likely to cause distress in almost anyone'. The range of stressors has increased significantly in recent years and includes traumatic hospitalizations for cancer treatments such as for autolgous bone marrow transplantation, severe asthmatic attacks, etc., as well as events that were traditionally associated with this condition such as warfare, kidnappings, torture and rape. In clinical practice the stressors most frequently associated with PTSD are traffic accidents and this is not determined by the severity of the physical injury sustained.

Controversies in PTSD

The concept of post-traumatic stress disorder (PTSD) is not without its critics, of whom Summerfield (2001) is the most vociferous. He points to the social utility of the diagnosis and argues that its emergence following the Vietnam War was driven by the anti-war movement and its desire to see attention moved from the soldier's background and personality towards an acceptance of the traumatogenic nature of war. Moreover, he and others draw attention to the expansion in the nature of the traumas that are now credited with causing PTSD, some of which, although upsetting, such as verbal sexual harassment, cannot compare with torture and rape. His view has been challenged by pointing to the neurobiological abnormalities that are associated with PTSD and the poor outcome in many when followed longitudinally. However, there are studies also showing that some people magnify or fabricate their symptoms deliberately for financial gain (see Chapter 12, p. 202) while others have symptoms maintained by the constant focus that is part of the legal process. In the latter this is not a conscious effort and when the legal case is resolved the symptoms diminish or resolve. This pattern is often found in those with unexplained or magnified pain following road traffic accidents. Interestingly, the prevalence of PTSD is no different among accident victims making claims when compared with those who are not.

A further criticism of PTSD concerns the classification of the syndrome. Some argue that the core symptoms such as intrusive thoughts are found in other disorders also such as depressive illness and that it would be best described according to the predominant symptoms. Moreover since the course of PTSD is variable, with depressive illness, drug misuse and panic disorder often emerging over time, it is arguably a heterogeneous condition and not a specific disorder (Breslau and Davis 1987). Complex PTSD, a proposed variant with symptoms overlapping those of borderline personality disorder, has its roots in repeated abusive traumas and includes both flashbacks or trauma-related nightmares and problems of emotional lability or dissociation (van der Kolk *et al.* 2005); developmental trauma disorder is similarly proposed for children who have responded to abusive trauma with emotional lability, dissociation and attachment problems, in addition to classic symptoms of PTSD. More recently the overlap with psychosis has been discussed. For example, women with auditory hallucinations and flashbacks following sexual abuse are now being classified as having PTSD (with or without personality disorder) rather than psychosis. A final consideration is the reliance upon memory to describe the stressful events that preceded the onset of symptoms, an attribute that is often unreliable even for highly traumatic and specific events such as atrocities witnessed by soldiers (Southwick *et al.* 1997).

Risk factors

The risk of developing PTSD is greatest in those who are vulnerable either because of personality dysfunction or where there is a prior history of psychiatric disorder. In addition the occurrence of other negative events prior to the trauma heightens the risk, as does the emergence of psychiatric symptoms prior to the trauma. Specific coping mechanisms are associated with a higher risk and these include the identification of an external locus of control, i.e. feeling powerless over one's life, emotion rather than problem-focused coping and disengagement from the stress. The occurrence of an acute reaction immediately following the event also increases the risk of subsequent PTSD (Briere *et al.* 2005).

Central to the diagnosis of PTSD is the fact that the event must be outside the realms of 'normal' experience. The nature of the stressor itself plays an uncertain role since it is the perception and processing of the stressor which determines the likelihood of developing PTSD. For this reason even relatively 'minor' accidents may sometimes be followed by marked symptomatic change. Undoubtedly, however, the greater the real threat to life, the greater the risk – thus victims of violent rapes, torture, kidnapping and serious physical injury are at special risk even though this may be delayed for months after the event. PTSD can also develop by proxy, such as witnessing the maiming or killing of others. Certain occupations carry a special risk, including body handlers and army personnel, firefighters and ambulance staff. However, PTSD is not inevitable and some, even those exposed to severe trauma, seem to adjust well. Those exposed to man-made rather than natural disasters are at greater risk. Shame, often experienced after rape, appears to potentiate the risk.

The biological basis of PTSD

The neurobiology of PTSD is complex and still evolving. Neuroendocrine studies have focused on endogenous opioid depletion, abnormal cortisol secretion and catecholamine excretion. Changes to activation of the areas of the brain concerned with memory encoding and retrieval have been described, as have abnormalities to the amygdala, the hippocampus, the lateral septum and the pre-frontal cortex. Noradrenaline is believed to play a role in inducing intrusive memories. However, few of the putative abnormalities have assisted in finding suitable treatments, with the exception of the SSRIs (see below), which may act indirectly as they have a modulatory effect on the noradrenergic system.

Epidemiology

PTSD is more common after man-made than after natural disasters and among civilian populations crime is the most likely trigger. So terrorist attacks are more likely to cause PTSD than earthquakes, and rape more so than a car accident. Studies in the USA suggest a lifetime prevalence of 1–9%, a not surprising figure in view of the high prevalence of traumatic events such as mugging, violence and traffic accidents. When assessments are made shortly after the incident the figure for those with psychiatric symptoms is much higher, but these are frequently self-limiting. For example a study of those living in the vicinity of the World Trade Center found the prevalence of PTSD 5–7 weeks after the 11 September 2001 attack to be 7.5%, and 9 months later, as a result of spontaneous resolution, the figure was 0.6% (Galea *et al.* 2002). In the general UK population there are no figures available but among army personnel deployed to Iraq the prevalence was 4.8% overall, with the rate being higher in deployed reservists in comparison with regular soldiers (Iversen *et al.* 2009).

Although traumatic incidents are more commonly experienced by men, women are more at risk of developing PTSD, possibly accounted for by the greater exposure of women to sexual offences such as abuse and rape or due to greater personal vulnerability.

Clinical features

Symptoms of PTSD are very common in the early days following a traumatic event but in this instance the diagnosis is not PTSD but 'acute stress reaction' (see above). Most of these symptoms reduce markedly over the subsequent weeks and a diagnosis of PTSD is made only if symptoms persist for at least 1 month. Inappropriate labelling at this early stage may only prolong the illness behaviour and may stimulate medico-legal action.

In many there may be a delay between the events and the onset of symptoms of up to 6 months but in a small proportion (1–4%) it may be delayed for several years. This is most likely when physical injury has occurred and the focus is not directed to the emotional reaction. The prognosis is also poorer.

Recognition of PTSD is often suboptimal. During assessment of anxiety and depression screening questions about traumatic events and intrusive dreams, memories and flashbacks related to the events are likely to be helpful.

Three broad symptom clusters are described in those with PTSD:

(a) intrusion

(b) avoidance

(c) hyper-arousal.

The intrusive cluster is regarded as the most unique to PTSD since symptoms from this group must be present to make the diagnosis. These consist of nightmares, flashbacks and intrusive thoughts of the experience which are very distressing. Flashbacks are often confused with intrusive memories and the term should only be used to describe the phenomenon of re-experiencing the event. Thus, the smell or action or emotional state at the time of the event may be recapitulated.

Avoidance results in numbing, inability to recall details of the trauma, restricted range of affect, depersonalization or derealization and active avoidance of reminders or symbols of the event.

Hyper-arousal is associated with anxiety, an increased startle response, insomnia, an increased sense of one's security or hypervigilance and irritability. In addition there may be survivor guilt and personal life may be seriously affected, with an inability to return to work due to debilitating anxiety or phobia.

Other symptoms include panic attacks, poor concentration, a sense of foreshortened future and mood disturbance.

Comorbidity

Comorbidity is the norm rather than the exception. This is unsurprising given the potential for trauma, in a susceptible person, to contribute to a range of conditions. Drug and alcohol problems are also commonly associated with PTSD as a poor coping response to intrusive symptoms. Some, particularly those who have suffered trauma in childhood due to abuse and/or neglect, are significantly disabled by low-grade symptoms from a range of diagnoses, co-occurring with PTSD.

Also, the symptom clusters and individual diagnoses fluctuate over time, with one or more often being dominant in different contexts. Intrusive symptoms of PTSD can re-emerge in the face of new stressors such as events that resemble the triggering traumas.

As well as developing psychological symptoms, physical syndromes are often also dominant and include chronic pain, gastrointestinal disorders including irritable bowel syndrome, fibromyalgia and chronic pelvic pain, the latter especially in women who were victims of child sexual abuse. Other unexplained physical symptoms include nausea, shortness of breath and headache.

Case 3

Mr. G. worked as a driver for a company. He was involved in a road accident in which a pedestrian who walked in front of his van was killed. While upset by this he returned to work 1 week later. The following week he was involved in another fatal accident when a car driving at high speed at 2 a.m. on the wrong side of the motorway hit his van in a head-on collision. The driver of the other vehicle was killed and Mr. G. was seriously injured. He was unconscious for 1 hour and required hospitalization for treatment of a fractured tibia. He tried to return to work but was unable to due to panic when he was a passenger, low mood and exhaustion due to insomnia. He also experienced regular nightmares and ruminations about the accident. He blamed himself, even though he was not at fault, and he frequently returned to the site of the accident so as to try and recall the event and was preoccupied by his limited recollection of the event. At the time of referral he was experiencing symptoms every day and was 6 months post-accident. In light of the symptoms of PTSD and low mood he was commenced on an SSRI antidepressant and referred for CBT. He was initially poorly adherent to treatment. Under pressure from his psychiatrist, his employers and his family he became more diligent. His symptoms gradually improved over the subsequent 5 months and he returned to work.

Comment

This man met the criteria for PTSD. He was already vulnerable, having experienced a similar event a few weeks previously. His poor adherence to treatment impaired progress while his amnesia for the event caused added distress and impaired his processing of the incident itself.

Treatment and prognosis

An empathic response to the patient is the first requirement for successful management. Among those with PTSD anger may often be dominant and this will be directed at the third party who caused the event. Even when the events are naturally occurring rather than man-made, anger may be directed at the hospital receiving the victims or at those organizing the rescue. Frustration may be felt at the changes in income or living standards that have ensued and the patient will usually wish to articulate this. The lost opportunities and the change in personal life may be a source of mourning, as in any major loss, and this should be acknowledged.

Pharmacological interventions consist mainly of SSRI antidepressants. Their effect is not just on comorbid depression but also on the core symptoms of PTSD, thus bringing about a global improvement in the patient's condition.

As well as the SSRIs, other agents such as the TCAs are used without specific licence particularly when depression supervenes although they also reduce the intrusive symptoms. While there are numerous open trials and case reports of the efficacy of clonidine, alprazolam, meclobomide, buspirone and lithium there is no evidence for their efficacy from double-blind studies.

Psychological interventions consist largely of behavioural and cognitive models. Treatment involves imaginal exposure and relaxation techniques and cognitive approaches that aim to modify the dysfunctional thinking about the event. Up to 20 sessions with an experienced therapist may be needed.

Eye movement desensitization and reprocessing (EMDR), first described in 1989, is one of the newer treatments described in the literature. The theory is that the distressing images and thoughts can be diminished if they are paired simultaneously with a series of rapid eye movements induced by the therapist. Successful RCTs have resulted in EMDR (up to 12 sessions) along with CBT being recommended in NICE guidance. A systematic review has found that trauma-focused interventions such as EMDR or cognitive therapy are superior to more general psychological treatments (Bisson and Andrew 2007). Other therapies include hypnotherapy but it is believed that exposure in imagination is the key element in successful outcome with the approach.

Prevention

The role of critical incident stress debriefing (CISD) assumed increasing importance in the wake of large-scale terrorist attacks and traumatic incidents during warfare. Indeed most hospital emergency plans incorporate CISD as part of the official response and failure to provide the same is frequently incorporated in negligence suits against official organizations such as the army, police force, etc. CISD consists of a single session in a group setting that involves reviewing the event and the emotions associated with it. Recent studies have shown that not only is CISD unhelpful but it may cause harm by interfering with the natural healing and processing that occurs for most people subjected to severe trauma. A recent Cochrane review concludes 'Compulsory debriefing of victims of trauma should cease' (Rose et al. 2004).

Prognosis

The current literature on the prognosis of PTSD is variable and inconclusive. The prognosis depends on a number of factors such as the presence of abnormal personality and the duration of symptomatology before treatment is instituted. Some remain chronically incapacitated and between 9 and 33% still have a definite psychiatric disorder several years later (Tarsh and Royston 1985). A majority fail to return to work and those who do so return at varying intervals after settlement of litigation. The prognosis is generally better after traffic accidents than after burns, head injuries or disasters.

Finally, it should be realized that families often become over-protective and frequently reinforce avoidance behaviour, thereby causing entrenchment and reducing the capacity for psychological rehabilitation. One of the influences on this is the lengthy litigation process, and attempts at hastening settlement should be encouraged so as to facilitate early reintegration at work and in the community at large.

Bereavement

Bereavement, due to loss of a close relative or friend, is a particular response to a stressor and includes both normal and problematic responses. For most people the grieving process is uncomplicated albeit emotionally painful and will have resolved by 6–12 months, with a re-adaptation to life without the deceased. For some grief is complicated (Birtwistle and Kendrick 2001) by not occurring at all or by being excessively protracted. In addition some people develop physical problems or behavioural problems such as substance misuse, depressive illness and anxiety symptoms.

Normal grief

The earliest descriptions of grief continue to hold good to the present day with their focus on the four stages of the process; although these do not imply any sequential phasing but are overlapping and intermixing. The first or numb phase describes the initial reaction of shock or disbelief, lasting for hours or even weeks. A second or yearning period is characterized by pangs of sadness and pining during which anger and/or self-blame may occur as well as crying, sighing and disturbance of sleep and appetite. Disorganization is prominent in the next period when the full realization of the death occurs, resulting in despair, withdrawal and apathy. Finally with resolution the person adapts to life without their loved one and hopelessness declines. At this point there is a gradual return to social activity, although many people describe ongoing feelings of loss.

Other features described by those who are bereaved include seeing or hearing the deceased, especially when among crowds (illusions), deriving comfort from talking to the deceased and feeling that he/she is looking after family members left behind.

Abnormal grief

A small proportion of those bereaved describe either protracted grief or no grief at all and in this group professional help is required with the aim of preventing the later development of major emotional problems. Failure to experience any grief is rare and in most instances the absence of emotion may stem from actively avoiding reminders of the deceased or striving to conceal emotion through fear of losing control.

Those who continue to describe acute symptoms of grief such as yearning and despair often require antidepressants and diagnostically they are regarded as then having a depressive episode. As well as depression, some describe symptoms of anxiety but these almost always co-exist with depressive symptoms and should be treated as such. The misuse of alcohol is an occasional further complication of bereavement; for most the increased use of alcohol post-bereavement is a temporary aid to sleeping and to reducing the 'edge' of the grief. Most studies report an increase in suicide and attempted suicide following the death of a spouse or parent.

Grief in other situations

The circumstances of the death can also affect the response and pathological reactions are particularly associated with a number of these including:

- death of a child, baby or sibling
- pre-natal loss of a baby through stillbirth, abortion or miscarriage
- violent death
- unexpected death
- where the bereaved is responsible for the death
- death by suicide or murder
- where post-mortem or inquest is involved
- when the body is not recovered
- when there is uncertainty as to whether death has occurred, e.g. disappearance.

Risk factors for abnormal reaction

A number of factors, apart from the circumstances of the death, are associated with abnormal reactions and foremost among these is whether the funeral was attended, although whether this has a causal role or whether it is an early symptom of an abnormal reaction is uncertain. Those who have many previous bereavements and a history of psychiatric disorder are also at increased risk as are those who were excessively dependent or ambivalent in their relationship with the deceased. Being male, under the age of 65 and lacking social supports also increases the risk, and where the relationship does not allow for full participation in the mourning process, e.g. extramarital or same sex relationships, 'disenfranchized' grief can occur.

Management

For most the grieving process takes place spontaneously and without any recourse to counsellors. Unless there are grave reasons, the bereaved should be supported to attend the funeral, touch the deceased and say goodbye if they wish. The use of hypnotics in the early stages of bereavement can help although there are no trials showing that the normal grieving process is not interfered with.

Where grieving has failed to occur or where it has remained unresolved, so that the person is still tearful, unable to visit the grave or look at a photograph, professional intervention may be necessary. Using the facilitating techniques the expression of emotions should be encouraged and support given whilst the stages of numbness, anger, guilt or blame are worked through. During therapy it may also be appropriate to give permission to reduce the frequency of visits to the cemetery or to remove the clothes and other possessions of the deceased.

Continued grief may indicate a need for antidepressants if the criteria for depression are reached.

Bereavement counselling may be necessary in situations of loss other than those of a loved one, including physical losses such as amputations, mastectomy, etc.

Summary

- Adjustment disorder is defined by the presence of a stressor and by a symptom cluster which improves with time as a new level of adjustment is reached, or when the precipitating stress is removed.

- Medication, such as antidepressants, has little part to play in treatment.

- Acute stress reactions resemble PTSD except that they occur in the early period following a traumatic incident and commonly resolve spontaneously.

- Post-traumatic stress disorder occurs in the face of extraordinary stress.

- Support and treatment of the primary symptom cluster is the mainstay of management.

- Psychological debriefing may be harmful.

- The prognosis is variable and some remain permanently incapacitated even after litigation has been completed.

- Bereavement may be complicated by being absent or by being protracted.

References

Birtwistle, J., and Kendrick, T. (2001). The psychological aspects of bereavement. *Primary Care Psychiatry*, **7** (3), 91–95.

Bisson, J., and Andrew, M. (2007). Psychological treatment of post-traumatic stress disorder (PTSD), Cochrane Database of Systematic Reviews, **3**.

Blacker, C. V R., and Clare, A. W. (1988). The prevalence and treatment of depression in general practice. *Psychopharmacology*, **95**, 514–517.

Breslau, N., and Davis, G. C. (1987). Post-traumatic stress disorder. The stressor criterion. *The Journal of Nervous and Mental Disease*, **175**, 255–275.

Briere, J., Scott, C., and Weathers, F. (2005). Peritraumatic and persistent dissociation in the presumed aetiology of PTSD. *American Journal of Psychiatry*, **162** (12), 2295–2301.

Brown, G. W., and Harris, T. (1978). *The Social Origins of Depression. A study of Psychiatric Disorder in Women*. London: Tavistock.

Casey, P. R. (2009). Adjustment disorder: epidemiology, diagnosis and treatment. *CNS Drugs*, **23** (11), 927–938.

Casey, P. R, Dillon, S., and Tyrer, P. J. (1984). The diagnostic status of patients with conspicuous psychiatric morbidity in primary care. *Psychological Medicine*, **14**, 673–681.

Galea, S., Ahern, J., and Resnick, H. (2002). Psychological sequelae of Sept. 11 terrorist attacks on New York City. *New England Journal of Medicine*, **346**, 982–987.

Iversen, A. C., van Staden, L., Hughes, J. H., *et al.* (2009). The prevalence of common mental disorders and PTSD in the UK military: using data from a clinical interview-based study. *BMC Psychiatry*, **9**, 68.

Jones, R., Yates, W. R., and Zhou, M. H. (2001) Readmission rates for adjustment disorders: comparison with other mood disorders. *Journal of Affective Disorders*, **71** (1), 199–203.

Read, J., von Os, J., Morrison, A. P., and Ross, C. A. (2005). Childhood trauma, psychosis and schizophrenia: a literature review with theoretical and clinical implications. *Acta Psychiatrica Scandinavica*, **112**(5), 330–350.

Rose, S., Bisson, J., and Wessely, S. (2004). Psychological debriefing for preventing post traumatic stress disorder (PTSD) (Cochrane Review). In: *The Cochrane Library*, Issue 1. Chichester: John Wiley.

Southwick, S., Morgan, C., Nicolaou, A., *et al.* (1997). Consistency of memory for combat-related traumatic events in veterans of Operation Desert Storm. *American Journal of Psychiatry*, **154**, 173–177.

Spitzer, R. L. (2007). In Horwitz, A. V., and Wakefield, J. C. (eds.), *The Loss of Sadness*. New York: Oxford University Press.

Summerfield, D. (2001). The invention of post-traumatic stress disorder and the social usefulness of a psychiatric category. *British Medical Journal*, **322**, 95–98.

Tarsh, M. J., and Royston, C. (1985). A follow-up study of accident neurosis. *British Journal of Psychiatry*, **146**, 18–25.

van der Kolk, B. A., Roth, S., Pelcovitz, D., Sunday, S., and Spinazzola, J. (2005). Disorders of extreme stress: the empirical foundation of a complex adaptation to trauma. *Journal of Traumatic Stress*, **18**, 389–399.

Wessely, S., Bryant, R. A., Greenberg, N., *et al.* (2008). Does psycho-education help prevent post traumatic psychological distress? *Psychiatry*, **71** (4), 287–302.

Further reading

Casey, P., Dowrick, C., and Wilkinson G. (2001). Adjustment disorders: faultline in the psychiatric glossary. *British Journal of Psychiatry*, **179**, 479–81.

Suggested reading for patients

David, M., Eshelman, E. R., and McKay, M. (2008). *The Relaxation and Stress Reduction Workbook*, 6th edn. Oakland, CA: New Harbiner Publications.

Schiraldi, G. R. (2009). *The Post traumatic Stress Disorder Source Book. A Guide to Healing, Recovery and Growth*, 2nd edn. New York: McGraw-Hill.

Useful addresses

Victim Support, Cranmer House, 39 Brixton Road, London, SW9 6DZ, UK.

Assist (Assistance, Support and Self-Help in Surviving Trauma) Helpline 01788560800.

Federation for Victim Assistance, Ireland +353667119830.

Useful websites for patients

www.uktrauma.org

www.trauma-pages.com

http://www.rcpsych.ac.uk/mentalhealthinfo/problems/ptsd/posttraumaticstressdisorder.aspx

http://www.rcpsych.ac.uk/mentalhealthinfoforall/problems/bereavement/bereavement.aspx (this website contains information on support organizations for those bereaved)

Anxiety disorders

Learning objectives

Anxiety as a symptom
Anxiety as a trait
Generalized anxiety, panic, depersonalization, social anxiety and phobic disorders
Pharmacological and psychological approaches to treatment
Obsessive compulsive disorder and its management

Anxiety can be mild and transient or incapacitating and chronic. It is one of the commonest emotions seen by practitioners in primary care. Anxiety is a universal emotion which is unpleasant and associated with psychological feelings as well as bodily sensations such as palpitations and sweating. The roots of anxiety lie in our phylogenetic ancestry where it served as a warning of danger and threat.

Anxiety as a normal response

Anxiety is first and foremost the normal response to threat or stress. Thus most people, prior to an interview or other stressful situations, will experience feelings of psychological tension along with somatic symptoms. This anxiety will, in most, improve performance and be of benefit. If, however, the level of anxiety is excessive, as indicated by impaired performance, a short-term intervention can be helpful. The point at which anxiety interferes with performance varies from individual to individual and with the particular circumstances, e.g. a person who is ill-prepared for an examination may experience higher levels of anxiety than one who is better prepared. The relationship between anxiety and performance is illustrated by the Yerkes–Dodson curve shown in Figure 5.2 (p. 34).

Much of the general practitioner's role is to help patients view anxiety as a brief, and sometimes unpleasant, but normal and self-limiting condition in response to a stressful situation. Deciding on a specific diagnosis, if any, is also important. Formal therapy or medication is indicated for severe or persistent problems.

Anxiety as a symptom

Anxiety can be present in all psychiatric conditions to a greater or lesser degree. In schizophrenia, for example, there is normally little difficulty recognizing that anxiety is secondary to other symptoms. In conditions such as depressive illness anxiety is present in almost 70% (Kessler *et al.* 2005a). Depression may, however, be misdiagnosed as anxiety and consequently inappropriately treated. Such misdiagnosis is not surprising since there is debate within psychiatry about the separation of these two disorders. On the one hand some believe that both can be clearly distinguished on the basis of their symptoms whilst the opposing view is supported by findings from therapeutic trials and from natural history studies.

The anxiety/depression conundrum

The debate about the separation of depression from anxiety disorders is further complicated by the fact that in primary care the diagnosis 'mixed anxiety with depression' is commonly used and it is said to affect 1 in 7 of the general population. On the other hand it has always been recognized that even in severe depression anxiety symptoms are prominent. So, when is the label 'mixed anxiety and depression' most appropriate as distinct from 'depression'? A further diagnosis often made in primary care is anxiety with secondary depression, a combination that is not formally recognized as a diagnostic entity.

The ICD classificatory system enhances this confusion, since depression is included under the affective disorders group while mixed anxiety and depression is classified with the anxiety disorders in a group termed 'Neurotic, stress related and somatoform disorders'. On the other hand DSM does not mention mixed anxiety and depression at all. A diagnosis of mixed anxiety and depression is made only when, according to ICD-10, neither component reaches the threshold for a single diagnosis of either depression or generalized anxiety. If either cluster reaches the threshold for a specific disorder, then the mixed diagnosis should not be made and instead the primary diagnosis would depend on the threshold syndrome. If the threshold for both anxiety and for depression were reached then the diagnosis would depend on which was primary.

In this regard, three considerations will assist the doctor in determining whether the anxiety or the depression is primary:

- the timing of the onset relative to other symptoms
- the previous history of the patient
- the age of the patient.

The timing of symptom onset is crucial and if anxiety predates the depressive symptoms then a primary diagnosis of anxiety with secondary depression may be more appropriate, while if both developed in tandem or depressed mood preceded the anxiety, a primary mood disorder is more appropriate. With respect to age, there is evidence that generalized anxiety seldom occurs for the first time in those over the age of 35 and all such individuals should be regarded as likely to have 'masked' depressions and be managed accordingly. Finally if the person has a prior diagnosis of either generalized anxiety or depression this should also be borne in mind when deciding on the current syndromal diagnosis.

Anxiety as a trait

This refers to the habitual tendency of the individual to be anxious and to worry. It describes a lifelong personality trait and is distinct from generalized anxiety (see below), which is a description of a syndrome/illness. When severe, the trait of anxiety may be a manifestation of an anxious or avoidant personality disorder. In addition to persistent worrying and tension, the patient with anxious personality disorder frequently has strong feelings of social inadequacy and fear of criticism and rejection with a consequent unwillingness to become involved in relationships or occupations.

Generalized anxiety disorder (GAD), as a time-limited disorder, may be superimposed on those with anxious traits, with anxious or avoidant personality disorders or on those with neither of these underlying features. The treatment principles are, however, similar once anxiety affects performance irrespective of the underlying vulnerabilities.

Anxiety as a disorder

Anxiety disorders are classified into three groups – generalized anxiety disorder (GAD), panic disorder, and phobic anxiety. Some further divide panic disorder into panic with and without agoraphobia and contend that panic disorder underpins all agoraphobia. However, most clinicians regard agoraphobia as separate and hence classify it with the phobias. The relationship between anxiety and depression is considered above (the anxiety/depression conundrum).

Some authorities also question the validity of panic as a diagnostic entity and point to the instability of the diagnosis over time. Many patients develop other disorders, especially depressive illness or agoraphobia. Others become dependent on alcohol after years of drinking to self-medicate. Some also argue that panic is nothing more than a severe form of GAD. In spite of these misgivings, which we share, the disorder is classified in ICD-l0 and in DSM-IV.

Epidemiology

GAD is found in about 8% of primary care attendees (Wittchen 2002) but among the general public about 3% develop the condition during a single year while the lifetime risk is 5%. There is a 2:1 female excess in GAD seen in primary care and in the general population whereas among psychiatric inpatients the ratio is equal. The lifetime prevalence for panic disorder is about 4.8% (Kessler *et al.* 2006) although the point prevalence is much lower at about 1% and there is an excess in females. The prevalence of phobias varies with the sampling frame but in the general population an estimated 5–10% of the population have disabling fears although only a minority seek help. Social anxiety disorder (also called social phobia) has received a lot of attention recently and figures from the USA suggest that around 7% of attendees in primary care meet the criteria for this condition while up to 13% in the general population develop it at some point during life. For all phobias there is a female excess and all social classes are represented. The 1 year period prevalence in the general population is between 8 and 18% (Kessler *et al.* 2005a) while the lifetime prevalence of all phobias is over 25% (Kessler *et al.* 2005b). They typically begin in adolescence or early adulthood and the young are therefore over-represented although the natural history is largely unstudied since few present for treatment. Thus the possibility that at least some spontaneously resolve with the passage into adulthood seems likely.

Aetiology

The aetiology of anxiety disorders is not well understood. Various neurotransmitter systems have been investigated including the GABA, alpha 2 adrenergic and 5HT 1A systems. Genetic contributions may also play a part since up to 50% of monozygotic twins are concordant for the disorder, especially panic disorder. Cognitive theorists hypothesize that those with anxiety disorders are responding to incorrectly perceived dangers. For phobias learning theory is invoked and it has been demonstrated that the fear response becomes attached to another stimulus through conditioning (see below).

Generalized anxiety disorder

The core feature of GAD is generalized and persistent anxiety which is not confined to any one situation. Feelings of nervousness, fear, tension and light-headedness are common and terms such as 'being like a taut wire' and 'feeling like bursting' are often used by patients to describe their feelings. Other physical symptoms include palpitations, sweating, hypersensitivity to noise, headaches and gastrointestinal discomfort. Fears that a family member will have an accident or anxious foreboding (a general feeling of fear which is unfocused) are also common and there may be a tendency to worry about everything. Sleep difficulties, especially initial insomnia, are common, often severe and may be the presenting complaint.

Case 1

Mr X, a 22-year-old student, was sent by his parents because of worries about his impending degree examination. He had always done well and was one of a family of six, all of whom had professional qualifications. He admitted to feeling tense and getting overwhelming feelings of panic when he thought of the volume of work he had to get through. On closer questioning he admitted that he had felt similar tension before exams in the past, all of which he had been successful in. It was explained that his tension was a natural reaction to the pressure he was under and as similar feelings in the past had not incapacitated him he was not offered any further treatment apart from diazepam 2 mg per day over the examination period. He was successful in his exams and returned 2 months after the results still feeling keyed-up and having episodic palpitations, sweating and dizziness. His pleasure from life was normal and he looked forward to his future career with excitement. Appetite, concentration and sleep were normal and he denied feeling depressed although his symptoms 'got him down'. A diagnosis of generalized anxiety disorder was made at this point and his symptoms resolved with instruction in relaxation exercises.

Comment

The decision not to 'treat' at first referral was appropriate although the doctor should have been alerted to the family pressure and expectations which might render him vulnerable to ongoing anxiety symptoms. Diagnosis and treatment were appropriate when he developed pathological anxiety. For the future, encouragement to distance himself from his family at such times should be recommended.

Panic disorder

The principal features of panic disorder include the sudden onset of attacks of palpitations, sweating, breathlessness, etc., which overwhelm the patient and are associated with intense feelings of fear. This may lead to the belief that a myocardial infarction or cerebrovascular accident is occurring. Secondary fears of dying, of losing control, or of going mad are common. The crescendo of fear may lead to the person leaving the situation in which the panic has occurred; this can result in phobic symptoms developing. The attacks are classically not related to any particular situation and they are generally unpredictable, although some patients recount a variety of scenarios which induce panic. Panic disorder can therefore accompany both GAD and more specific phobic problems. It can also be a presenting feature of depressive illness as illustrated by Case 2 below.

Case 2

Mr X, a 52-year-old man with a 6 year history of panic attacks, was referred. These were especially bad in the mornings and in consequence he would wake up early. He had difficulty in beginning his day's work as managing director of his firm and he attributed this to tiredness from the sleep disturbance and from the almost continuous panics. He denied depression but admitted to feeling hopeless about his symptoms ever resolving. He had no previous contact with the medical profession and had a supportive wife and children. He was by nature punctilious. He could not recall any precipitating event or any untoward stresses at the onset of his symptoms. He had earlier been prescribed tranquillisers with some slight improvement in his symptoms. A diagnosis of depressive illness was made and he responded dramatically to a tricyclic antidepressant.

Comment

The age of onset along with the diurnal swing in the symptoms should have been sufficient to make the correct diagnosis initially. Even where depression is denied, there is often a change in intensity of other symptoms, in this case anxiety, throughout the day. Where anxiety is part of a depressive illness, treatment of the former brings only temporary relief.

Phobic disorders

The aetiology of phobic anxiety is best understood in terms of classical conditioning. It is recognized that many phobias begin after a traumatic event, e.g. fear of dogs after being bitten. Using this model, the bite is the unconditioned stimulus and fear the response. Fear then becomes linked to all dogs (the conditioned stimulus) and may generalize further to all furry animals or to some other similar stimulus. In classical theory extinction of the response occurs if the conditioned stimulus (the dog) is presented repeatedly without the unconditioned stimulus (the bite). This is the basis for exposure as a method of treatment. There is no evidence that genetic factors play a part in the development of phobias since the necessary twin and adoptive studies have not been carried out. However, some phobias, such as social anxiety disorder and illness phobias, are more common in families in which these conditions already exist although the respective role of environment or genes is yet to be clarified. Personality variables such as dependence may be important in the aetiology of agoraphobia and social anxiety disorder.

Phobias are classified into five types as follows.

Agoraphobia

Agoraphobia is the most disabling of the phobias. It can involve fears of open spaces but more often of being enclosed, of crowds and of leaving home. In its most severe form the sufferer is completely housebound. If the person deals with their phobia by remaining housebound (complete avoidance) then the physical and psychological symptoms of anxiety may be virtually absent. Some people, especially if assisted by family members, adapt to this way of life. Agoraphobia is more common in women than in men and begins in late adolescence and early adulthood. There is some evidence for a link with dependent personality disorder. Without treatment it runs a fluctuating course and may persist for years being interspersed with episodes of depression, which itself may need treatment.

Social anxiety disorder

Also known as social phobia, this disorder was first described as a discrete entity in the 1960s. It is next in frequency to agoraphobia. The condition is slightly more common among boys and often has its onset in the early teens. Social anxiety is classified into two types – generalized, in which there is excessive fear in a wide variety of social situations outside the family circle, which may include writing or using a keyboard in public, and non-generalized, in which the anxiety is circumscribed to only one or two isolated situations such as answering the door. Social anxiety differs from shyness, which does not prevent the person from carrying out their usual activities. The simple question 'Do you feel embarrassed in front of others?' may point to this diagnosis and further evaluation of the extent to which functioning is impaired will be required to clarify the diagnosis. Without treatment its course is chronic.

Case 3

Mrs X, a 28-year-old lady with a lifelong history of fear of meeting people, was referred for treatment. Her list of fears, compiled in a hierarchy from most to least disabling, was as follows: meeting people who were strangers, meeting people whom she knew, signing cheques in public places, e.g. banks, queuing in the supermarket, eating in public, drinking in public, and speaking on the telephone. This lady had always had this constellation of symptoms with little exception. Her husband was sympathetic but constantly encouraged her to carry out these activities. A diagnosis of social anxiety disorder was made. She was referred to a social anxiety group and benefited from this significantly.

Comment

The treatment of social anxiety disorder was beneficial. Some might also consider the use of those SSRIs which are licensed for use in this condition but this was not discussed in this instance. The possibility of a pharmacological approach was reserved in the event of failure of psychological techniques, which in this patient did not arise.

Animal phobias

Animal phobias begin in childhood and rarely present for treatment. Spider phobia is both classic and common. The sufferers are normal in personality and function well in every other respect. They rarely develop other symptoms such as depression and there is no free-floating anxiety, unlike agoraphobia or social phobia. There is some evidence that fear of snakes and possibly of spiders arises as a result of genetic imprinting.

Miscellaneous phobias

These include fears of blood and injury, of storms, of heights, of particular forms of travel and a host of other situations. They run a continuous course and begin any time throughout early adulthood. They resemble animal phobias in other respects.

Illness phobia

Illness phobias are distinct in that the focus of fear is internal. They include fears of any illness – often those which have had recent publicity. There is often intense worrying and rumination about the feared disease. They are equally common in both sexes and are very similar to hypochondriasis. If ruminations are present they may be linked to obsessive compulsive disorders.

It is important to bear in mind that phobias, like free-floating anxiety, do not begin for the first time in middle adulthood. They can arise as a symptom of a primary depressive illness and the treatment is then of that disorder.

Differential diagnosis

The most common confusion arises in relation to *depressive illness* where anxiety is a prominent feature. The age of the patient along with details of other symptoms of depression will clarify the diagnosis. As a general rule if the anxiety symptoms develop in tandem with depressive symptoms, then it is best to classify and treat as depression. On the other hand pre-existing GAD can be exacerbated by particular stressors and depression may follow. (See also p. 52: The anxiety/depression conundrum.) Generalized anxiety must also be distinguished from *alcohol withdrawal* since patients often conceal the amount they consume and withdrawal symptoms during periods of relative abstinence mimic anxiety and panic attacks. The episodic nature of these will also aid in concealing alcohol abuse as the true cause. *Benzodiazepine withdrawal* also gives rise to psychological and physiological anxiety and unless specifically enquired about may be missed. It is also important, in GAD, to ask screening questions to rule out diagnoses such as PTSD, OCD, body dysmorphic disorder and anorexia nervosa.

Treatments

In general no formal treatment is required for trait anxiety. On the other hand if the anxiety is leading to avoidance behaviour or significant symptoms then it is best thought of as GAD or another specific diagnosis, and treatment may be indicated.

Psychological – general

The consultation in primary care can provide an excellent opportunity for initial intervention. For mild anxiety an *explanation of the cause* and reassurance that the symptoms are not due to organic disease may help the patient from unnecessarily worrying that the symptoms are organic in origin. A common fear is of collapsing during a panic, although this rarely occurs. Other concerns are that heart disease will result from the symptoms or that a severe psychiatric illness will ensue. Often the relief from simple reassurance is temporary and in all but the mildest of conditions more active treatments including behavioural exposure are needed. Where the symptoms have been precipitated by a known cause, e.g. marital conflict or work-related problems, various psychological therapies (see Chapters 16 and 17) may be offered in primary care. More psychodynamic exploration of the conflicts causing the disorder may require referral to qualified psychotherapists. However, such exploration is not generally the preferred approach except in specific patients. There is ample evidence that used inappropriately or inexpertly psychotherapy can worsen symptoms and cause long-term damage. Cognitive behavioural approaches are preferred.

Behavioural and cognitive behavioural treatment

After explanation, the next approach to treatment for the general practitioner should be *relaxation techniques* or basic CBT approaches. These may well be within the competence of many general practitioners. Demonstrating relaxation methods to the patient, essential for improving the likelihood of a positive outcome, may require more time than the traditional appointment allows.

The general approach is the progressive relaxation of different muscle groups throughout the body and is outlined in Appendix 1 of this chapter. In addition, this approach may be combined with imagery – the use of pleasant images to facilitate and maintain relaxation. Those GPs who are trained in hypnotherapy can also use this to facilitate relaxation.

Practical advice about *restructuring the patient's timetable*, so as to avoid unnecessary stress, e.g. rushing, is given along with guidance on *distraction* when tension is developing. This may take the form of exercise such as jogging or deep breathing, of concentrating on the surroundings or of mental activities such as doing calculations, reciting a poem or prayer, etc. The patient may also be advised to avoid *coffee or alcohol*, at least for a time, since these sometimes worsen pre-existing anxiety.

In cognitive approaches anxiety-provoking stimuli are induced by the therapist and the patient is taught to control his anxiety simultaneously. Insight is given about the abnormal thinking which leads to tension and ways of controlling the unhelpful thoughts outlined. Cognitive therapy is based on the theory that distorted perception of dangers and of situations underpin the anxiety symptoms and by learning to identify these faulty thinking patterns the symptoms can be brought under control.

Cognitive therapy should only be used after adequate training. GPs and other primary care workers can attend 'CBT in the 10 minute consultation' and other courses to gain basic CBT skills. It may be beneficial especially in those with GAD, social anxiety and panic disorder and is useful for those who decline formal therapy or are on the waiting list for the CBT focused mental health teams. In other jurisdictions, such as Ireland, community-based psychological services are less well developed and these interventions can often be resourced only by referral to the psychiatric services or to generic counselling services.

For phobias, the treatment of choice is *systematic desensitization*. First, this involves training in progressive relaxation as described above although there is debate about the necessity for this initial step. Then hierarchies of situations provoking anxiety are con-structed followed by graded exposure to these situations. For example, a social phobic may describe answering the telephone as the least fearful, then answering the door, then eating in public, and so on. By counterposing these anxiety-provoking stimuli, either in imagination or ideally in vivo, with relaxation, the anxiety is extinguished. Throughout the exposure the patient self-monitors the level of anxiety and this is fed back at the end of the session to demonstrate the reduction that occurs with repeated exposure (Appendix 2 of this chapter). Graded exposure beginning with the least fearful situation and systematically working through the hierarchy is generally preferred to flooding. In the latter the patient is allowed to experience extended exposure to highly anxiety-provoking stimuli from the start.

There is some evidence that training a relative to participate in treatment is advantageous, particularly if they are unwittingly supporting avoidance behaviour. Indeed the role of the relationship is an important determinant of outcome, especially in agoraphobia (Hafner, 1977). The phobia can preserve the delicate balance within the marriage between the dependent patient and the controlling spouse. Treating the phobia may disturb this balance and is sometimes resisted by one or both parties. Before commencing therapy it is essential to assess the commitment of both parties to this.

Many patients enquire about *self-help groups* and whilst there is no conclusive evidence that they are unhelpful, some groups may unwittingly support those with low motivation who prefer not to address their fear.

Pharmacological

Tricyclic antidepressants were shown to be beneficial when benzodiazepines fell from favour, but are not commonly used now for the treatment of anxiety disorders. They have largely been replaced by the *SSRIs* in the management of GAD although the starting dose should be lower than the antidepressant dose and then titrated upwards. A disadvantage is that there is often an initial worsening of symptoms and it may take several weeks for a noticeable response (Katzman 2009). The NICE guidance to general practitioners states that long-term SSRIs may sometimes be required for GAD (NICE 2009).

The *benzodiazepines* were the mainstay of treatment of GAD for several decades because they provided rapid symptomatic relief. Due to the risk of dependence their use has waned. Generally they are best avoided but there are three scenarios in which they may be used – in each careful monitoring by the prescriber is essential:

(1) during a crisis for up to 3 weeks with tapering doses and regular reviews with return to normal functioning supported by psychosocial strategies;

(2) as a part of cognitive behavioural programme where they may be helpful in overcoming initial intense fear of situations; there should be a period at the end of the programme when they are not prescribed and exposure continues without the aid of benzodiazepines;

(3) where the patient is given a small number of tablets, perhaps no more than 10 per month, to be used only when essential; often this is reassuring to the patient and they are not used, serving an 'insurance policy' role instead.

In general it is best to use a medium- or long-acting preparation since the short-acting benzodiazepines are more likely to cause withdrawal symptoms. In light of the danger of possible litigation against doctors for contributing to benzodiazepine dependence, close monitoring is essential.

Pregabalin is also licensed for the treatment of GAD in dosages of 150–600 mg/day. As a non-benzodiazepine it has a favourable profile concerning physical dependence.

Beta-blockers such as propranolol were first reported as successful in treating anxiety neurosis in 1966 and since then there have been several studies verifying this. Their anti-anxiety property relates to their peripheral activity and they are therefore most useful in those presenting with somatic symptoms, with no direct effect on psychic anxiety. There is little to choose between various preparations but propranolol (40–160 mg) or oxprenolol may be preferred because of the paucity of side effects associated with them.

Low-dose *major tranquillizers* such as quetiepine may occasionally be used in severe cases unresponsive to other treatment although they are not licensed for this purpose.

Buspirone is a different anxiolytic without the risk of dependence. There is a delay in its onset of effects of up to 10 days making it inappropriate for use with short-term severe anxiety but it may have a place in those chronically anxious people who fail to respond to other measures. There is evidence that it loses its effect when given to those who have previously responded to benzodiazepines. It is not recommended for benzodiazepine withdrawal.

In general panic disorder is treated in a manner similar to GAD with the exception that beta-blockers and buspirone are not useful. There is a delay in the onset of effect and as with GAD the initiating dose should be lower than that used in depression. Early reduction of medication results in relapse and it may need be continued for 6–12 months. There is evidence that *monoamine oxidase inhibitors* (MAOIs) are similarly effective in the treatment of panic disorder although they are unlikely to find widespread use because of the potential for serious drug interactions.

Medication has little use in the long-term treatment of phobias, with the exception of social anxiety disorder. Paroxetine and escitalopram are the only SSRIs with a licence for its treatment along with venlefaxine (extended release). Beta-blockers may indirectly benefit those with the non-generalized form by reducing tremor and palpitations, as may the benzodiazepines. Musicians often use beta-blockers for performance anxiety. Overall both pharmacological and psychological treatments produce significant improvement although additional studies are required to demonstrate specific indications and benefits of pharmacological over psychological treatments. For the other phobias benzodiazepines may be used prior to commencing behaviour therapy to reduce anxiety levels and facilitate engagement with the specific exposure process.

Depersonalization and derealization

Depersonalization refers to an unpleasant state in which the patient feels detached and 'outside' themself. A variant, derealization, is the feeling that objects seem far away or unreal. These are not psychotic symptoms as is sometimes mistakenly assumed but uncommon manifestations of overwhelming anxiety. Primary depersonalization or derealization can occur in the absence of other obvious anxiety symptoms but are uncommon. Primary depersonalization and derealization are difficult to treat and are often persistent.

More commonly depersonalization and derealization are secondary to some other disorder, usually depressive illness or severe generalized anxiety. In these circumstances the treatment is of the primary disorder. These phenomena may occur in healthy people at times of tiredness, hunger or intense transient emotional states and they are then short-lived. Epidemiological studies have found that up to 70% of the general population experience these symptoms on an occasional basis and children may also experience them. A brief trial of an anxiolytic or antidepresssant with anxiolytic properties may help in some. Otherwise there is no specific treatment except to support the patient.

Obsessive compulsive disorder

Obsessive compulsive disorder (OCD), once thought to be a rare disorder, has been shown to be more common than was previously thought, affecting about 2–3% of the population. A word of caution must be extended against the lay use of the word 'obsessed', which is generally used to describe being preoccupied by some issue or worry. This is quite a different usage from the medical meaning of the term obsessive compulsive.

Once thought to have its origins in abnormalities of the Freudian defence mechanisms, its putative causes have now moved definitively to the biological sphere. Brain imaging studies, whether functional or structural, have found a decrease in size of the caudate nuclei and also abnormalities to the frontal lobes and the cingulum. Studies of serotonergic function have found differing results but an abnormality of this system is suggested by the superior effect of serotonergic drugs over other neuroleptic agents in treating OCD. Family studies of OCD show that 35% of first-degree relative of OCD patients themselves have OCD although whether this is genetically or environmentally determined is uncertain.

In addition to this possible genetic aetiology obsessive compulsive symptoms may occur in those with a history of past trauma, particularly abuse and attachment problems. For this reason it is not uncommon for those with PTSD, borderline personality disorder and other related problems to have comorbid OCD.

The predominant symptom is of a subjective compulsion to carry out some action or to dwell on some thought or abstract subject. Resistance occurs in the early stages of the illness but frequently disappears as the condition becomes established. Obsessional rituals may take the form of handwashing, touching doors, carrying out routine behaviours in a certain order, etc. with cleaning, avoiding and checking rituals the most common. The carrying out of the rituals often leads to slowness and this is known as obsessional slowness. Sometimes the behaviour may be preceded by an obsessional rumination, e.g. repeated handwashing following thoughts of contamination. The content of ruminations may vary from a preoccupation with words, or numbers, to intrusive blasphemous or sexual thoughts, or to violent images. The patient is aware that these are his own thoughts and can therefore be distinguished from thought insertion, which is a psychotic symptom seen in schizophrenia. Ruminations are especially distressing to the patient since many feel that they augur madness. Associated symptoms include anxiety, depersonalization and secondary depression.

There is no doubt that some sufferers have obsessional premorbid personalities with the typical features of punctiliousness, perfectionism, rigidity and cautiousness. However, most of those with obsessional personalities do not develop obsessive compulsive disorder.

Obsessional symptoms are seen most commonly not in obsessive compulsive disorder, but as part of a depressive illness or sometimes in schizophrenia also.

Differential diagnosis
Schizophrenia
One important difficulty lies in distinguishing obsessive compulsive disorder from schizophrenia since the obsessional symptoms frequently resemble passivity feelings or thought insertion. A careful mental state assessment is essential to make this distinction.

Depressive illness
Since obsessional symptoms often occur in depressive illness care must be taken to exclude this condition.

Obsessional personality disorder
Those with obsessional personalities (see Chapter 9) often have rituals which resemble obsessive compulsive disorder. The distinction lies in the severity and intrusiveness of the symptoms.

Management

Optimum treatment is a combination of pharmacotherapy and cognitive behaviour therapy (Storch and Merlo 2006) and in persistent cases pharmacotherapy may be required indefinitely, even when behavioural techniques have also been used. Several antidepressants have been shown to be effective in the treatment of OCD, even in the absence of depression. In particular the tricyclic clomipramine and the SSRIs fluoxetine, paroxetine, escitalopram and sertraline have been found to bring about a dramatic relief of symptoms although recommended doses of the SSRIs are much higher than those used in treating depression.

Ruminations are the most difficult to manage and for these a behavioural procedure called thought stopping is used, where the patient is instructed to ruminate, then to stop the offending thought and change to a more appropriate one. The switching may be facilitated by pulling on an elastic band attached to the wrist or by some other method, designed to distract. This is practised several times in the session until the patient has learned to control the ruminations. For obsessional rituals, response prevention is the method of choice. Gently restraining the patient from carrying out the action will initially cause anxiety to increase and an overwhelming urge to ritualize but eventually this urge will decrease and with it the rituals. Obsessional fears of contamination are best dealt with by exposure to dirt and desensitization.

Occasionally depression supervenes during behaviour therapy and this may need treatment with antidepressants. Where the obsessional symptoms are part of another condition such as depressive illness or schizophrenia the management is of the underlying condition.

Prognosis

At its most severe this is an extremely disabling condition. For this reason, before the advent of behaviour or cognitive therapy, leucotomy was on occasions used when all else failed. These therapies have radically altered the prognosis and now up to 70% of those treated can expect to improve. Those with obsessional personalities or those whose symptoms are chronic have inevitably a poorer outlook but the intensity of symptoms may fluctuate.

Summary

- Anxiety may be a normal response to stressful situations but it may occur as a symptom of some other syndrome, e.g. depressive illness, or may be a disorder in itself.
- Treatment is required only if anxiety is considered to be pathological. Attempts to reduce the normal anxiety response will impair performance.
- Cognitive behaviour therapy is the treatment of choice for phobias, panic and generalized anxiety disorder.
- Antidepressants are also useful adjuncts and are significantly better than tranquillizers, especially in the management of anxiety disorders.
- Depressive illness is frequently misdiagnosed as an anxiety disorder.
- In general practice the prevalence of anxiety disorders takes second place to depressive illness and adjustment reactions.
- Depersonalization and derealization most commonly occur in severe anxiety and/or depression. As primary disorders they are uncommon.
- Obsessive compulsive disorder is uncommon but debilitating. The main thrust of treatment is with cognitive behaviour therapy and anti-obsessional antidepressants.

References

Hafner, R. J. (1977). The husbands of agoraphobic women: assortive mating or pathogenic interaction. *British Journal of Psychiatry*, **130**, 233–239.

Katzman, M. A. (2009). Current considerations in the treatment of generalised anxiety disorder. *CNS Drugs*, **23** (2), 103–120.

Kessler, R. C., Chiu, W. T., Demier, O., *et al.* (2005a). Prevalence, severity and co-morbidity of 12-month DSM-IV disorders in the National Co-morbidity Survey Replication. *Archives of General Psychiatry*, **62**, 617–627.

Kessler, R. C., Berglund, P., Demler, O., *et al.* (2005b) Lifetime prevalence and age-of-onset distributions of *DSM-IV* disorders in the National Co-morbidity Survey Replication. *Archives of General Psychiatry*, **62**, 593–602.

Kessler, R. C., Chiu, W. T., Jin, R., *et al.* (2006). The epidemiology of panic attacks, panic disorder, and agoraphobia in the National Co-morbidity Survey Replication. *Archives of General Psychiatry*, **63**, 415–424.

National Institute for Health and Clinical Excellence. (2009). Partial update of CG22: Anxiety: management of generalised anxiety disorder and panic disorder (with or without agoraphobia) in adults in primary, secondary and community care.

Storch, E. A., and Merlo, L. J. (2006). Obsessive-compulsive disorder: strategies for using CBT and pharmacotherapy. *Journal of Family Practice*, **55** (4), 29–33.

Wittchen, H. U. (2002). Generalised anxiety disorder: prevalence, burden and cost to society. *Depression Anxiety*, **16** (4), 162–171.

Suggested reading for patients

Butler, G. (1999). *Overcoming Social Anxiety and Shyness: A self-help guide using Cognitive Behavioural Techniques*. London: Constable and Robinson.

Hyman, B., and Pedrick, C. (2010). *The OCD Workbook: Your Guide to Breaking Free from Obsessive Compulsive Disorder*, 3rd edn. Oaklands, CA: New Harbinger Publications.

Leahy, R. (2006). *The Worry Cure: Seven Steps to Stop Worry from Stopping You*. London: Piatkus Books.

Wehrenberg, M. (2008). *The 10 Best Ever Anxiety Management Techniques: Understanding How Your Brain Makes You Anxious and What You Can Do To Change It*. New York: W.W. Norton.

Useful websites and contact numbers for patients

No Panic Helpline (UK) 0808 808 0545

Helpline (Ireland) 01 272 1897

http://www.nopanic.org.uk

http://psychology.iop.kcl.ac.uk/cadat

http://www.fearfighter.com

http://www.rcpsych.ac.uk/mentalhealthinfoforall/problems/obsessivecompulsivedisorder.aspx

Appendix 1: Deep muscle relaxation

The patient is seated on a comfortable reclining chair or lying on a couch. The room must be quiet and the doctor aims to convey a feeling of relaxation himself. The whole routine takes about 20 minutes. The therapist begins:

Anxiety and tension are frequently associated with tense muscles. By using these exercises which I will demonstrate to you, you will be able to distinguish tension from relaxation and you will learn to relax yourself when this tension occurs. We will work through all the muscle groups, first tensing them and then relaxing them. We will begin with the right arm. I want you to make a tight fist, bend your wrist and then your elbow up to your shoulder. Get these as tight as you can so that you will be aware of the tension and pain in them. When they are as tight as possible begin to slowly unbend your arm so that it lies beside you, then your wrist, and finally your fist so that your palm is facing downwards. When you hear the word 'relax' let the remaining tension leave your arm so that it feels loose and relaxed.

Pause for about 10–15 seconds, during which the word '*relax*' is spoken once.

I want you to make the fist again and bend your wrist and elbow like you did the last time, but now tensing your muscles even more. When they are as tight as possible begin to slowly relax them, concentrating on how different your relaxed arm feels from the tension of a moment ago. Now try to relax your arm, forearm and fingers even more than before. [Pause] Let all the tension flow out through your fingers.

This sequence is continued for the other arm and forearm. For the shoulders tension is achieved by extending the neck and pulling the shoulders up round the neck, relaxation by allowing the head to fall forward and the shoulders to drop.

For the forehead the patient is instructed to frown and to tightly shut the eyes. Relaxation is achieved by smoothing the forehead and opening the eyes. The jaws are then clenched and the tongue pressed against the roof of the mouth and then slowly released.

The chin is pressed firmly against the upper sternum and then released. To control breathing a deep breath is inhaled which is then forced out against a fixed diaphragm and closed throat. The patient is then told to note the feeling of pressure in the intercostal muscles. He is then told to expire slowly and to continue to breathe slowly and evenly.

The stomach muscles are contracted and then relaxed whilst the patient is instructed to concentrate on the feeling of tension and then relaxation. The shoulders and buttocks are pulled together whilst the back is arched. They are then slowly released so that the patient is limp and heavy. The knees are pushed into extension as far as they will go, followed by the ankles and toes being extended as far as possible until a feeling of tightness is noted in the thighs, calves and feet. Relaxation then follows with the knees going into a position of slight flexion and falling slightly apart.

For each of these muscle groups it is important to repeat the exercise so that '*a little more tension than the last time*' is felt. Words like '*calm*', '*relax*' and '*loose*' are used repeatedly.

When the patient is fully relaxed it is useful to ask the patient to conjure up some relaxing picture and to think about this for a few moments. This is followed by a pause of about 1 minute so as to allow the patient to enjoy the feeling of complete relaxation and freedom from tension.

The patient is instructed to carry out these exercises twice each day. When he is fully conversant with them, they can be modified according to individual needs. The breathing and shoulder/neck routines are especially useful for controlling situational anxiety, e.g. in a queue. For the practised patient the tension routine may be omitted and the instruction to '*relax*' given straight away.

Appendix 2: Self-monitoring

'*I want you to mark off on the line below what your present level of overall tension and anxiety is.*'

No anxiety _____ The most anxious I could feel

0   10

Over the period of therapy, the decrease in anxiety will be plainly in evidence and can be utilized in giving the patient insight.

Mood disorders

Learning objectives

Description and epidemiology of various mood disorders
Vulnerability and triggers
Biological and psychological aspects of risk
Specific issues relating to mood disorders in general practice
Depression at special times
Bipolar disorder
Improving Access to Psychological Therapies (IAPT) initiative
Pharmacological interventions – which antidepressant?
Lifestyle and physical interventions

Depressive illness is one of the most frequent psychiatric disorders diagnosed in general practice. In this setting it has many faces, making it difficult to diagnose. It can be severe, resulting in hospitalization, or relatively mild and transient. It may present with agitation or psychomotor retardation; or it may be masked behind physical symptoms or anxiety. The term 'masked' does not imply deliberately concealing symptoms due to stigma or fear but refers to a lack of awareness of depression due to the prominence of other symptoms. These are sometimes referred to as 'depressive equivalents'. Occasionally the individual does not have the language to express how they feel and this is termed alexithymia.

Its high prevalence, significant impact on functioning, frequent recurrence and the emerging range of treatment options makes it the most important condition to manage well.

Classification of affective disorders

Unipolar depression (also termed depressive episode) is the term used to describe a single episode of depression and when it recurs it is termed recurrent depressive disorder.

Bipolar illness refers to depressive illness intermixed with mania or hypomania, called bipolar I and II respectively. Bipolar L is the term used instead of manic depression.

Dysthymia is a chronic, low-grade depressive condition which usually begins in early adulthood and is generally refractory to treatment. It is associated with long-standing personality difficulties and some classify dysthymia as another category of personality disorder. When an acute episode of depressive illness is superimposed on dysthymia the term 'double depression' is invoked.

The traditional subdivisions of depressive illness into categories, i.e. neurotic/psychotic and reactive/endogenous, although still used by some have been abandoned by many clinicians and also by the official documents on classification, i.e. ICD-10 and DSM-IV (see Chapter 4). The neurotic/psychotic dichotomy was based on the type of symptoms described. An alternative and separate classification was derived from the presence or absence of precipitants, i.e. reactive/endogenous. Provided both are used independently these differing systems still have some utility. However, over time both were used interchangeably so that neurotic and reactive became synonymous, as did psychotic and endogenous.

This caused confusion in labelling and therapeutic inertia in relation to those designated neurotic/reactive who were not believed to respond to antidepressants. It is now recognized that stressful events can precipitate a full-blown and sometimes severe depressive illness.

The decision to have a separate category for adjustment disorder (see Chapter 5) and to classify depressive illness by severity of symptomatology alone was hailed by many as an advance. However, adjustment disorders have not been frequently utilized as a diagnosis in general practice. We believe that GPs, while needing to be vigilant for mood disorders, should be wary of overdiagnosis and might utilize the following terms in certain situations:

- normal adaptive reaction – when symptoms are significant immediately (weeks) following a life event (a normal coping response) although some might argue that a normal adaptive reaction should not be given a specific label; on the other hand letting somebody know that their reaction is normal and likely to resolve quickly may be useful for both physician and patient;

- adjustment disorder – when the reaction to an event is excessive or prolonged and the symptoms do not amount to a depressive episode;

- dysthymia – when some depressive symptoms are present for long periods, beginning in early adulthood, but do not reach the threshold for depressive episode.

The dispute over depressive episodes and other similar entities such as adjustment disorders is an excellent example of how the current psychiatric classification systems, which are primarily based on symptom numbers and duration, cannot produce discrete pathological entities.

Bipolar disorder is also going through a process of re-classification; the European system (ICD-10) recognizes bipolar disorder as a single entity whilst DSM-IV has subdivided it into bipolar I and II. There are now moves to increase the number of sub-categories further to incorporate milder forms of hypomania as well as those hypomanic episodes that are triggered by antidepressant treatment.

The description in this chapter is based on the dominant ICD-10 and DSM classification systems. However, some commentators continue to view depression as part of a spectrum of mood variation, intimately connected to social context (Dowrick 2009).

Depressive episode, recurrent depressive disorder and bipolar disorder

In Britain depressive episode is the same as unipolar depression, the term used in the USA. It is colloquially known as depressive illness or simply depression.

Prevalence

Depression is part of the continuum from normal mood, through transient low mood and mild depression to severe depressive episodes. Doctors and psychologists have defined the cut-off (using ICD-10 or DSM-IV) for making a diagnosis of depressive episode in terms of symptom numbers. There is still ongoing debate about the cut-off and about the legitimacy of the diagnosis of mild depression, further highlighting the imperfections of the current system of classification.

Using various approaches to case identification among general practice consulters a 1 year prevalence of between 3 and 17% has been found although there are very wide cross-national differences. For example a recent study using the same methodology in all 15 centres world-wide found the rate for current major depression lay between 1.6% in Nagasaki and 26.3% in Santiago. Manchester had a prevalence of 17.1% (Simon *et al.* 2002). Although it is tempting to ascribe these cross-national differences to differing risk factors and therefore to regard it as a true finding, this study found that in the centres of high prevalence, which included Manchester, milder cases were being identified whilst in the other centres the illness was of greater severity. However, variability in single-country studies is more likely to be accounted for by demographic, urban/rural and methodological differences. Other studies have suggested a 1 year prevalence of around 10%. The lifetime risk is about 10% for men and 20% for women although a recent Swedish study spanning 17 years found a much higher probability risk of 25% for men and 45% for women up to the age of 70.

Bipolar disorder (formerly manic depression) is much less common and has a lifetime risk of around 1%. The sex ratio is also slightly different, with a female/male ratio of 3/1 for unipolar depression and of 1.5/1 for bipolar disorder. The mean age of onset at 30 is a little earlier too.

There is no established link with social class and depressive illness although there are associations with vulnerability factors such as unemployment. In general it predominates in women under the age of 45 and in men over the age of 55. The more severe episodes peak in the elderly.

Bipolar II disorder is a relatively recent addition to the current diagnostic categories, and has been the subject of much less research. One study found a prevalence for this disorder of around 10% in the general population (Angst *et al.* 2003) and there is also evidence that it is under-diagnosed, being mistaken for depression in around 30% of those so diagnosed (Piver *et al.* 2002). This group of conditions, ranging from classic manic-depression through to depression with mild forms of hypomania, are referred to as bipolar spectrum, in a manner analogous to the broad group of depressive disorders that spans psychotic depression through to dysthymia.

Aetiology

Depression can be seen from many perspectives. Similarly the causes have been investigated in different ways. We suggest that an integrated model of aetiology is preferable. Depression can be seen as a disturbance in function resulting from psychosocial factors, mediated through biochemical processes, whose extent depends on genetic make up.

1 Life stressors

It is accepted from a wide body of research that major events have an impact on mood and can trigger both depressive illness and bipolar disorders. Events such as bereavement and childbirth have long been known to provoke depressive episodes and terms such as postnatal depression and prolonged grief reaction were used descriptively in recognition of this. Naturalistic studies have shown that such episodes have a similar long-term prognosis to those which appear to be unprovoked. Moreover, all life events, but especially unpleasant ones, have been implicated. Included amongst the most stressful are those already mentioned, but also moving house and loss of a job. There was a mistaken view that severe psychotic depression occurred without any precipitants – i.e. that it was endogenous. This has been disproven, and even hypomania may be provoked by stresses.

2 Vulnerability and personality

Research has shown that certain factors increase the likelihood of becoming depressed in the face of a life stress. These include the absence of a confiding relationship, unemployment, caring for young children and the loss of a mother in childhood (Brown and Harris 1978). The importance of outlets and of support from family and friends is obvious from this work and should be borne in mind by the GP who is involved in the work of prevention. In some vulnerable individuals personality attributes increase the likelihood of becoming depressed. For example those of obsessional disposition may be at risk of developing depression in response to 'change' events. However, no one personality type is consistently associated with depression. In particular, the difficulty of assessing personality in the presence of depression must be remembered (see Chapter 9). The supposed association between depression and pyknic body build has been disproven.

3 Psychological causes

Freud proposed that depression was analogous to mourning and even where there was no obvious loss the depression was a response to a symbolized loss. However, investigators have found that fewer than 10% of those experiencing recent losses develop a depressive illness. This indicated the innate capacity of most individuals to respond adaptively to loss-based stressors.

Other theorists have emphasized the importance of emotional deprivation or maternal loss in causing depression. These 'attachment problems' have been associated with many psychiatric conditions such as alcoholism, antisocial personality, etc., so although important they seem to be non-specific.

The theory of 'learned helplessness' has attracted much attention but is not satisfactory as a specific explanation for depression. The theory states that depression develops when rewards and punishment are no longer dependent on the actions of the individual and the lack of control over whether these are received. Beck (1967) suggested that depressive cognitions may be central to depression and are important factors in maintaining the disorder once established. These negative cognitions refer to oneself, one's past experiences, and the future and are termed the 'cognitive triad'. This theory has led to the cognitive approaches to treatment described below.

4 Neurochemical

Neurochemical shifts from average levels in normal subjects are understood to mediate depression. There is no specific neurochemical abnormality responsible. The most acceptable hypothesis derives from the observation that antidepressants exert their central neurochemical effect on the 5-hydroxytryptamine (5HT) and noradrenergic receptors. Suggestions that the reduced availability of 5HT at synapses is the core to depressive illness have been countered by theories that it is due to the reduced sensitivity of the postsynaptic receptors. The possible role of noradrenaline (NA) has also been investigated and findings of depletion of NA and of an increase in the number of presynaptic receptors have been reported. Newer antidepressants act by raising central catecholamine levels, particularly 5HT and noradrenaline. The roles of sodium, calcium and magnesium have also been subject to testing and their involvement remains to be clarified.

The 'time-keeper' hormone, melatonin, has also been a focus of attention, mainly because of the seasonal variation in depression in some patients and the diurnal changes in symptoms. So far, the results are unconvincing. Since a variety of neuroendocrine imbalances have been found in those with mood disorders it is possible that this dysregulation is the result of more fundamental abnormalities elsewhere. Of particular interest are the adrenal and thyroid axes as well as growth hormone. The predominance of depression among women and the special risk following childbirth suggest a hormonal cause, but there is no convincing evidence for this. It is more likely that psychosocial stressors cause a generalized dysregulation, especially in genetically vulnerable individuals.

5 Genetic
The genetic basis for unipolar depression, although present, is weaker than in bipolar depression, with a concordance among monozygotic twins of about 50% and among dizygotic twins of 10–25%. For bipolar I disorder there is no doubt about the increased risk among the relatives of affected patients or of the higher concordance for the condition among monozygotic twins (up to 90%) than dizygotic twins (up to 25%). Moreover 50% of bipolar I patients have at least one parent with a mood disorder, usually depressive illness, and if one parent has bipolar I disorder there is a 25% chance that a child will be similarly affected. Molecular biology has enabled greater study of the exact mode of inheritance for these disorders and although no certainty as yet exists, associations for mood disorders, especially bipolar I, with chromosomes 5, 11 and the X chromosome have been reported.

Presentation in general practice
General practice is the most common health service setting in which depression is diagnosed. Two main forms of presentation can be identified.

Physical symptoms
Patients sometimes describe physical symptoms such as anorexia, loss of energy, aches and pains and stomach problems rather than depression itself. Disturbed mood might be attributed to the physical symptoms. Symptoms of anxiety including palpitations, tremor and sweating are very common in depression. Pain may predominate: either without discernable cause or a lowering of threshold. It is not surprising that these will often be the prime focus of the patient's attention rather than the accompanying emotional changes. There are a number of reasons why the patient may present with somatic symptoms, including low IQ, a (mistaken) belief that the doctor only wants to hear about physical symptoms and absence of psychological mindedness. Doctors need to be vigilant about the possibility of mental illness and ask screening questions if depression is suspected. Cultural factors also have a bearing and many ethnic groups present mainly with physical symptoms. Some people appear depressed but only admit to physical symptoms. A range of diagnoses associated with medically unexplained symptoms are described in Chapter 12.

Case 1

Mrs X was a 62-year-old lady who presented to her family doctor with a 2 year history of 3 stone weight loss and tiredness. She felt low and had both anorexia and insomnia (initial and late), but related these to her physical symptoms. She had married a few years earlier and had a good relationship with her husband. She did domestic work for a neighbour and was free from any worries, financial, family or otherwise. She had no previous contact with the medical or psychiatric services and seemed to have been well adjusted all her life. Extensive investigations by the local physician included blood picture, barium studies and endoscopies, which were all normal. Failure to improve resulted in a second round of investigations similar to those already done. Again the results were negative. She was referred by her general practitioner to the psychiatric services at this point, to determine whether a psychiatric disorder could account for her symptoms. A diagnosis of depressive illness was made and she responded to a tetracyclic antidepressant. At the time of writing she had been returned to the care of her general practitioner and was symptom-free. Attempts to discontinue her medication after 1 year resulted in a recurrence of the symptoms but increasing it again led to an improvement. A detailed family history revealed a number of relatives with significant depression and it was recommended that she remain on this medication indefinitely.

Comment

This lady illustrates the severity of physical symptoms which may accompany depressive illness, particularly in older adults. The likely reason for the diagnosis being missed initially was the absence of any stressors and her good premorbid personality. It is important to remember that many patients have depressive illnesses without obvious precipitants and who in all other respects are well adjusted. The dictum that 'she is not the type' is a dangerous myth! The possibility of misdiagnosing this lady as having somatization disorder is also a concern. The presence of classic biological symptoms of depression, along with older age, makes this a very unlikely diagnosis.

Emotional symptoms

Those who articulate emotional difficulties make the doctor's work easy and this mode of presentation is becoming more common. The patient will describe depression, anxiety and tearfulness and may also recognize an obvious cause for these. Anxiety is common in depressive illness and, when this is the presenting symptom, anxiety may mistakenly be regarded as the primary diagnosis. The age of the patient together with assessment of sleep, mood and other symptoms should clarify the diagnosis. Among general practice patients diurnal changes in mood may not be obvious but changes in the level of anxiety with morning worsening should alert the doctor to the possibility of depression.

Other emotional problems

Presenting with some other problem, e.g. loss of libido, excessive drinking, forgetfulness or relationship problems, may also occur and, may initially lead the doctor to suspect a sexual difficulty, primary alcohol abuse, dementia or personality disorder rather than depression unless a careful history is obtained from the patient. A history from another family member may be a useful aid to distinguishing depression from these other diagnoses.

Difficulties in making the diagnosis

It has been shown that between a third and a half of those patients with emotional disorders are not identified and prevalence rates as low as 3.5% have been described. However, it has also been demonstrated that over time most significant depression is identified in primary care (Kessler *et al.* 1999).

There are several explanations for the failure to recognize psychiatric illness in general and depressive illness in particular. First, some patients do not consult despite obvious distress. In particular, men may have difficulty in expressing their emotional difficulties or may be reluctant to discuss them. Men also consult GPs less frequently. It has been suggested that the predominance of alcohol abuse among men results from their tendency to use it for symptomatic relief rather than attending their doctors for appropriate treatment. The majority of people with significant symptoms do, however, consult their doctors; but they may not present all the classic symptoms.

Amongst consulters the reasons for non-detection are four-fold.

- First, the *knowledge* and *interest* of the doctor have inevitable implications for detecting depressive illness (see Chapter 2).
- *Sociodemographic factors* may be a source of bias with males, those from high socio-economic groups, the young, the elderly and the unmarried being less likely to be labelled as psychologically unwell than their female, separated and less well off counterparts.
- The manner in which patients present their symptoms is of crucial importance and complaints of physical symptoms, such as insomnia, tiredness, palpitations, etc., may reduce the probability of being correctly diagnosed. On the other hand those who normalize their symptoms are also less likely to be diagnosed with an emotional disorder (Kessler *et al.* 1999).
- Finally, there is the difficulty of confusing depressive illness with anxiety or adjustment disorder because of the symptom overlap.

Whether those who are diagnosed are more severely ill than those whose illness remains undetected is as yet uncertain but the latter are often less obviously depressed and may have an associated physical illness which distracts from the emotional difficulties.

Symptoms

Depression

The symptoms of depressive illness are listed in Table 7.1. The prominence of anxiety has already been emphasized. Psychotic symptoms are rare among people in general practice with depression; for those presenting with psychosis it is an important differential diagnosis. The content of the psychotic symptoms is negative, gloomy and often centres on catastrophe and evil. Hallucinations are heard in the second rather than the third person.

Hypomania

Hypomania represents a milder form of mania in that psychotic symptoms are absent or the level of impairment is less. Hypomania and mania are uncommon and may be confused with schizophrenia. When hypomania/mania occur simultaneously with depression the clinical picture is of tearfulness, overactivity and irritability alternating with elation and it is termed

Table 7.1. Common symptoms of depression, hypomania and mania

Mild/moderate depression	Hypomania
Gloom/tearfulness	Elation or lability
Irritability	Irritability and hostility
Anxiety: free-floating and phobic	Disinhibition
Depersonalization	
Agitation or retardation	Overactivity
Insomnia: early, middle or late	Insomnia
Hypersomnia	
Aches and pains	
Anorexia or overeating	
Impaired concentration	Impaired concentration
Lack of confidence	Grandiosity
Inability to cope	
Overvalued ideas of guilt, reference, hypochondriasis	Overvalued ideas of reference
Obsessional rituals or ruminations	
Severe depression	Mania
Inability to cry	
Inability to feel	
(loss of emotional resonance)	
Delusions of guilt	Delusions of grandiose identity or ability
Delusions of persecution	Delusions of persecution
Delusions of reference	Delusions of reference
Hypochondriacal delusions	
Nihilistic delusions	
Auditory hallucinations, 2nd person critical	

dysphoric hypomania (or mania) or a mixed affective state. Management of the mixed affective states is with major tranquillizers in the first instance, until a clear picture of either depression or more commonly of hypomania (or mania) emerges.

Differential diagnosis

1 Anxiety

The pre-eminence of anxiety in depressive illness is another source of diagnostic confusion. Questions about accompanying symptoms such as sleep, appetite and mood changes will clarify the diagnosis as will the presence of morning intensification of anxiety or depression. In general practice the diagnosis 'anxiety with depression' is commonly used to indicate co-occurring depressive and anxiety symptoms. For this diagnosis to be made both must begin simultaneously. Technically this diagnosis should be used for those with anxiety and with depressive symptoms which do not reach the threshold for major depression. In practice GPs use it commonly for those with comorbid anxiety and depression.

2 Personality disorder

When depression with anxiety or irritability is ongoing, personality disorder is a possibility. However, in the absence of any history that the symptoms and behaviour have been present since early adulthood the diagnosis of personality disorder is incorrect and serves only to 'justify' the failure of treatment rather than help the patient. There may of course be a co-existing personality disorder.

3 Normal adaptive reactions and adjustment disorder

The first consideration is whether the symptoms are appropriate to the current situation in which the person finds himself/herself. The presence of symptoms per se may not be abnormal when they occur in response to a specific stressor and can often be explained to the patient as a normal adaptive response to a stressor. No intervention is required other than general support. It should be noted that some practitioners use the term 'adjustment reaction' to describe these brief understandable reactions although this is not a formally recognized term in either DSM or ICD.

Adjustment disorder (see Chapter 5) is often difficult to distinguish from normal adaptive reactions but once functioning is impaired adjustment disorder is the appropriate diagnosis.

Adjustment disorders are also difficult to distinguish from depressive illness since most of the aetiological factors are common to both conditions, i.e. life events. There is also symptom overlap. Following a life event, even if depressive symptoms reach criteria for depressive episode, this diagnosis is not usually made. Instead, adjustment disorder is the appropriate diagnosis. These are self-resolving conditions and apart from support and symptomatic treatment of insomnia or anxiety no further treatments are required (see Chapter 5).

Thereafter, for those with depressive symptoms that persist beyond two weeks and meet the criteria, technically a depressive episode should be diagnosed. However, there is a caveat, which is that the current classifications set a low threshold for making a diagnosis of depressive episode (called major depression in DSM) when in fact these symptoms often resolve spontaneously. The current criteria may lead to an overdiagnosis of depressive episode in primary care, with the consequent prescription of antidepressants, when a diagnosis of adjustment disorder would be more appropriate.

4 Bipolar disorder

When manic or hypomanic symptoms are present the possibility of bipolar disorder must be considered. A state resembling mania/hypomania can be induced by illicit substances and schizophrenia also has to be considered. Sometimes manic and depressive symptoms occur simultaneously, termed a mixed affective state.

Atypical depression

This disorder has achieved prominence recently and the term is used to describe those who exhibit hypersomnia, overeating, evening worsening of symptoms, anxiety and irritability. Symptoms are often long-standing. Sometimes a depressive episode may be superimposed on the grumbling long-term symptoms and this is known as 'double depression'. The best evidence for treatment suggests that a combination of SSRIs (sertraline) and CBT achieves the optimum outcome but that response to CBT alone is similar to that of placebo. This must be considered against a background of very few intervention studies. There is anecdotal evidence that the long-term use of a variety of antidepressants, including the MAOIs, may be beneficial. This is seen in case vignette 2 below. For the general practitioner the importance of this condition lies in the unusual symptom pattern and the consequent likelihood of the diagnosis being missed.

Case 2

Mr X was a 45-year-old married man with a 5 year history of not coping with work, low self-esteem and anxiety. The difficulties at work resulted in occasional days off but there was no other noticeable effect. He felt his education at an expensive boarding school had been wasted and that he had learned little while there. He felt that his wife had made all the major decisions and he regarded himself as weak despite having risen to senior management in his firm and being materially affluent. His anxiety was the most crippling aspect of his problems and prevented him going on holiday or even planning the following weekend. Anxiety was especially bad in the mornings and he believed it caused him to wake early each morning and to be excessively irritable at work. He felt depressed about his state but did not describe any diurnal swing to his mood state. He tended to overeat and was most contented when he went to bed, sleeping for up to 9 hours each night (2 hours more than usual). He had been well until 5 years earlier. His mother was not supportive and his only sister lived a bohemian existence in another country and he had little contact with her. His wife was supportive but she was disorganized about the house and he found this difficult, being a tidy and well-organized man. He failed to respond to SSRI and tricyclic antidepressants in therapeutic doses prescribed by his general practitioner. A diagnosis of atypical depression was made and MAOIs were prescribed (phenelzine 45 mg BD). He made a good recovery, which is not always the case, and his view of himself, his education and his future altered completely. His MAOIs were reduced to 15 mg BD and he remains symptom-free.

Comment

The symptoms were by and large those of atypical depression. This patient illustrates the long-standing nature of depressive illness and the effect it can have on the patient's view of himself. Because of the predominance of anxiety and unusual symptoms such as overeating these patients are often regarded as having personality disorders and remain untreated. A guide is the age of the patient and a clear-cut history of a change in behaviour from normal.

Effects of untreated depression

The effects of untreated depression are potentially serious: mortality from suicide of 15% has been reported in older studies of those with severe depression. Much lower rates of suicide have been reported in a more recent study with follow-up for up to 6 years, being lowest in those with mild depression (0.5%), followed by moderate depression (1%) and highest in severe depression (2%), with men having over twice the risk of suicide compared to women (Kessing 2004). Marital disharmony consequent upon irritability, loss of libido or excessive emotional dependence may lead to eventual marital breakdown. The effects upon the bonding process with the newborn of depressed mothers are potentially life-long and may increase the propensity to depressive illness among these children in adult life. Many sufferers also have handicapping phobias secondary to their illness, leading to isolation and restriction of outlets and some may abuse alcohol in order to obtain symptomatic relief. It is therefore important to recognize and offer treatment for depression. Engagement and follow-up for those initially declining treatment may be effective in limiting the negative impact.

Assessing depression in general practice

After, or indeed while, a diagnosis is established a more comprehensive assessment may be completed over a number of consultations to include:

- risk of self-harm
- severity
- aetiology
- comorbidity
- concerns, expectations and ambitions
- investigations.

(The approach to arriving at a diagnosis and formulation in primary care is described in Chapter 3.)

Thoughts of being better off dead or not wanting to wake up are common and associated with cognitions of hopelessness. More specific ideas for suicide need to be taken seriously and reviewed; those with specific plans or intent are likely to need specialist assessment (see Chapter 11).

Aetiology is best assessed in general practice by focusing on social factors as a part of listening to a patient's narrative and can, if sensitively carried out, be valued by him/her. Discussion of predisposing factors such as traumas or abandonment can help patients understand the origins of their depression.

Patients will normally disclose precipitating events, but may need prompting to discuss perpetuating stresses such as relationship problems, illiteracy, housing, employment and financial difficulties. Family history should also be explored.

Comorbidity is common in depression and should be investigated thoroughly, particularly in those resistant to treatment. Brief screening questionnaires can be used, as can some screening questions for a variety of comorbid disorders. These include:

- the AUDIT (Saunders *et al.* 1993) questionnaire for alcohol
- enquiry about drug use
- nightmares or flashbacks (PTSD)
- repeated cheking, excessive cleaning/organizing (OCD)
- deliberate weight loss and bingeing (eating disorders)

- non-suicidal self-harm, aggression and anger, relationship problems (personality issues)
- panic, hyperventilation (panic disorder).

The use of these brief questions will allow a comprehensive evaluation of the person's psychiatric status. More complete questioning should be carried out in any suspected second disorder.

Eliciting concerns, expectations and ambitions is important. The first critical step, as discussed in detail in Chapter 3, is to reach a shared agreement about diagnosis. Some patients find it useful to be given a definitive diagnosis: either to validate a sick role, or because it makes sense of such varied symptoms. Others resist depression as a diagnosis, but would agree they are 'stressed' or 'down'. Fears include being 'locked up', or having to take medication forever. These concerns need to be elicited before formulating a management plan.

Perhaps more importantly, and in line with a 'recovery' and solution focused approach, it can be very useful to have discussions about the patient's individual hopes for the future. This can link back to previous strengths and activities associated with enjoyment and achievement as well as exploring new possibilities. Just asking, 'if in the future you have made a good recovery, what will you be doing and what will you have succeeded in achieving?' can help clarify an individual's goals. For some, depressive cognitions will make this step difficult at this time but there is no evidence that it is harmful.

Severity of depression can be assessed in a number of ways:

- symptoms (symptom numbers, severity of individual symptoms and whether psychotic symptoms are present)
- impact of functioning
- recurrence and chronicity.

Severity of symptoms (Table 7.1) can be further assessed using specific scales such as the General Health Questionnaire (GHQ) (Goldberg and Hillier 1979), Hospital Anxiety Depression Scale (HADS) (Zigmond and Snaith 1983) and Beck Depression Inventory (BDI) (Beck et al. 1961). These scales can contribute to making a diagnosis, and monitoring progress; they are also used as part of the Quality and Outcomes Framework for rewarding quality care in the UK. However, they perform differently in clinical practice as compared to research settings. In the former there is a risk of symptom exaggeration so as to obtain particular treatments. They should always be used in conjunction with a full diagnostic interview and never as a replacement.

Patients with tiredness or weight loss may need early investigations. Also, when depressive illness fails to respond to adequate treatment it is important to rule out the common physical causes of depressive illness, especially thyroid disease and malignancy.

Dexamethasone suppression tests are disturbed in some patients with depressive illness and measurement has been advocated by some. These are unlikely to be helpful to the general practitioner since they are normal in most of those with depression.

Depression at specific times

Postnatal depression

This refers to the occurrence of depressive illness, usually in the 12 months following childbirth although the symptoms may sometimes have preceded childbirth. Symptoms are similar to those at other times of life but the feelings of uselessness and inability to cope centre on the patient's role as a mother. In its severe form, known as puerperal psychosis, the presence of delusions may place the baby and also the mother at risk of physical harm. Admission to hospital is necessary in these circumstances. A mother and baby unit provides the optimum setting for the management of depression following childbirth.

There is uncertainty about the time period within which the birth of a child may be considered a precipitant. Whilst stressors are no longer believed to be specific to childbirth this does not exclude the importance of helping the depressed mother adjust to her new role as mother or to the stresses inherent in tending a baby. The pharmacological treatment of the symptoms is, however, similar to that used in all patients with depressive illness and the long-term prognosis is similar to that of depressive illness in general. Certain antidepressants are recommend while breastfeeding (see p. 85). Antenatal depression is also common and also has specific pharmacological treatments. The roles of the midwife and health visitor are critical, particularly with respect to early diagnosis. Psychosocial treatments are being investigated at present for use with or without antidepressants simultaneously.

The menopause

The menopause has traditionally been believed to be associated with an increase in emotional problems, especially depressive illness. A number of studies are now available which refute this belief and in fact depressive illness is a condition which predominates in younger women. There is no doubt that women do suffer emotional difficulties at this time but these may be due to the change in status as children leave home, to the loss of family and friends through bereavements which often gather momentum in the middle years and perhaps to previously untreated depression which is augmented at times of personal stress. Attempts to relate symptoms to hormone levels or to treat them with replacement therapy have been inconclusive.

Case 3

Mrs X was a 72-year-old woman who had become a widow 1 year earlier after a happy marriage of 42 years. Her husband had died of renal failure and she had been prepared for his death for several weeks. She had no prior contact with the psychiatric services and had a supportive family of four daughters. She and her husband had lived with her older daughter and family and relationships were excellent. At the time of his death she grieved normally – she went to his funeral, cried, visited his grave regularly and prayed for him. After 18 months she still cried for many hours each day, had trouble getting to sleep and had little interest in meeting her friends. She had lost about 1 stone in weight and was unable to concentrate. Her family had taken her on holiday but she got little pleasure from this. Her usual GP felt that she would improve with time and advised her to join a local widows' group. This she did but took little interest in the meetings. She was diagnosed with depression complicating bereavement by a locum whom she had visited for a 'tonic'. She described a close relationship with her late husband although she viewed herself as being independent. She responded over time to SSRI antidepressants and bereavement counselling. Over 3 months she returned to her usual activities and at the time of writing was off all medication (she was treated for 12 months) and was symptom-free. She still spoke of her loneliness for her husband but got comfort from praying for him each morning, from visiting his grave every month and from her dreams about him.

Depression in the elderly and delusional depression – see **Chapter 15**

Depression and physical illness – see **Chapter 12**

Treatment

Once a diagnosis has been agreed it is useful to give information about the illness. It is important not only to be honest but also to correct some of the myths which exist.

(1) Emphasize that it is an illness which explains the multiple symptoms they may have. A simple description of the neurochemical abnormalities may be useful to help explain why they feel so bad, but it is also helpful to emphasize the role of psychosocial factors which they may have already articulated.

(2) The likelihood of recovery should be explained. Many patients may believe it is up to them to change: changing behaviour can be helpful and is a part of many psychosocial treatments, but it is important not to increase feelings of failure and ensure that self-care is supported by practitioners.

(3) When discussing medication, distinguish between tranquillizers and antidepressants regarding dependence.

(4) Draw attention to the possible and likely side effects of antidepressants and explain the delay in onset of antidepressant effect in order to improve adherence. There are many good leaflets about depression, medication and talking therapies. Websites can be useful to represent psychotropic treatment as a means of placing patients in a better position to help themselves by emphasizing the improvement in negative cognitions that will occur with treatment (see p. 95).

It can be useful to divide treatment options into four complementary areas:

• practical support and advice
• psychological therapies
• antidepressants
• physical treatment.

General practitioners should not ignore the important part they can play in the consultation by being empathetic, doing 'micro therapy' and encouraging follow-up.

Practical support and advice

For many years many GPs have provided practical support and advice to patients with mental health problems, including depression. While this has not been emphasized in guidelines it is valued by patients. There is little objective evidence for or against. General practitioners' talk and advice lies in that hinterland between the role of friend and therapist. Difficult judgements need to be made about how emotionally involved to become, whether to disclose any personal details and whether physical contact is helpful. Each of these natural and potentially beneficial behaviours has potential risk: dependence and inappropriate attachment, as well as feeling emotionally drained or emotionally exposed. There is also the danger of having accusations of inappropriate behaviour levelled at one. More practically, in addition to the kind of 'micro therapy' discussed in Chapter 20, relatively simple advice and support can be given to include:

- healthy diet
- limiting drug and alcohol use
- exercise (for which some evidence exists)
- talking things through with family and friends
- taking out time to relax and having time to oneself
- specific relaxation, meditation
- addressing relationships
- adjusting work patterns.

These are in many ways similar to the conversations of everyday friendships and yet advice from a practitioner is imbued with authority and additional meaning. We therefore need to exercise caution and options should probably be explored as possibilities rather than presented as definitive advice.

Psychological therapies

Chapters 16, 17 and 18 outline a range of therapy modalities. For depression there is now evidence to support several approaches; the recent NICE guidelines (2009) emphasize the effectiveness of CBT over counselling or interpersonal therapy (ITP); however, the effect sizes are not very different. When discussing therapy it is now appropriate to look at the range of options rather than simply referring for counselling. It is important to consider both modality and setting.

Some people wish to gain ongoing support from GPs and other practitioners. This may be appropriate. Others may request and require more structured therapies such as solution-focused and problem-solving interventions. These can also be incorporated into consultations but are best supported by training and supervision.

Increasingly, following the Improving Access to Psychological Therapies (IAPT) programme in the UK, patients with depression can be referred, normally within practices, to assessment and intervention sessions where the range of treatment options listed in Table 7.2 can be discussed. Five steps in the process of recognition and treatment have been outlined by NICE in its guidelines. Step 1 refers to the recognition of depression in primary care while step 5 refers to inpatient psychiatric care or the involvement of mental health service crisis teams. Steps 2 and 3 are also located in the primary care setting and involve both pharmacological and psychological therapies and it is here that the IAPT services are relevant.

For those with recurrent depression who are taking antidepressants, the use of cognitive therapy or of mindfulness therapy should be considered especially if the person has a strong preference for psychological approaches.

Table 7.2. Components of stepped care (steps 2 and 3)

Step 3	**Interventions run by the IAPT service**
	Up to 20 sessions CBT with qualified therapist
	Up to 20 sessions IPT or counselling psychotherapy, or similar
Step 2	**Interventions run by the IAPT service**
	Assessment
	Guided self-help for stand-alone interventions below
	Large group psycho-education (e.g. stress control)
	Small support groups and courses – e.g. bereavement, anger management, mindfulness, anxiety management
	User-facilitated support groups
	Computerized self-help – e.g. Beating the Blues
	Up to six sessions of cognitive behavioural therapy (e.g. behavioural activation, anxiety management), counselling, solution-focused therapy
	Case management, medication support (telephone-based) for those choosing anti-depressants, 'watchful waiting', follow-up for those with a non-IAPT service psychosocial intervention following initial assessment
	Psychological interventions and activities run by others
	Independent sector counselling (accredited), e.g. Cruise, Relate
	Support for drug and alcohol and other addictive problems (e.g. AA, Gamblers Anonymous) or other local services
	Other activities
	Exercise referral schemes
	Third-sector-run interventions and groups
	Adult education course, e.g. literacy
	Stand-alone self-help interventions
	Internet-based CBT (e.g. Moodgym and Living Life to the Full)
	Self-help books (bibliotherapy), Prescribe a Book Scheme
	Exercise

Cognitive therapy

This is the current favoured psychological therapy for depression although there is a question as to whether it is superior to other psychological therapies in primary care (Bortolotti *et al.* 2008). Aaron Beck first described the technique and immediately it was the subject of controlled trials with antidepressants and on its own. It is based on the idea that the way we think affects our feelings and behaviour. Cognitive therapists also suggest that, due to illness, negative cognitions reinforce and maintain the affective symptomatology. Therapy aims to examine these cognitions and the assumptions about confidence, self-worth, etc., that accrue from them. Chapter 16 provides more detail.

Pharmacological treatments

The importance of antidepressants for treating depressive illness in general practice has been emphasized by placebo-controlled trials in this setting, especially for moderately severe depression (Simon 2002).The THREAD study shows modest benefits of prescribing SSRIs to those with new episodes of mild to moderate depression that has lasted for 8 weeks. However, the additional benefit of prescribing, over and above supportive care, is relatively small, and may be at least in part a placebo effect (Kendrick *et al.* 2009). Even more doubt has been expressed by others claiming the apparent effects are due to placebo (Kirsch *et al.* 2008).

It is important to prescribe antidepressants in therapeutic doses and for up to 1 month before changing to another. The antidepressant groups are listed in Table 7.3.

Table 7.3. Antidepressants in common use

	Sedative/ alerting	Starting dose (mg)	Minimum therapeutic dose (mg)	Maximum therapeutic dose (mg)
Tricyclics				
Amitriptyline	Sedative	50–75	100	200
Imipramine	Mildly sedative	50–75	100	200
Clomipramine	Mildly sedative	50–75	100	200
Lofepramine	Mildly sedative	70 BD	210	280
SSRIs				
Fluoxetine	Neither	20	20	80
Fluvoxamine	Neither	100	100 TID	300
Paroxetine	Neither	20	20	50
Sertraline	Neither	50	50	200
Citalopram	Neither	20	20	60
Escitalopram	Neither	10	10	20
Phenylpiperazines				
Trazodone	Sedative	150	200	60
SNRIs				
Venlafaxine	Neither	75	75	375 (taken in divided doses)
Venlafaxine XL	Neither	75	75	225 (XL is taken once per day)
Duloxetine	Neither	60	60	120

Table 7.3. (cont.)

	Sedative/ alerting	Starting dose (mg)	Minimum therapeutic dose (mg)	Maximum therapeutic dose (mg)
NaSAS				
Mirtazepine	Sedative	15	30	45
NaRIs				
Reboxetine	Slightly alerting	4 BD	8	12
Melatonergic antidepressants				
Agomelatin	Neither	25	20	50
Tetracyclics				
Mianserin	Sedative	30	60	120?
Maprotiline	Mildly sedative	75	75	150
MAOIs				
Irreversible				
Tranylcypromine	Alerting	10 BD	30	60
Phenelzine	Alerting	15 BD	45	60
Reversible				
Moclobemide	Neither	300	150 BD	600

The elderly and those with idiosyncratic reactions should be prescribed lower doses but these are the exception. The usual practice is to begin with the recognized starting dose and to increase this to the therapeutic dose after 5–7 days. Despite claims that patients do not tolerate these doses, especially when tricyclics are used, warning of the possible side effects and of the delay in onset enhances adherence.

Several studies have shown that many patients believed to be chronically depressed had not received the minimum therapeutic dose. However, more general practitioners now report prescribing in accordance with British National Formulary guidelines in relation to dosage and duration (Kerr 1994). The increased use of SSRIs has largely reduced this problem since the starting dose is for many also the minimum therapeutic dose.

The general practitioner should be familiar with one or two antidepressants from each group and develop a flexible approach to prescribing.

Choosing an antidepressant

The SSRI antidepressants have revolutionized the treatment of depression due to their favourable side-effect profile and the ease with which a therapeutic dose can be reached. For these reasons they have become the antidepressant of first choice in primary care.

However, there are other considerations that might influence the treatment decision. Yet it is commonly the case that many doctors have little experience of prescribing, or of seeing prescribed, other antidepressants. Such a limited perspective might not serve our patients optimally and so the factors that should be taken into account when choosing an antidepressant for an individual patient are outlined below, although the list is not exhaustive.

1 Efficacy and effectiveness

The first consideration when choosing any treatment is its efficacy and effectiveness. Both are different – efficacy refers to the benefits of a particular drug when compared to placebo in randomized controlled trials, i.e. in a controlled environment. This is obviously of importance in establishing that the treatment is beneficial. Effectiveness, on the other hand, measures how well treatment works in clinical practice and is more difficult to measure than efficacy due to lack of controls and the presence of factors that militate against effectiveness, such as comorbid substance misuse.

The *efficacy* of SSRIs compared to tricyclic antidepressants is generally equivalent, with significant advantages also attaching to the SSRIs in terms of discontinuation due to poor tolerability (NICE 2009). Among the SSRIs, fluoxetine has the highest discontinuation rate. However, a meta-analysis for these guidelines identified amitryptiline as non-significantly superior to SSRIs for those being treated as inpatients, a group most likely to have severe depression.

For *effectiveness*, on the other hand, measurement is more difficult and investigators have examined this using measures such as the proportion achieving a therapeutic dose, the duration of treatment and rates of treatment compliance.

Since the SSRIs are generally prescribed at the full therapeutic dose from the beginning, it is likely that, on this measure, they will be superior to TCAs and this has been demonstrated to be correct using a general practice database (Donoghue and Hylan 2001). That study also found that patients prescribed SSRIs were seven times more likely to adhere to treatment than those prescribed TCAs. Other studies have found that those taking SSRIs are more likely to have a longer initial course of treatment and are less likely to request an alternative.

In clinical settings, several studies have found benefits from tricyclics as compared to SSRIs in those with severe depression or with melancholia or who were being treated as inpatients. However, studies of inpatient prescribing habits have found that while TCAs dominated in the 1990s these have since been replaced by third-generation antidepressants such as mirtazepine and venlefaxine. In general SSRIs are used less frequently for inpatients than for outpatients.

In summary, SSRIs have advantages over TCAs both in a controlled setting and in clinical practice, with the exception of those with severe depression, for whom TCAs appear to be superior.

2 Speed of onset of antidepressant effect

With most antidepressants the period from commencing treatment to showing an antidepressant response is more than 2 weeks and can be up to 6 weeks. Such a delay is problematic for a number of reasons, including the danger of discontinuing treatment. However, there is some evidence that the newer SSRIs (escitalopram), the SNRIs (venlefaxine and duloxetine) and mirtazepine (NaSSA) have a more rapid onset of effect than others. However, most of this information has been gleaned in post-hoc analyses. Moreover, in some the benefit may not stem from the antidepressant effect but from improvements in associated symptoms such as anxiety, insomnia, aches and pains, etc. The best evidence for an early antidepressant effect at present rests with escitalorpam. However, even improvement in associated symptoms should not be ignored if patients themselves feel these benefits.

3 Side-effect profile

While discontinuation of antidepressants is more likely among TCA users, it is tempting to forget that SSRIs have side effects also that may have an impact on the choice of antidepressant.

Nausea and anorexia can occur with the SSRIs and with the SNRIs. If severe this might cause weight loss and affect adherence. Fluoxetine is especially likely to cause weight loss in the early stages of treatment and this may persist even with the onset of the antidepressant effect. If the patient is already experiencing significant anorexia and/or weight loss then consideration should be given to prescribing an antidepressant that increases weight such as a tricyclic or mirtazepine. Most other antidepressant groups are weight-neutral and these should also be considered.

Postural hypotension is important since it can cause dizziness and, if severe, falls. The tricyclic antidepressants and trazadone are most commonly associated with this side effect although lofepramine is less likely to cause this than the other TCAs. The SSRIs do not affect blood pressure, with the exception of citalopram (and possibly escitalopram), which can cause a slight drop in blood pressure. At higher doses reboxetine may cause a drop. The other antidepressants are not linked to postural reductions in blood pressure.

4 Comorbid physical illness

Hypertension – the SNRIs and reboxetine should be used with caution in those with hypertension while SSRIs, mirtazepine and TCAs are not associated with elevation of blood pressure.

Diabetes – there is limited or no information on some antidepressants such as reboxetine or trazadone and the SNRIs appear to have no impact. Tricyclic antidepressants are associated with hyperglycaemia and are best avoided. On the other hand the impact of mirtazepine on diabetic control, despite its tendency to increase weight, is unknown and in non-diabetic controls it does not impair glucose tolerance. MAOIs such as phenelzine can cause severe hypoglycaemia. Thus the SSRIs seem to be the first choice and fluoxetine has a favourable effect on diabetic control, reducing insulin requirements and weight. SNRIs are also likely to be safe while TCAs and MAOIs are ideally avoided.

Epilepsy – all antidepressants have epileptogenic potential but the least problematic are the SSRIs. The risk is dose-related but there seems to be no differences between the available products. The TCAs on the other hand are best avoided while SNRIs and mirtazepine should be used with care.

5 Interaction with other medication

All tricyclic antidepressants have the potential to interact with SSRIs and cause a serotonin syndrome. Cimetidine also increases the plasma levels of TCAs. TCAs and MAOI are also best avoided due to the possibility of hypertensive crises but in specific circumstances, such as in managing refractory depression, the combination is sometimes used judiciously. Among the SSRIs there are few differences between preparations. All interact with St. John's wort. Most also increase plasma levels of some antipsychotics, carbamazepine and some benzo-diazepines. They should be used with caution in those taking NSAIs and with warfarin. Reboxetine can interact with erythromycin and ketoconazole. Venlefaxine should be used with caution in those taking cimetidine, clozapine or warfarin. SSRIs in combination with other antidepressants could induce a serotonin syndrome.

6 Pregnancy

Ideally antidepressants should not be prescribed in pregnancy. However, untreated depression during pregnancy is associated with a number of problems for the mother and for the baby. These include poor weight gain, poor self-care in the mother, use of alcohol and nicotine and difficulties forming a relationship with the baby. There is also an increased risk of postnatal depression and ultimately of suicide. The decision on whether to continue or commence an antidepressant during pregnancy is made in consultation with the doctor based on a risk/benefit assessment. The decision on whether to use antidepressants during pregnancy could be assisted by obtaining the latest information on the risks of the various preparations from the manufacturers or from a pharmacist and providing this to the patient. The following is a guideline only.

First trimester: it is important to realize that no antidepressant is licensed for use in pregnancy. As the tricyclic antidepressants have been available for over 50 years they have the advantage of having most safety information available. With use in the first trimester there is no evidence of anatomical or behavioural teratogenecity. Similar results have been found for most of the SSRIs, apart from paroxetine, which has been shown to be associated with an increased risk of cardiac malformations and with anancephaly. No adverse effects have been demonstrated with citalopram, escitalopram or with those belonging to other groups (venlefaxine – SNRI; mirtazepine – NaSSA; trazodone – phenylpiperazine) although more data are required.

Later in pregnancy: there is evidence of discontinuation symptoms in the newborn baby if tricyclics are taken up to the time of delivery. These include irritability, convulsions and sleeping and feeding problems but all are reversible. It is important that these medications be discontinued gradually in the weeks immediately preceding parturition. The use of fluoxetine in the third trimester is associated with reversible perinatal consequences such as irritability and feeding problems.

7 Breastfeeding

There is always a dilemma about whether to breastfeed or to prescribe antidepressants. This is especially acute for the woman who may fear for the safety of her newborn child if exposed to antidepressants in breast milk. On the other hand the risks to the baby when the mother has depression cannot be ignored as the baby's relationship with her may be compromised and in severe depression there may be a threat to life. There is now some information available concerning the presence of antidepressants in breast milk to assist in making this decision. Among the SSRIs the first choice is sertraline, followed by paroxetine or citalopram, while flowxetine is contra-indicated as it is detected in breast milk in doses above 20 mg and there are case reports of infants exhibiting somnolence and irritability, although without adverse long-term effects. However, the sample sizes in these studies are small. The information concerning escitalopram is scant but case studies suggest that there is no accumulation.

Venlefaxine is found in breast milk in very small amounts (3.2%) but without any side effects in the short or long term, while case studies of mirtazepine suggest no accumulation.

Among the tricyclic antidepressants there is no evidence that amitryptiline, imipramine or their metabolites accumulate in the serum of newborn infants. However, cloimipramine has been found but it decreases over time and no long-term adverse consequences have been reported. It is recommended that infants be monitored for drowsiness if the mother is taking tricyclics.

8 Prominent insomnia and anxiety

Anxiety and insomnia are symptoms that are commonly associated with depressive illness. Indeed some find these symptoms more disabling than the low mood. Thus their early resolution is very desirable. All antidepressants reduce anxiety and insomnia once the antidepressant effect occurs. However, with the SSRIs, especially fluoxetine, these symptoms may worsen in the initial period of treatment, with the danger that medication will be discontinued. Paroxetine is the exception as it may cause sedation. When there is significant insomnia, two possible approaches to treatment should be considered. The first is to add a benzodiazepine for symptomatic relief of anxiety and insomnia for short-term use until the antidepressant effect becomes obvious. The second is to choose an antidepressant with anti-anxiety properties that emerge early in treatment. For this a tricyclic antidepressant such as amirtyptiline, cloimipramine or dothiepin might be considered. Paroxetine and mirtazepine are alternatives in light of their sedating effect, although it is only present in mirtazepine at the starting dose of 15 mg and it diminishes as the dose increases.

9 Age – less than 18 years

The only antidepressant licensed for use in those under the age of 18 is fluoxetine and this should only be used after psychotherapeutic interventions have failed, according to the NICE Guidelines (2009). Even then the medication should be used in conjunction with psychotherapy and the patient should be closely monitored. This recommendation came about as a result of studies showing an increase in suicidality in young people taking SSRIs. The guidelines concluded that, apart from fluoxetine, the risks outweigh the benefit. These considerations do not apply when SSRIs are used to treat other conditions such as OCD (see also Chapter 14).

10 Toxicity in overdose

In light of the association between suicidal behaviour and depressive illness, concern about the toxicity of prescribed treatments, if taken in overdose, looms large. This will first require an assessment of short-term suicide risk (see Chapter 11) in the patient. If such a risk exists then even the prescription of a safer drug such as an SSRI could be fraught with problems since the person may, instead of overdosing, hang himself. There is in these circumstances the risk of a false sense of security.

If, however, the risk is not immediate but the possibility of a more long-term or uncertain risk exists, then an SSRI is definitely a safer option. There is no doubt that TCAs taken in overdose are more toxic than other antidepressant groups, although lofepramine is the exception to this since it is less cardiotoxic. More recently venlefaxine has been shown to have similar toxicity. However, placed in the context of the totality of suicides, TCAs alone are responsible for 2–4% of deaths.

The question of whether antidepressants trigger suicidal thoughts and/or behaviour is considered in Chapter 11. Prescribing for the elderly will be discussed in Chapter 15.

Dealing with poor treatment response

The basic principles when dealing with poor or partial treatment response are as follows:

(a) Has the patient adhered to treatment?

(b) If non-adherence is due to side effects change to another drug in that class or to a new class

(c) Has the patient received a therapeutic dose?

(d) Has the patient had a trial of suitable duration (at least 4 weeks)?

(e) Is the patient consuming alcohol or other depressogenic substances?

(f) Is the mood change due to a depressive illness or is there an alternative diagnosis?

(g) Are there psychosocial factors contributing to perpetuation of the mood disturbance?

(h) Is the depression more severe that at first appears, e.g. psychotic or melancholic in type?

(i) Are there significant comorbidities?

The answer to these questions will determine whether treatment should continue being delivered by the general practitioner with antidepressants or whether other options should be considered, including referral to specialist psychological services or to a psychiatrist for other treatments such as ECT, lithium augmentation, etc.

Combination drug therapy

Treatment-resistant depression is defined as any depressive episode which fails to respond to antidepressants. In clinical practice it refers to depressive illness that has failed to respond to a number of antidepressants in therapeutic doses. It does not include those unwilling to take or intolerant of antidepressants. The management of treatment-resistant depression rarely falls entirely to the general practitioner since failure to respond to treatment is one of the common reasons for referral to the psychiatric services. A number of drug combinations have been found to be helpful and are listed in Table 7.4 although the evidence base for these is weaker than for monotherapy. Lithium augmentation has the strongest supportive evidence and the serum levels required are less than for prophylaxis (0.4 mmol/L or above).

Table 7.4. Drug combinations useful in treating resistant depression

Lithium plus any antidepressant
An MAOI plus a tricyclic (tranylcypromine, imipramine or clomipramine should not be included in the combination)
Lithium plus amitriptyline plus an MAOI
Mirtazepine and venlafaxine or an SSRI
Fluoxetine and olanzepine

The effects are often noticed early in treatment and a trial of 6 weeks is sufficient. Augmentation of the current antidepressant regime with T3 is used occasionally.

L-tryptophan was used to augment the tricyclics or some combinations. This has now been taken off the market and is only available on a 'named patient' basis.

Physical treatments

Electroconvulsive treatment (ECT)

ECT is not routinely used in treating depression but can be successful as an emergency method where life is at risk from either suicide, starvation or dehydration or where psychotic features are present.

It can be used in an outpatient setting also if depression is prolonged, severe and resistant to antidepressant treatment; a positive outcome is most likely when the typical biological symptoms are present. It does not prevent relapse and for this reason antidepressants are prescribed in conjunction and are normally continued for at least 9 months. There is little definite evidence that brain damage occurs even with repeated usage of ECT.

Transcranial magnetic stimulation (TMS)

A recent development has been the use of repetitive transcranial magnetic stimulation (rTMS) in which a controlled, rapidly fluctuating magnetic field is generated using a hand-held coil. The left prefrontal cortex is targeted and preliminary studies suggest that it may be a safer and more acceptable alternative to ECT. However, its benefits are equivalent to those of antidepressants or with brief-pulse unilateral ECT but not to those obtained from bilateral or high-dose unilateral ECT. It is not recommended for those who are suicidal or psychotically depressed. It is not routinely available at centres in Britain or Ireland.

Deep brain stimulation (DBS)

DBS involves the implantation of an electrode in the area of the brain relevant to the illness (Parkinson's disease, OCD or depression). A battery-operated transmitter, like a pacemaker, delivers electrical impulses through a hair-thin wire with the electrode at the end. DBS does not damage healthy brain tissue although it is more invasive than other physical treatments. It has the advantage of being able to reach deep brain structures in a targeted way and so can be illness-specific. It is not routinely available.

Vagus nerve stimulation

Vagus nerve stimulation is more invasive than TMS and less so than DBS. Its use so far has been in the treatment of refractory epilepsy but some have suggested that it might be useful in the treatment of refractory depression. Its benefits in epilepsy stem from the effect of internal stimulation of the vagal nerve by inhibition of neural processes in the brain. Its use in depression is still experimental.

Lifestyle interventions

Diet has long been thought to affect depression; in particular the omega-3 fatty acids play a role in brain structure and function. This has led to an increasing interest in the role of these in the treatment of both unipolar depression and bipolar disorder. Of itself there is no evidence that fatty acids as monotherapy are effective. Most studies have investigated these as adjuncts to standard antidepressants and benefits have been shown in both depression and bipolar disorder in some but not in all of the studies as well as a possible prophylactic effect in perinatal depression (Pawels and Volterrani 2008).

Exercise is also recommended as an adjunct in the treatment of depression. However, contrary to the recommendations of NICE, the benefits are uncertain and a Cochrane systematic review (Mead *et al.* 2009) examining 23 studies found large benefits but only in the trials that were least well-designed. For the trials with adequate randomization and concealment the effects were not significantly different from cognitive therapy or from placebo. The results of a large pragmatic HTA-funded trial of exercise prescription in primary care are awaited. In summary, the lifestyle interventions, while popular, have limited evidence to support their benefits.

Alcohol is known to be a depressant and this must be avoided in those with depression, while patients must be encouraged to get adequate sleep.

Prophylaxis in unipolar depression

Those with a single episode of depression require antidepressants for 6 months or more. Those with recurrent severe unipolar depression may derive benefit from long-term antidepressants for 2 or more years. If these fail, then lithium should be considered although it may be less successful than in those with bipolar illness. The rule of thumb for prescribing long-term antidepressants is the occurrence of three or more episodes of depression in 5 years, although even less frequent episodes may require prophylaxis if the symptoms during episodes are very severe and there are other risk factors for recurrence such as a family history of mood disorders.

Prognosis and recovery

The prognosis for those with unipolar depression varies enormously and both recovery and recurrence depend on a range of factors. Full recovery can take several months although symptomatic improvement occurs relatively quickly and is often noticed within 2 to 3 weeks of beginning treatment. This delay is often due to the lag in social recovery and discussion with the patient will often reveal that although sleep, appetite and mood disturbance have gone, the patient still feels unable to cope totally with housework, employment or many of the other aspects of life which involve social functioning. This has important implications for practicalities about such matters as returning to work, or resuming social engagements, etc. A careful balance is required between encouraging resumption of social roles and pushing individuals into situations which they find stressful.

The outcome of individual episodes of depressive illness is good and full remission can be achieved in about two-thirds of patients provided they are treated adequately. However, there is also a high relapse rate even among those treated in primary care, with 25% having a recurrence over the subsequent 5 years (Wilson *et al.* 2003). Spontaneous remission occurs in some but overall treatment has been shown to reduce time to remission. Recovery is more likely in those with less severe and less prolonged illness at diagnosis.

Recent work has shown in primary care setting that increasing age, social adversity and physical symptoms can all contribute to continued depression. There are large differences between statistics on the likelihood of sustained recovery, ranging from 2 to 73 % in the recent THREAD study, where recovery was more likely for women, people who are married or cohabiting, had few somatic symptoms and received their preferred treatment (Dowrick *et al.* 2010). Furthermore, remission rates among patients in aversive social contexts are consistently much lower irrespective of treatment (Brown *et al.* 2010). There are potentially significant implications from those results with respect to discussing the need for treatment.

A small but important group, less than 15% of those with severe depression, become chronically ill despite aggressive treatment. Outcome is governed by a number of factors, including the inherent biological process of the illness, the presence or absence of personality disorder and the adequacy of the support the patient receives from family, friends and social environment. The role of primary care in the management of those with complex or enduring depressive illness is discussed in Chapter 19.

Prophylaxis in bipolar disorder

\Lithium is the longest-established and most widely used prophylactic although there are problems associated with its use, including its limited effectiveness in about one-third of patients, especially in those with rapidly cycling disorder (four or more episodes of mania or depression in 1 year). In addition sudden discontinuation can provoke rebound mania, although this can be lessened if withdrawal is gradual over a period of 2–4 weeks. Earlier concerns about treatment resistance to its prophylactic effect following discontinuation have receded. Although recent studies suggest that lithium may be less teratogenic than was previously thought provided levels are carefully monitored and kept within the therapeutic range, great care must still be exercised when the possibility of pregnancy arises. It can be reinstated in the second trimester and should be discontinued again before delivery. Careful monitoring is required as renal function changes during pregnancy and toxicity may occur. Lithium salts are excreted in breast milk and bottle feeding of the newborn is to be preferred. Abnormalities of thyroid function are not absolute contraindications to lithium prophylaxis but do necessitate closer monitoring. Although there have been claims of renal damage occurring even with doses in the therapeutic range, it is now believed that these have been exaggerated and that they are unlikely unless renal function was compromised at the outset of treatment or toxicity occurred.

Generally speaking lithium is required for life and there are now numerous studies showing that despite many years of treatment, discontinuation of lithium results in relapse. Its narrow therapeutic window and associated toxicity make it a less than ideal drug for prophylaxis (see Table 7.5). In addition compliance has been shown to be poor and patients often complain of feeling slowed up. However, lithium has the strongest evidence base supporting its value in prophylaxis.

For optimal prophylaxis blood levels between 0.6 and 1 mmol/L are required but some studies find better control is achieved at levels above 0.8 mmol/L. Occasionally, control may be achieved in the lower range of 0.4–0.6 mmol/L. There is little to choose between once-daily and multiple dosing in relation to prophylaxis but polyuria is less frequent with single dosing. Blood levels should be checked as close to 12 hours following the last dose as possible, and every 3 months once lithium has been established, although before levels have been stabilized weekly checks are required. Prior to commencing lithium, thyroid and renal function should be checked, the latter by measuring urea and electrolytes and creatinine clearance. Cardiac function should be checked by ECG if cardiac problems are suspected. Checks of these functions should be carried out annually thereafter.

Lithium levels may be elevated in those taking thiazide diuretics, ACE inhibitors and non-steroidal anti-inflammatory agents. Toxicity may also occur in those with nausea/vomiting or other conditions leading to salt/water depletion.

If lithium is contraindicated as a prophylactic agent carbamazepine is an option. However, some have suggested that its efficacy may fade over time. Side effects include dizziness, blurred vision, ataxia, rashes and GIT disturbances and these are dose-related. It can also precipitate Stevens-Johnson syndrome, blood dyscrasias and toxic epidermal necrolysis. In addition it is metabolized by the cytochrome P-450 enzymes and may reduce the effectiveness of other drugs metabolized in the same pathway by enzyme induction, including other anticonvulsants and the oral contraceptive. It can also be teratogenic and folate is recommended in women contemplating pregnancy.

Sodium valproate is a commonly used mood stabilizer and it is the preferred choice in rapid cycling bipolar disorder. It is well tolerated and the commonest side effects are nausea, ataxia, GIT disturbance and tremor. Weight gain may also occur due to increased appetite. Due to its impact on liver function it cannot be used in those with liver disease or with a family history of hepatic conditions. It may elevate the plasma levels of other anticonvulsants and increase the anticoagulant effects of warfarin. It too is teratogenic and folate supplementation is required.

Lamotrigine has been found to be effective in bipolar disorder and is licensed for prophylaxis, especially where depressive episodes have predominated. The most common side effects are headache, nausea, diplopia, dizziness and ataxia. It can cause skin rashes and serious reactions such as angio-oedema and Stevens-Johnson syndrome, while exposure of the fetus to lamotrigine in the first trimester can lead to teratogenesis, making folate supplements essential in those contemplating a pregnancy. Its metabolism is induced by carbamazepine and valproate.

Blood levels for the anticonvulsants are less important in the prophylaxis of bipolar disorder than they are for lithium, and therapeutic levels have not been established. A full blood count, renal, liver function and cardiac evaluation are required prior to commencing therapy with carbamazepine. Since leucopenia is a rare but dangerous side effect a white cell count is advisable at regular intervals. Before commencing valproate and during the first 6 months of treatment liver function should be monitored. Full blood count, liver and renal function should be assessed before lamotrigine is introduced but there is no requirement for further evaluations thereafter. Unlike lithium discontinuation, there is little evidence of rebound mania when anticonvulsants are withdrawn.

Other recent developments include the licensing of several atypical antipsychotic agents as mood stabilizers. These include olanzepine and quetiepine. Weight monitoring is essential, especially with olanzepine as it is associated with significant weight gain. At baseline, blood glucose, lipids and weight should be measured and 1 month later when taking olanzepine, but 3 monthly checks are appropriate for other antipsychotic agents.

The reader is referred to the NICE Guidelines for details of the physical monitoring of those on mood stabilizers (2006).

In general combination treatments that include lithium and another mood stabilizer are more effective than monotherapy although side effects and toxicity increase. Lithium remains the first choice for long-term prophylaxis in bipolar disorder but for rapid cycling or for treatment-resistant bipolar disorder, then anticonvulsants, especially valproate, alone or in combination are the preferred options. Antipsychotic agents also have a role in these difficult-to-treat groups.

Table 7.5. Adverse effects of lithium

Side effects	Toxic effects[a]
Fine tremor[b]	Nausea and vomiting
Thirst and polyuria	Ataxia and impaired coordination
Hypothyroidism	Dysarthria
Teratogenesis	Coarse tremor
Weight gain	Muscle twitching
Emotional dulling	Fits
Leucocytosis	Nephropathy
Nephrogenic diabetes insipidus	Confusion
Rashes, especially psoriasis	Hyper-reflexia and nystagmus
Cardiac arrhythmias	Coma

[a] These occur when the serum levels exceed 1.3 mmol/l but may occur with levels in the therapeutic range in some patients.

[b] This may be treated with propranolol.

When is prophylaxis required

Many patients inquire about the requirement for prophylaxis in bipolar disorder. In general, if there have been three or more episodes of depression/mania over a 2 year period, long-term prophylaxis is required. However, a decision to offer prophylaxis may be made on pragmatic grounds if, for example, the first episode of mania was very severe, in either duration or impact. Prophylaxis is generally for life, except in special circumstances such as pregnancy. Those who might be poorly adherent to treatment could be recommended a depot antipsychotic although this is not the routine or preferred option.

Relapse prevention in bipolar disorders

Many support groups advocate self-management in recognizing early-warning symptoms of relapse, particularly manic episodes. There is now clear evidence from randomized trials that such interventions work and they function best when they are a central plank of treatment and follow-up. The training can be delivered by a mental health professional or by a patient trained in the techniques.

The elements include:

(1) identifying the 'relapse signature' for each pole of the illness for that particular patient. The 'signature' consists of a constellation of symptoms occurring concurrently rather than a single symptom which might be too non-specific

(2) having access to a mental health team that will respond with flexibility and urgency, otherwise the window of opportunity to prevent relapse will be missed

(3) having a mental health team that trusts the patient's early-warning signs (Morris 2004).

Prognosis in bipolar disorder

Among those with bipolar illness the periods between episodes tend to shorten in the early years of the illness but subsequently increase. Those with rapid cycling disorder have individual episodes in quick succession and have a poorer prognosis than slow cyclers. Before the introduction of modern treatments the episodes remitted spontaneously in many cases. In general bipolar disorder can be controlled provided treatment is adhered to.

Summary

- Depressive illness is present in about 10% of consulters and next to adjustment disorder is the most common mental health problem seen in general practice.

- It is important to identify depressive illness and treat it but not to over-diagnose.

- A significant proportion of depressed patients are unrecognized because of the mode of presentation, which is often with physical complaints.

- The aetiology of depressive illness is multifactorial and includes a combination of risk factors and triggers such as life stresses, absence of supports, physical illnesses and genetic predisposition, the latter especially in bipolar disorder.

- Some patients do not have any obvious precipitant to their episodes of illness, but most can identify ongoing stressors and specific precipitants.

- Before medication is prescribed, time should be taken to explain the nature of the illness, the treatment and its side effects to the patient. This may improve adherence.

- There has been an expansion in the available drug and psychosocial treatment options in recent years and the GP should familiarize himself with their uses and risks.

- Untreated depressive illness has a morbidity which affects both the patient and his family. Collaborative treatment is required.

- The prognosis for treated depressive illness is good but a small proportion (less than 15% of those with severe depressive illness) become chronically incapacitated.

- Bipolar disorder is much less common than unipolar disorder.

- A range of medications are available to stabilize mood.

References

Angst, J., Gamma, A., Benazzi, F., *et al.* (2003). Toward a redefinition of sub-threshold bipolarity: epidemiology and proposed criteria for bipolar-II, minor bipolar disorders and hypomania. *Journal of Affective Disorders*, **73**, 133–146.

Beck, A. P. (1967). *Depression: Clinical, Experimental and Theoretical Aspects.* New York: Harper and Row.

Beck, A. T., Ward, C. H., Mendelson, M., *et al.* (1961). An inventory for measuring depression. *Archives of General Psychiatry I*, **4**, 561–71.

Bortolotti, B., Menchetti, M., *et al.* (2008). Psychological interventions for major depression in primary care: a meta-analytic review of randomized controlled trials. *General Hospital PsychiatryI*, **30**(4), 293–302.

Brown, G. W., and Harris, T. O. (1978). *The Social Origins of Depression.* New York: Free Press.

Brown, G. W., Harris, T. O., Kendrick, T., *et al.* (2010). Antidepressants, social adversity and outcome of depression in general practice. *Journal of Affective Disorders*, **121**(3), 239–246. Epub ahead of print.

Donoghue, J., and Hylan, T. R. (2001). Antidepressant use in clinical practice: efficacy versus effectiveness. *British Journal of Psychiatry*, **179**(suppl 42), s9–s17.

Dowrick, C. (2009). *Beyond Depression. A New Approach to Understanding and Management*, 2nd edn. Oxford: Oxford University Press.

Dowrick, C., Flach, C., and Leese, M. (2010) Estimating probability of sustained recovery from mild to moderate depression in primary care: evidence from the THREAD study. *Psychological Medicine*, (PM09/8004) epub ahead of print.

Goldberg, D. P., and Hillier, V. F. (1979). A scaled version of the General Health Questionnaire. *Psychological Medicine*, **9**(1), 139–145.

Kendrick, T., Chatwin, J., and Dowrick, C. (2009) Randomised controlled trial to determine the clinical and cost-effectiveness of selective serotonin reuptake inhibitors plus supportive care, versus supportive care alone, for mild to moderate depression with somatic symptoms in primary care. The THREAD Study. *Health Technology Assessment*, **13**(22), 1–159.

Kerr, M. P. (1994). Antidepressant prescribing: a comparison between general practitioners and psychiatrists. *British Journal of General Practice*, **44**, 275–276.

Kessing, L. V. (2004). Severity of depressive episodes according to ICD-10: prediction of risk of relapse and suicide. *British Journal of Psychiatry*, **184**, 153–156.

Kessler, D., Lloyd, K., Lewis, G., and Gray, D. P. (1999). Cross-sectional study of symptom attribution and recognition of depression and anxiety in primary care. *British Medical journal*, **318**, 436–439.

Kirsch, I., Deacon, B. J., Huedo-Medina, T. B., *et al.* (2008) Initial severity and antidepressant benefits: a metaanalysis of data submitted to the Food and Drug Administration. *PLoS Medicine*, **5**(2), e45.

Mead, G. E., Morely, W., Campbell, P., *et al.* (2009). Exercise for depression. *Cochrane Database of Systematic Reviews*, **3**,

CD004366. DOI: 10.1002/14651858. cd004366.pub4.

Morris, R. (2004). The early warning symptom intervention for patients with bipolar affective disorder. *Advances in Psychiatric Treatment*, **10**, 18–26.

National Institute for Health and Clinical Excellence. (2009). Depression in adults. *Clinical Guide 90*. London: National Institute for Clinical Excellence.

NICE (2006). The mamangement of bipolar disorder in in adults, children and adolescents in primary and secondary care. *Clinical Practice Guideline Number 38*. London: National Institute for Clinical Excellence.

Pawels, E. K., and Volterrani, D. (2008). Fatty acid facts part 1. Essential fatty acids as treatment for depression, or food for mood? *Drug News and Perspectives*, **21**(8), 446–451.

Piver, A., Yatham, L. N., and Lam, R. W. (2002). Bipolar spectrum disorders. New perspectives. *Canadian Family Physician*, **48**, 896–904.

Saunders, J. B., Aasland, O. G., Babor, T. F., *et al.* (1993). Development of the Alcohol Use Disorders Identification Test (AUDIT): WHO collaborative project on early detection of persons with harmful alcohol consumption. II. *Addiction*, **88**, 791–804

Simon, G., Goldberg, D. P., Von Korff, M., and Ustun, T. B. (2002). Understanding cross national differences in depression prevalence. *Psychological Medicine*, **32**, 585–594.

Simon, G. E. (2002). Evidence review: efficacy and effectiveness of antidepressant treatment in primary care. *General Hospital Psychiatry*, **24**(4), 194–196.

Wilson, L., Duszynski, K., and Mant, A. (2003). A 5-year follow-up of general practice patients experiencing depression. *Family Practitioner*, **26**, 685–689.

Zigmond, A. S., and Snaith, R. P. (1983). Hospital Anxiety and Depression Scale. *Acta Psychiatrica Scandinavica*, **67**(6), 361–370.

Further reading

Lehtinen, V., Casey, P., Wilkinson, C., Vazquez-Barquero, J. L., and Wilkinson, G. (1998). Problem solving and group psycho-education for depression: multicentre randomised controlled trial. Outcomes of Depression International Network (ODIN). *British Medical Journal*, **321**(7274), 1450–1454.

Suggested reading for patients

Bates, T. (1999). *Depression: The Common Sense Approach*. Dublin: New Leaf.

Jamison, K. R. (1997). *An Unquiet Mind. A Memoir of Moods and Madness*. London: Picador.

Last, C. G. (2009) *When Someone you Love is Bipolar: Help and Support For You and Your Partner*. New York: The Guilford Press.

O'Connor, R. (2010). *Undoing Depression: What Therapy Doesn't Teach You and Medication Can't Give You, 2nd edn. New York: Berkley Books.*

Rupke, S. J., Blecke, D., and Renfrow, M. (2006). Cognitive therapy for depression. *American Family Physician*, **73**(1), 34–37.

Williams, M., Teasdale, J., Segal, Z., and Kabat-Zinn, J. (2007). *The Mindful Way through Depression: Freeing Yourself from Chronic Unhappiness*. New York: The Guilford Press.

Wolpert, L. (1999). *Malignant Sadness*. London: Faber and Faber.

Useful websites for patients

Royal College of Psychiatrists' information on depression: www.rcpsych.ac.uk/info/dep.html

Online support for those affected by bipolar disorder: www.pendulum.org

Online psychological services and information about major depression: www.psychology.net.org/major.html

Up-to-date information about depression: www.allaboutdepression.com

Useful addresses

The Association for Post Natal Illness (provides information and offers one-to-one support from mothers who have been through postnatal depression), 25 Jerdan Place, Fulham, London, SW6 1BE. UK. Tel: 020 7386 0868. Email: info@apni.org. Website: www.apni.org.

Aware (provides information and support to people affected by depression in Ireland and Northern Ireland), 72 Lower Leeson Street, Dublin 2, Ireland. Helpline: 00 353 1 67661666. Tel: 00 353 1 661 7211. Email: info@aware.ie. Website: www.aware.ie.

Depression Alliance (UK) (information, support and understanding for people who suffer with depression and for relatives who want to help), 35 Westminster Bridge Road, London, SE1 7JB. UK. Tel: 020 7633 0557. Fax: 020 7633 0559. Website: www.depressionalliance.org.uk.

Depression Alliance (Scotland), 3 Grosvenor Gardens, Edinburgh, EH12 5JU, UK. Tel: 0131 467 3050.

Depression Alliance Cymru (Wales), 11 Plas Melin, Westbourne Road, Whitchurch, Cardiff, CF4 2BT, UK. Tel: 02920 692891.

Psychosis

Learning objectives

Aetiology, symptoms and prognosis for schizophrenia
Categories of persistent delusional disorder
The role of the GP in providing mental health care
Best practice for delivering physical care for individuals with psychotic illness

The psychoses are recognized as the most serious mental health problems affecting working-age adults. Primary care has an important role in initial diagnosis, in ongoing physical and mental health care and in promoting social inclusion and supporting carers. A number of diagnoses make up the group, including schizophrenia, schizo-affective disorder and delusional disorder. Mania is considered in Chapter 7 and organic psychosis in Chapter 15. Working across organizations and sectors is the key to aiding better health and social outcomes.

Schizophrenia

Kraepelin and Bleuler are the founding fathers of the concept of schizophrenia and Bleuler described the core symptoms, known colloquially as the four As: ambivalence, altered associations, autism and blunted affect. Many of the symptoms described by them, such as delusions and hallucinations, were known to occur in other conditions and the core symptoms were sufficiently ill-defined and subjective to make validation of the condition unsatisfactory. In more recent years Schneider identified and described the first-rank symptoms, hence refining the diagnosis and validating the condition, facilitating clinical diagnosis and research into treatments.

Since the development of community rather than institutional approaches to management, the importance of overcoming stigma and ensuring engagement in mainstream activities such as work, leisure and relationships (social inclusion) has been recognized as being of major importance. The condition remains relatively common and, although there is now recognition that recovery is possible, it remains for many a devastating illness which requires an ongoing multidisciplinary approach to treatment.

Prevalence

The lifetime risk of developing schizophrenia is about 1% whilst the annual prevalence is between 2 and 4/1000. The number of new cases each year lies between 0.2 and 0.5/1000. There is a slight excess of men over women and the age of onset is earlier in men, with a peak age of onset between 15 and 25 and a decade later in women. It is very rare before the age of 10.

The prevalence of patients with psychosis varies considerably from practice to practice. Prevalence is increased in urban areas and in practices where GPs have an interest in mental health (Kendrick *et al.* 1991), varying from a relatively high point of 6.1 per thousand to 1.7 per thousand in one study. The numbers of patients with chronic psychosis per practice ranges from 1 or 2 per practice in suburban, single-handed practices to over 100 patients in large inner-city group practices.

A cohort study in south east London illustrates the level of contact with GPs (Melzer *et al.* 1991; Conway *et al.* 1994). A year after discharge from hospital patients with schizophrenia had poor social adjustment and 55% still had psychotic symptoms. Ninety-four per cent were in contact with the health services, 55% of whom had been in contact with a GP in the previous 3 months. However, 3 years later contact had reduced to 26% for GPs in the previous 3 months. Ten per cent were in contact with their GP only. In a contrasting survey of 16 suburban practices with an interest in mental health, 90% of patients were in contact with the practice, compared to 73% in contact with psychiatrists or CPNs (Kendrick *et al.* 1994).

Aetiology

Genetic

The importance of a genetic contribution to this illness has been apparent since the early part of the twentieth century although it is clearly identifiable in only a minority of cases. The magnitude and type of this contribution is still a matter for debate. A number of genetic mechanisms have been investigated with ambiguous results and these include both monogenic and polygenic modes as well as genetic heterogeneity. It is generally believed that genes contribute to vulnerability rather than making illness certain or even likely. Almost half of all chromosomes have at some point been associated with schizophrenia; the most common associations are with the long arms of chromosomes 5, 11 and 18 and the short arm of chromosome 19 and the X chromosome. The risk where both parents have the condition is about 35%, where one parent is affected 12% and a second-degree relative 2.5%. For twins, the concordance increases likewise. For monozygotic twins it lies between 35 and 60% and for dizygotic twins between 9 and 26%, whilst for a non-twin sibling the risk is about 8%. Genetic studies into the traditional subtypes (hebephrenic, catatonic and paranoid) have found no evidence that they breed true although there may be a slightly lower risk of schizophrenia in the relatives of those with the paranoid type.

Family

Older theories particularly of the antipsychiatry school focused on the role of family psychopathology in the genesis of the condition. The most popular theory, dubbed the 'double bind', suggested that the dissonance between the verbal and non-verbal cues which the child faced in his day–to-day life made schizophrenia the inevitable and indeed the only 'sane' response. This view with its legacy of blame and guilt has never been scientifically proven and has been abandoned. An equally judgemental view, referred to as 'schism' and 'skew', described the balance of dominance within the family which was thought to be at risk of producing schizophrenic members. This theory has also been relegated to the archives. The importance of the family, however, has not been ignored and there is now a convincing body of opinion, backed up by research, that prognosis is determined, in part, by family behaviour described as 'expressed emotion' (EE) (see under psychosocial interventions).

Personality

The existence of an association between schizoid premorbid personality and schizophrenia is a commonly held belief. Recent evidence has questioned this and suggests that many schizophrenics who show evidence of schizoid personality may in fact have incipient schizophrenia. Also, only a minority of those with this type of personality disorder develop schizophrenia. Further problems arise with regard to schizotypal personality disorder, which is regarded in the DSM classification system as a personality disorder (Chapter 9), whilst the World Health Organization Classification (ICD-10) includes this as a variant of schizophrenia.

Environment

The recognition that many sufferers with this illness belong to poorer socio-economic groupings suggested that there may be some risk factor in these groups which predisposed. Closer scrutiny of their family background showed that this was mainly the effect of the illness with the associated 'social drift' downward, rather than any inherent pathogen in the social environment per se. However, the fact that the children of immigrants have a three to five times greater risk of developing schizophrenia as compared to the indigenous population suggests that environmental factors may be operational.

As with depressive illness, many schizophrenic episodes follow upon major psychological trauma although the type of event has been shown to be non-specific. Those episodes which have a definite precipitant have a better prognosis than those which arise spontaneously. However, such events would not act as a trigger unless there was a prior vulnerability to the illness.

Another approach to environmental causes has focused on the observation that significantly more people with schizophrenia are born in the winter months than at other times of the year, thus raising the possibility of pathogens such as viruses. The possible causal role of birth trauma or temporal lobe dysfunction has been suggested also. Other authorities contend that schizophrenia may be a reflection of a wider neurodevelopmental disorder since it has been found in some studies to be associated with 'soft' neurological signs.

Biological theories

There has been considerable interest in the specific areas of the brain that may be the primary site of pathology in schizophrenia. These include the basal ganglia, the frontal cortex and the limbic system. Several post-mortem studies have found a decrease in size of other areas including the amygdala, hippocampus and the parahippocampal gyrus and these findings are replicated by the findings of MRI studies in living patients. Studies focusing on the basal ganglia have found an increase in D2 receptors but have failed to establish whether this is the result of medication or the underlying neuropathology of the condition. As the basal ganglia are connected to the frontal cortex this area has inevitably become a focus for investigation.

The theory that abnormalities in dopamine turnover or in dopaminergic receptors are responsible for this disorder has been expounded for more than 25 years. The simplest theory is that schizophrenia results from too much dopaminergic activity. In particular D2 receptors have been linked to the positive symptoms and D1 to the negative symptoms. Other receptors such as D5 being related to D1 and D3 and D4 to D2 receptors amplify this picture as increases in D4 receptor share been found in post-mortem samples from schizophrenia patients.

Other receptors have also been the subject of investigation of the source of positive and negative symptoms. Serotonin turnover, especially that linked to $5HT_2$ receptors, has been implicated in the negative symptoms of schizophrenia. A decrease in function in the prefrontal cortex, the area with the highest density of $5HT_2$ receptors, and an increase in size of the lateral ventricles may be associated with negative symptoms. Recent imaging studies have shown a decrease in the size of the temporal and limbic areas of the brain, changes that may play a part in the positive symptoms of schizophrenia.

Brain imaging

The earliest imaging studies, i.e. CT studies, showed enlargement of the lateral and third ventricles and a reduction in cortical volume. Other studies have shown cerebral asymmetry, altered brain density and reduced cerebellar volume. However, these abnormalities have also been reported in a variety of psychiatric and organic brain disorders. Attempts to clarify whether the brain changes are static or progressive are inconclusive. Overall, what these investigations have demonstrated is that schizophrenia is an illness associated with structural abnormalities. However, the magnitude of these changes is small and so imaging is unhelpful in making the diagnosis in clinical practice.

MRI studies have amplified the findings from CT studies in identifying a reduction in volume in the hippocampla-amygdala complex and the parahippocampal gyrus in those with schizophrenia. Some have also found differences between the right and left hemispheres although others have not. The greater sophistication of positron emission tomography (PET) and magnetic resonance spectroscopy (MRS) is also now being used to further our knowledge of the neurobiological aetiology of schizophrenia but as yet without any definitive conclusion.

Symptoms

The prodrome and duration of untreated psychosis

There is increasing interest in the early phase of schizophrenia and the duration of untreated psychosis, (DUP). Duration of untreated psychosis is defined as the length of the period from symptom onset to referral for treatment. There is some evidence that this influences the prognosis. In most studies this is of the order of 1–2 years, due to the subtlety of the symptoms. These may include poor concentration, social withdrawal and unusual ideas not tantamount to psychosis. There is now a move towards developing prodromal intervention services that identify high-risk groups in the hope either of preventing transition to psychosis or of commencing treatment during the prodrome. The evidence that transition to psychosis can be prevented is equivocal (Marshall and Rathbone 2006) although there may be some benefits in relation to cost-effectiveness (Valmaggia *et al.* 2009). Others describe a 'critical period' of 2–5 years from the onset of symptoms when intervention is crucial if deterioration in social and cognitive function is to be prevented.

The acute phase

In the absence of biological markers, the most common approach in clinical practice is to base the diagnosis of schizophrenia on the presenting symptoms. These acute symptoms are related to both perception and thought content. The abnormalities of perception most commonly consist of auditory hallucinations in the third person, and somatic hallucinations and less frequently in the olfactory, gustatory or tactile modalities. The disorders of thought content manifest as delusions of persecution or reference, delusions of control (also called passivity) and delusional mood. At times abnormalities of the form of thought are found and

Table 8.1. First-rank symptoms of schizophrenia

- Thought insertion
- Thought withdrawal
- Thought broadcasting
- Primary delusions
- Passivity of thoughts, actions or impulses
- Echoe de la pensée
- Third-person auditory hallucinations discussing the patient or commenting on his actions
- Somatic hallucinations

these present as incoherence as thoughts slide and merge into one another. Perplexity of mood may also occur, as may depressed mood, although the latter is most commonly seen after the acute phase has passed. If persistent it requires treatment in its own right. Many of these symptoms may occur in other conditions such as mania, making a definitive diagnosis difficult at initial presentation.

In an attempt to overcome this difficulty, Schneider proposed a set of symptoms, known as symptoms of the first rank (Table 8.1), which he believed to be pathognomonic of schizophrenia, in the absence of any organic cause (Mellor 1970). This has considerably improved the reliability with which the diagnosis is made although the occurrence of some of these symptoms in severe depression or mania makes them less than perfect as defining features. Nevertheless, they have gained widespread acceptance in European clinical practice. There are other criteria in use, especially in the USA, but these have found less usage in clinical practice.

Ongoing illness

The striking feature is the personality change which afflicts those who remain unwell. Negative 'symptoms' predominate; volition is reduced, interest in social encounters is diminished and personal hygiene is often poor. It is these symptoms which relatives find most difficult to understand and often attribute them to laziness. Behaviour may be stilted with mannerisms and/or stereotypes. Hallucinations and delusions may occur, as in the acute syndrome, but the latter are often fixed and systematized. Affect is blunted, making rapport difficult, and formal thought disorder is often gross. An unexpected but common finding is age disorientation, and some patients display intellectual deficits when tested psychometrically.

Syndromes of schizophrenia

The older classification of schizophrenia into the *simple, paranoid, hebephrenic* and *catatonic* subtypes has largely fallen into disuse, due in part to the overlap between them when presenting clinically. Also the picture may vary between episodes. Apart from the paranoid type, with its better prognosis and the lower risk to relatives, these classifications are of doubtful validity. In particular, caution should be exercised when making a diagnosis of simple schizophrenia since it is based on the absence of features rather than on positive symptoms and some sources recommend its abandonment.

Not all those who have an episode of classic schizophrenia progress to the chronic residual state. This led to the use of the term *schizophreniform* to describe those patients whose illness had a precipitant, an acute onset, prominent depressive features and clouding of consciousness. This term is still in use.

Schizoaffective psychosis is a controversial label for a condition interposed between schizophrenia and bipolar disorder in which typical schizophrenic and depressive or manic episodes succeed each other, or occur concurrently. The prognosis is better and its proponents suggest lithium as the preferred maintenance treatment. Many believe that as depression and excitement are commonly part of schizophrenia their presence does not warrant this label and that this additional term confuses rather than clarifies. However, it is a useful term for those presenting with symptoms of both schizophrenia and bipolar disorder and is included in both ICD-10 and DSM-IV.

Differential diagnosis

Mania

Acute schizophrenia with its attendant excitement and delusions may be difficult to distinguish from mania. The presence of first-rank symptoms is helpful, although manic patients sometimes have these symptoms also. The content of the delusions is not helpful in making the diagnosis. It may only be possible to make a definitive diagnosis in retrospect, having considered the course of the illness.

Drug-induced psychoses

Drug-induced psychoses present with schizophrenic-like symptoms and a drug screen should be carried out in every young person having their first psychotic episode. Nevertheless, even those that are drug-induced may exhibit the same course as schizophrenia with relapses and remissions, or with negative features. The risk is particularly high in those using cannabis (Moore *et al.* 2007), amphetamines or ecstasy.

Acute and transient psychotic disorder

Brief psychotic disorders can occur in response to major emotional stressors and are of sudden onset. Consciousness may be clouded and although psychotic symptoms are present the full range of schizophrenia symptoms are lacking. Clinically these are very difficult to distinguish from those with a schizophrenic illness of acute onset. Treatment is with antipsychotic agents and hospitalization is usually required. There is a risk of depressive symptoms in the immediate post-psychotic phase. Treatment is required until symptomatic recovery is complete and close monitoring in the follow-up period is required for indications of relapse or for the emergence of a typical schizophrenic illness, an occurrence in an unknown percentage of such patients. Recent studies show that although about one-third remain symptom-free without medication over a 12 year follow-up period, there is a variable course for the remainder and the outcome is better than in schizophrenia and similar to depressive psychosis.

Borderline personality disorder

Some young people, often with histories of abuse and abandonment, with emerging borderline personality disorder, first come to the notice of health services during crises which include vivid auditory and visual experiences. Sometimes they are true hallucinations but more normally on close questioning they are images or sounds in the head. These are referred to as micropsychotic episodes and they are usually brief, but for some can persist for weeks and months at a time.

Depressive illness

The apathetic and withdrawn state of the chronically ill patient may resemble that of severe depressive illness. A detailed history of the previous episodes and, especially, of the level of functioning between these should clarify the diagnosis.

Management of schizophrenia

Decisions about the management of schizophrenia should take the patients' and, if relevant, the carers' views into account. Social, psychological and medical treatments all have their place although pharmacotherapy is almost always required. As services specialize, patients may fall under the care of many teams over time, including early interventions, home treatment, assertive outreach and primary care liaison services. The stresses, as well as therapeutic potential of home environments and hospital wards, should be considered when deciding about admission.

Acutely disturbed behaviour

The use of intramuscular, intravenous or oral haloperidol and lorazepam in combination is the most effective method of achieving rapid tranquillization. Sometimes zuclopenthixol acuphase is used to achieve rapid sedation but this is almost always in a hospital setting since the maximum dose is set at a low threshold. For those with less severe acute disturbance olanzapine or other oral medication is often given, particularly when adherence is not a problem.

First-episode psychosis

Patients with obvious psychosis may present to the GP alone and are sometimes brought to the surgery by their family. The immediate concerns are to distinguish drug-related or organic psychosis from the first episode of a 'functional' psychosis, and to engage the patient in treatment. Reducing the 'duration of untreated illness' is a key aim of management and GPs may benefit from education about the advantages of this. All such cases should be referred to the now well established Early Intervention Services, although GPs find that some patients will not accept a referral. Sometimes a specialist assessment can be carried out in primary care and be less stigmatizing for first contact; a shared assessment, taking into consideration the needs and strengths of the family, resulting in follow-up and treatment from the specialist team and continued involvement of primary care, is a satisfying process to aim for.

The mainstay of treatment is with major tranquillizers, which are instituted immediately the diagnosis is made. There is little to choose between the various phenothiazines or the butyrophenones in terms of efficacy but the spectrum of side effects may influence this decision. In particular, the butyrophenones such as haloperidol are more likely to cause extrapyramidal symptoms but are less sedative than the phenothiazines. Doses of up to 2000 mg of chlorpromazine orally, or its equivalent, may be required initially and anticholinergic agents should not be given unless side effects develop as these lower blood levels. During this period, the patient is best managed in a tranquil environment since overstimulation may provoke a recrudescence of disturbance.

The older medications have now been largely replaced by the newer atypical antipsychotic agents as the first-line treatment for schizophrenia. These have fewer extrapyramidal side effects, lessening the necessity for antiparkinsonian medications. The agents available at present include risperidone, haliperidone, olanzepine, quetiapine, amisulperide and ziprasidone. With these treatments the positive symptoms definitely improve and possibly the negative symptoms. A recent review found that overall there is little difference in efficacy between the first- and second-generation antipsychotic agents in treating positive symptoms. However, the second-generation medications are more effective for negative symptoms and within that group clozapine is superior to the others. Extrapyramidal side effects are more common with first-generation antipsychotics and both groups are associated with the metabolic syndrome and QT prolongation (Tandon *et al.* 2008).

Following discharge, medication is continued for 2 years in the patient having a first episode. Where there have been prior episodes, treatment is generally for life. If there is a likelihood of non-adherence to treatment, depot preparations may be necessary (see below).

Antidepressants and at times ECT may be required if depressive symptomatology supervenes and persists. This is now believed to be an inherent part of the illness and not due to medication as was formerly suggested.

Case 1

Miss X was a 22-year-old girl in her third year at university. During her last year she had become anxious and even agitated at times and felt she could not cope. She felt inordinate pressure was being put on her by her tutors and that she was not liked by them. One day she threw a chair at one of them and was referred for counselling. She became increasingly distressed and finally decided to return home the month prior to her exams. When seen by her local general practitioner she was agitated, claiming that people were sending messages to each other about her by telepathy and that there was a plot going on to prevent her getting her degree. She believed she heard people laughing at her through the wall of her bedroom and felt one of these was the tutor. Her general practitioner made a diagnosis of schizophrenia, having also obtained a urine sample immediately after she returned from university which was negative for illegal substances. He liaised with the early intervention service, treated her with olanzapine, saw her the next day for review and when her symptoms settled after a few days referred her to the early intervention team for confirmation of the diagnosis and for ongoing treatment. At the time of writing she was symptom-free, functioning normally and had returned to university.

Comment

This girl's increasing disturbance was heralding a schizophrenic illness. Her family were reluctant to have her treated as an inpatient but assured the general practitioner that if she did not begin to respond within 2 days of commencing treatment they would then not object to admission. She herself agreed and responded rapidly. Because of the acute onset the prognosis is good. Depot injections are not necessary since this girl adheres to treatment. She will be continued on medication for 2 years from the date at which she showed symptomatic improvement.

Management of treatment-resistant and residual schizophrenia

These are overlapping but distinct aspects of schizophrenia. Treatment resistance refers to ongoing acute symptoms, either positive or negative, that are unresponsive in whole or in large part to treatment. This feature may occur late in the illness after many relapses. On the other hand residual (formerly referred to as chronic) schizophrenia is a description of a subtype of the condition in which positive symptoms are present but of low intensity and the main features are the negative symptoms that have a particularly noticeable impact on social functioning. These are believed to be an inherent part of the illness especially in those with early and gradual onset.

Clozapine is the treatment of choice for both resistant and residual forms of the illness although if this fails then the strategies for further management diverge. In the treatment-resistant groups combination pharmacotherapy is used while in the residual schizophrenia group social and psychological interventions play a greater role.

Many patients require long-term medication and there is no therapeutic benefit in using depot in preference to oral preparations. The benefit of the former is due to their effect in reducing non-compliance. As a general rule, the risks of tardive dyskinesia are higher with depot than with oral preparations and this should be borne in mind when considering long-term treatment. The recent availability of risperidone and olanzepine in a depot format is a great advantage in this regard.

Clozapine is a dibenzodiazepine with an affinity for a host of receptors. It is finding use in the treatment of negative symptoms and in the treatment of those with resistant acute symptoms, estimated to occur in 5–25% of those receiving standard antipsychotic medication. Although it has the serious side effect of agranulocytosis, reported in up to 13/100 000 patients, it now has a significant part to play in the treatment of this difficult-to-treat group and it is estimated that 30–50% of patients unresponsive to other treatments show a positive outcome with this drug. A period of up to 6 months is required to achieve improvement.

Some psychiatrists prefer to administer this drug in hospital initially and until a dose of 300 mg per day has been reached. Monitoring can take place as an outpatient, consisting of weekly white cell counts for the first 18 weeks, then every 2 weeks for the remainder of the first year and then every 4 weeks thereafter as the risk of agranulocytosis is greatest in the first 18 weeks of treatment and after 1 year has the same risk as with standard antipsychotics. This monitoring is the responsibility of the psychiatric team and only when there is confirmation that there are no haematological side effects is the drug made available to the patient. This requires considerable administrative organization through the dedicated clozapine clinics. Other side effects of clozapine include nocturnal enuresis, sialorrhea, seizures, hypertension and vomiting. Increasingly robust shared care protocols are being developed for stable patients with blood tests being carried out in general practice.

Sertindole, an old preparation withdrawn from the market a number of years ago because of concerns about cardiac side effects, has again been relaunched for use in schizophrenia. It is useful for both the positive and negative symptoms but because of the possibility of QT prolongation most clinicians reserve it for those who are treatment-resistant or who have negative symptoms, the group for whom clozapine is currently prescribed. In addition, the requirement for ECG monitoring prior to commencing treatment, when a steady state is reached and thereafter, makes it a somewhat time-consuming drug to use.

Management of side effects

Anticholinergic agents should only be given when parkinsonism develops and the commonly used preparations include biperiden, benzhexol, procyclidine and orphenadrine. For acute dystonic reactions these will be required intramuscularly to abort the reaction. Thereafter, they should be continued regularly. Akathisia or 'restless legs' can be difficult to distinguish from agitation but in the former the patient is unable to control the movement. The treatment of choice is with diazepam, unless the offending drug can be reduced. Tardive dyskinesia is more serious than the other side effects because it may be irreversible. It is preventable by using the minimum required dose of drug and by avoiding antiparkinsonian agents. The effectiveness of 'drug holidays' in prevention is in dispute. When tardive dyskinesia is diagnosed, a reduction in medication may temporarily lead to a worsening of symptoms. Thereafter a number of drugs may be tried although none is universally successful. These include pimozide and tetrabenazine. Unfortunately many patients remain chronically symptomatic.

Psychosocial interventions

For those whose symptoms do not resolve, or who do not regain previous social functioning, psychosocial interventions are important. These should take account of the strengths of individuals and identify goals towards achieving social inclusion – relationships, leisure, housing, employment and education.

An important aspect of long-term treatment is the environment in which the patient lives. Understimulation will worsen the negative symptoms whilst overstimulation may precipitate relapse. Thus, a moderately stimulating milieu which includes occupational therapy is superior, on the one hand, to an unstructured long-stay ward and, on the other, to more intense treatments such as psychodynamic psychotherapy, which may provoke relapse.

Family work has an important role for some in reducing the risk of relapse. Several studies have found that families who are hostile, critical or over-involved, known as high EE (expressed emotion) families, contribute to relapse even when prior protection is given with medication. Low EE families are not associated with relapse. Education about the illness along with family therapy has been shown to reduce EE and the subsequent relapse rates.

Rehabilitation and recovery

Rehabilitation (de-institutionalization) is increasingly being recast as 'recovery'. Recovery, as defined by mental health users, refers to leading a satisfying and creative life within the confines of illness rather than any sense of cure. Many patients need help with the basic skills of everyday life, due to the illness itself and also due to the effects of being hospitalized or isolated from normal activities and networks. These including self-care, household management and social skills; traditionally the role of occupational therapists, support for these functions can also be provided by nurses, social workers or psychologists.

Recovery work needs to cut across all the key domains of social inclusion – relationships, leisure, civic participation as well as the traditional areas of accommodation and employment. Retraining for work may be feasible for those whose illness is under control and who have satisfactory social and personal skills. Volunteering or supported and therapeutic work can be important intermediate steps. There are now many innovative programmes supporting the introduction to mainstream work with excellent trial evidence for employment advisors within mental health teams increasing levels of employment; sadly practice lags well behind the evidence.

Accommodation is provided on the basis of the independence of the patient with long-term hospital care being needed only for the most incapacitated, and hostels, group homes and individual flats being better suited to the less impaired. Local authorities have a key role supporting people with mental illness to settle independently.

A key worker in the area of rehabilitation is the community psychiatric nurse, who is often the person most frequently in contact with the patient in the community. In countries with less well developed community services he or she becomes the critical link between the hospital and the community-based services; in the UK key workers (also called care coordinators) are not always nurses, and are part of a range of community-based teams (see Chapter 21). In addition to giving ongoing support and promoting further independence, the key worker also deals with

Case 2

Mr. X, aged 19, went to see his general practitioner for an annual medication review. The general practitioner was new to the practice and noted that X had not been seen for a year, but was taking olanzapine 10 mg. This followed an acute psychotic episode aged 17 when he had been seen by the child and adolescent mental health team. He had made a good recovery from the acute episode which had involved several weeks of sleepless nights, paranoid thoughts and some increasingly argumentative behaviour.

At the review he was feeling tired and lethargic and had put on weight during the last year. He was feeling unsure as to whether he had a mental health problem and was generally negative about his outlook for life, being unemployed and not in training or education. The general practitioner decided to discuss the case with the local psychiatrist and it was agreed that trial reduction of medication was appropriate, as most of his problems could be due to side effects. X had a sister who had had a psychotic episode and was under the mental health services, his mother was also believed to have mental health problems, but he had been brought up by his father and a stepmother.

He was fearful of becoming like his brother or mother. The medication was reduced to 5 mg and he was followed up monthly for a few months and after 6 months the medication was again reduced to 2.5 mg. His weight began to reduce; he gained energy and went back to college. He continued on 2.5 mg for a further year, having one brief episode of sleepless nights lasting a few days which resolved on its own. A year later it was agreed that his medication should be stopped altogether. There were no further episodes of mental health problems and after 2 further years, during which he had settled in a job, he was taken off the practice mental health register. During this time advice about relapses had been the main focus of conversations and had included liaison with his father.

Comment

This case illustrates the possibility of recovery following a first episode of severe mental illness and the role of the general practitioner in identifying individuals who are not engaged with specialist services. In this case it was important to come to a balanced judgement about both harms as well as benefits of medication. As models of recovery, particularly for first-episode psychosis, become standard in secondary care, it is time for primary care to develop both recovery and crisis plans for those individuals not under specialist services.

issues such as default from treatment and depot clinic appointments and may be the person to administer depot injections to those who cannot or will not attend the hospital for these. Most importantly they will support families and other carers, providing information on the illness and advice about managing behaviour; this is best done with the consent of and in collaboration with the patient in order to respect autonomy and confidentiality.

Outcome

A number of factors influence outcome. Onset during teenage years, insidious presentation, negative symptoms and poor premorbid personality augur badly for the future. Low IQ and a family history of schizophrenia are also associated with a poor prognosis. The features which are associated with favourable outcome are acute onset, precipitating stress, affective symptoms and late onset. Women have a slightly better prognosis than men. The adverse effect of belonging to a high EE family has been outlined above.

The prognosis of schizophrenia has improved considerably over the last 30 years, although it is still recognized as the most serious psychiatric disorder and most require long-term medication. Follow-up studies of patients discharged from hospital after acute episodes suggest that 25–33% make a complete symptomatic and social recovery whilst up to 25% remain psychotic, if followed up for 2 years. The remainder have an intermediate prognosis. The concomitant abuse of illicit drugs has an adverse effect on outcome since they have a destabilizing effect and result in frequent relapses and re-admissions to hospital.

Management of psychosis in primary care

GPs will most commonly come in contact with patients who have chronic psychosis when relatively well, either as the patient signs on at a new surgery or when presenting for minor physical problems. This is a useful time for the GP to get to know the person and to examine their ongoing as well as immediate physical health needs. GPs can be important advocates for a recovery-oriented approach to management and primary care workers may well be able to signpost people with stable psychosis to local mainstream services as a means of increasing social inclusion.

Management of relapse in primary care

A clearly flagged diagnosis in the records allows GPs to be alert to changes in mental state and to detect relapses early, perhaps when presenting for physical health issues. It is important to be alert to other problems such as drug misuse, which may be a form of self-medication, and also to comorbid depression. It may be possible to initiate treatment changes within the primary care setting, preferably in collaboration with the care coordinator or local psychiatrist.

The general practitioner will often be called to contribute to a Mental Health Act assessment (see Chapter 23) and their role can be very important because:

- they may be the only professional with prior knowledge

- they may know the family
- they can act as an independent advocate.

Proactive review of patients in general practice – general principles

It was not until the early 1990s that calls were made for general practitioners to be involved in proactive review of patients with long-term mental illness. Research demonstrated potential benefits but also showed that general practitioners resented work which was seen as duplicating that of secondary services and that financial incentives did not always result in high-quality reviews.

The GMS contract now provides incentives for the review of patients with psychosis and bipolar disorder through the active use of registers. The review has to consist of a 'physical health review', a 'medication review' and a 'review of responsibilities for care'. This will allow us to distinguish clearly between the review needs of those under specialist services and of those who are being looked after in primary care. Most but not all patients with chronic schizophrenia as well as many with bipolar disorder are under specialist care and on the CPA. Increasingly, as real shared care develops with specialists working also in primary care, reviews can be carried out jointly by GPs and psychiatrists. The differences between these reviews are summarized below.

Proactive review in general practice for those under specialist care

Those under specialist care often have little contact with primary care and may need encouragement to attend. The main benefits of the mental health review will be:

- improved physical health care
- familiarity with and trust in the primary health care team
- the GP meeting the patient while they are (relatively) well
- ensuring that shared care arrangements, including prescribing, are transparent.

This review can provide the foundation for close collaboration between patient, primary and secondary care, which will be of benefit in the event of relapse, crisis or worsening physical health.

Reviews for those not under specialist care

For those not under specialist services proactive reviews need to be broader and more regular, including annual screening for problems in a range of areas, including employment, accommodation, family issues and relationships, as well as assessment of mental state, physical health and medication review. Unmet needs which are revealed should be addressed, with ongoing care by the GP or referral to the psychiatric services. Mental health teams can support this care with practice-based training sessions and the provision of advice on best practice and on local services.

Systems within primary care

Care for psychosis, a long-term condition, requires systems to support it. This points to the importance of registers; these are created de facto by the accurate recording of diagnostic codes. A database of information for each patient should be consistent with specialist records

Table 8.2. Priorities for physical health care review

- Ask about the patient's concerns about physical health

- Consider needs for other chronic disease management

- Screen for common health problems with closed questions
  - cardiovascular
  - respiratory
  - gastrointestinal
  - dental
  - joint hearing and vision

- Physical examination
  - BP
  - BMI
  - visual acuity

- Lifestyle and health promotion assessment
  - smoking status
  - diet
  - exercise
  - alcohol and illegal drugs
  - smear and mammography
  - contraception and safe sex

- Side effects
  - weight gain

as laid out in Table 8.2. Electronic templates for storing data also prompt better care during proactive reviews.

Systems of review and recall are essential if registers are to be used to improve patient care. Ideally, patients with psychosis will be allocated a practice key worker, usually a GP, in order to develop trust and provide continuity. Systems for annual recall and review of people with psychosis, as a part of the Quality Outcomes Framework of the new contract, are now embedded in an annual cycle in general practice. There are additional incentives to encourage follow-up of those not attending an invitation for review. Local governance groups should focus on arrangements for how to respond when patients do not attend despite telephone calls and letters.

Can we justify a systematic approach?

There is no comprehensive randomized controlled trial demonstrating better health outcomes following a proactive approach to the care of physical health in this group of patients. Currently, however, the rates of diagnosis are lower than in the general population; preventive care treatment is lower still. A variety of methods of proactive physical review have met with mixed success; however, lessons for implementation have been learnt. That patients with severe and enduring mental illness believe GPs should focus more on physical care suggests the time has come for a more proactive approach.

Proactive care can be provided systematically or opportunistically. As most patients attend their general practice over a year the latter is theoretically possible. However, the reactive nature of general practice with consultations that are already rushed, combined with a reticent population, make it unlikely that opportunistic care alone will suffice.

Physical care for patients with mental illness

After years of tentative calls to encourage proactive physical health care for patients with long-term mental illness there are now real incentives in the UK. This section will outline the evidence, the issues for patients and practitioners in the consultation, and the organizational structures and processes required to improve physical health care. It applies primarily to those with psychosis but the principles apply to those with bipolar disorder without good function between episodes.

Increased morbidity and mortality

Estimates vary as to the increased risk of death for patients with long-term mental illness. International studies suggested standardized mortality ratios (SMR) from 150 to 700. The large Salford study of 6,952 psychiatric patients over a 15 year period estimated an SMR of 165 (Baxter, 1996). This was highest for patients with personality disorder with two times the mortality rate. Patients with chronic psychosis and severe affective disorders had approximately 60% increases, while those with other neuroses had 20% increases. The largest number of deaths was due to accidental and non-accidental injury in young people and to cardiovascular disease in the middle-aged and elderly. A more recent UK study of 370 patients with schizophrenia, however, suggests that SMRs for deaths due to natural causes may well be about 230.

A review of medical comorbidity in schizophrenia showed that only in rheumatological diseases and possibly carcinoma of the lung was psychosis protective. Ischaemic heart disease is increased for psychosis and affective disorders; this is primarily due to smoking in the case of psychosis and there may be a neuroendocrine link for depression. Other chest conditions are also more prevalent. While cognitive impairment is increased in schizophrenia, progressive dementia is not. Impairments are likely to be related to institutionalization, medication, untreated depression and an inherent part of the illness itself. Neoplasms do not appear to be particularly increased after controlling for other factors. HIV is more prevalent in most countries in patients with psychosis. Iatrogenic problems due to neuroleptics are common: tardive dyskinaesia is found in 3–62%; there is an increased prevalence of impaired glucose tolerance; seizures can be precipitated and clozapine causes blood dyscrasias. Hypothyroidism and electrolyte disturbances are common in patients on lithium. Antidepressants have a range of problems.

Engaging patients

In contrast to many patients with anxiety and depression, most patients with schizophrenia are not assertive when presenting bodily complaints and appear to have higher than average pain thresholds with late presentations of normally painful conditions such as appendicitis and peptic ulcer. Reductions in cognitive function and beliefs that they are not ill, as well as negative symptoms, contribute further to low attendance.

Case 3

Mr. X had lost contact with mental health services 4 years previously. His records showed a history of schizophrenia and he was reviewed by a general practitioner as a part of his annual mental health review. He was taking risperidone 3 mg and had some residual auditory hallucinations. He had done some voluntary work, but had stopped this recently and had very little contact with the outside world, apart from visiting his mother once a week and going to the shop to buy video games. He did not feel unhappy, but was keen to socialize. He was overweight with a BMI of 31, had raised blood pressure and smoked 30 cigarettes a day.

The general practitioner assessed his motivation for lifestyle change. It was clear that he had very little motivation to reduce his food intake or stop smoking, but was interested in doing more exercise. He was referred to a local voluntary-sector group, which ran weekly varied exercise classes for people with a range of mental health problems. He became very involved in the group, attending two to three times a week, and also went on a food hygiene training programme which was running at the centre. He attended one day concerned about his diet and over the next weeks worked with the practice nurse to make some significant changes to this. Surprisingly one day the practice nurse received a positive response when asked whether he was ready to attempt to stop smoking. Another person in the group had managed to quit and he suddenly realized that he would like some support to do the same. While he did not quit he reduced his smoking to 10 per day.

Comment

This vignette illustrates the potential for supporting people with SMI to change their lifestyle in order to promote health. It often requires great patience, with small rewards over time. The problems are similar to health promotion for the general population, but cognitive distortions and low levels of motivation make it more difficult in those with mental illness.

Some, particularly younger, patients with psychosis lack continuity and therefore trust with an individual GP. In this context, GPs need to ensure that the basic principles of good consulting are applied even more rigorously with this complex group of patients (see Chapter 3). The careful use of both closed and open questions, eliciting concerns, providing clear information and sharing decisions are all the more important in patients who are paranoid and may have associated cognitive impairment. The empathic and straightforward management of minor illnesses can provide a basis for developing the trust required for investigation of serious illness and preventive work.

Preventive care and smoking cessation

There are understandable reasons why preventive care is not taken seriously. Specialist mental health workers often lack the knowledge, practice nurses lack the confidence and some GPs are unenthusiastic about the prospects for health promotion. Others consider proactive physical care to be the least of the patient's problems or feel wary about putting therapeutic relationships at risk by discussing issues which are not of immediate concern.

However, patients are not all unconcerned about their physical health. Forty per cent of patients invited for a risk-factor profile were willing to attend and this was only a little less than the general population (Osborn 2000). Screening for high cholesterol and blood pressure is feasible. Ensuring adherence to lifestyle changes and medication may require more intensive work, including written information and collaboration with specialist mental health workers.

Smoking cessation for this group of patients has been shown to be successful; however, there are a number of tricky issues. Nicotine moderates symptoms. It is also thought to reduce parkinsonian effects of medication. Weight gain on cessation often deters patients. Although harms are understood the rewards of smoking are perceived as greater. The use of nicotine gum, with its lower rates of weight gain, is an option. However, this requires patients to minimize their intake of acidic drinks. A team in Melbourne have produced useful guidelines which suggest the need for some additional training for those involved in delivering smoking cessation. Assessment of the risks of cessation such as psychotic relapse, having knowledge of the relapse signature and side effects for each patient are important. Written plans and having group support available are useful. Patients should be seen 1–3 days after quitting to deal with any problems that arise and then weekly for a month to assess any changes.

There are many other areas of health promotion which should be considered in a structured way when reviewing the physical health of patients with long-term mental illness. These include those outlined in Table 8.2 and range from sexual health issues through to immunization against influenza. Practice nurses can easily be involved in the majority of this work.

Diagnosis and management of serious physical illness

Patients with psychosis may present few symptoms despite serious underlying conditions. They will require more proactive questioning for further symptoms as well as a low threshold for investigation. Patients with serious mental health problems often miss appointments. It is often worth asking the patient, when making an outpatient referral, if a copy of the referral and the subsequent appointment could be sent to the patient's care coordinator so that they can facilitate attendance. Patients with serious diagnoses often fail to attend for routine follow-up in general practice; liaison with specialists and having a named GP may help.

Working across the interface to support physical health

The importance of the relationship between primary and secondary care in achieving physical health is clear. Based on very practical experience Crews et al. (1998) have gone further and point out the importance of the three-way relationship between the specialist, generalist and patient.

In the UK the Quality Outcomes Framework incentivizes practices to invite patients for a physical review. Most will attend but some will not and at this point it is important for practices to involve secondary care. Many patients with long-term mental illness have developed trusting relationships with care coordinators. This trust sometimes does not extend to primary care. If these workers see the importance of physical health and introduce patients to their primary health care team, then trust can be extended to primary care.

An alternative system involves using the Care Programme Approach (or other specialist review system) as the basis for physical health checks. Instead of being invited to a care programme approach meeting, which they are unlikely to attend, the general practitioner could be sent letters requesting information about preventive physical care and chronic disease management for physical comorbidity. They could also be asked to invite the patient to an appointment with a GP or a practice nurse if there appears to be a need.

Formal communication

Formal communication has consisted traditionally of letters from GPs and discharges and outpatient letters from psychiatrists; the content of each has been subject to criticism. Key information for example about families and previous treatment from GPs and on care coordinators, medication, diagnoses, crisis plans and relapse signatures from specialists should be included. See Table 8.3 for examples of the data which should be shared.

GPs and care coordinators should update each other on important new issues as they arise. Electronic communication is still relatively unusual and will require the development of transferable coding systems in order to become an efficient mechanism for communication between teams. Eventually Primary Health Care Trusts and mental health teams may have immediate access to parts of the same records, allowing more seamless care.

Informal communication is particularly relevant during crises or relapses. The trust required for collaborative communication during crises, often involving urgent telephone calls, can be enhanced through joint working, particularly regular face to face discussion of cases.

Persistent delusional disorder

A group of disorders that previously had such names as paranoid psychosis, monosymptomatic delusional psychosis, delusional jealousy, etc. have been grouped together in the modern classifications under the rubric 'persistent delusional disorder' since they share the common features of delusions, in the absence of hallucinations or other psychotic symptoms. They are characterized by good preservation of personality, unlike schizophrenia.

Paranoid psychosis

The relationship between paranoid psychosis and both schizophrenia and paranoid personality is a matter of debate. Paranoid psychosis and its variants differ from schizophrenia in arising without the hallucinations or thought disorder that characterize the latter. It usually has an insidious onset and the delusions are often systematized. Even with treatment they often persist. Because personality is intact the patient is frequently able to continue to work and perform socially with the symptoms impinging only upon those who are close to the patient.

Delusional jealousy

A variant of paranoid psychosis is delusional jealousy (Othello syndrome). This may sometimes be associated with alcohol abuse. The patient constantly asks for 'proof' of his partner's fidelity, who may initially accede to these and other requests. This should be discouraged since it will offer only temporary respite from the doubts and queries and may reinforce the delusions. If the delusions fail to respond to treatment the couple may be advised to separate especially if threats of violence are being made by the patient.

Table 8.3. Information which should be recorded and shared

Socio-demographic data
Telephone number
Marital status: married, single, separated, widowed, divorced
Ethnicity: e.g. Asian, black, white, other
Housing type: council, housing association, rented, owned, hostel, no fixed abode
Home situation: lives alone – with help, lives alone – no help, lives with partner, lives with family, single parent
Number of children/dependants
Next of kin/address/telephone
Neighbour/main carer/address/telephone
Clinical data
Diagnosis
Date of first diagnosis
History of compulsory admission: y/n: dates and types
History of deliberate self-harm
Current risk of deliberate self-harm
History of harm to others
Current risk of harm to others
Risk of self-neglect
Substance misuse: e.g. alcohol, benzodiazepines, opiates, other
Specific indicators of relapse
Specific crisis response
Specific recovery plan
Psychotropic medication
CPA level
Responsibilities and recall
Frequency and responsibility for general reviews
Responsibility for psychotropic prescribing
Current specialist team
Current care coordinator
Other agencies/professionals involved
Date last physical review completed

Other delusional states

Delusions of love or erotomania (De Clerambault's syndrome) are also difficult to treat and the person at whom they are directed may be frequently harassed by the patient. Other monosymptomatic delusional states are associated with delusions that *bodily appearance is abnormal* (dysmorphic delusions), e.g. the ears are misshapen or that the body emits smells or harbours some serious illness or infection. The latter must be distinguished from severe depressive illness, which may be associated with similar delusions. At times of stress those with paranoid personality disorder may *decompensate* into a psychosis and immigrants are also vulnerable to short-lived psychotic episodes.

The treatment of all the above disorders is with antipsychotic medication, although forming a therapeutic relationship is often difficult since the recommendation that medication should be taken is often perceived as an indication that the doctor is colluding with those who disbelieve the patient or are his persecutors. Some authorities recommend pimozide in those with persistent delusional disorder, especially of the somatic and dysmorphic types. When agitation is severe, as may occur during periods of decompensation, then intramuscular sedation may be required.

Summary

- Schizophrenia has a prevalence of between 2 and 4/1000, with a slight excess among men.
- The cause is unknown, although there is a genetic component in some, and the concordance is higher among monozygotic than among dizygotic twins. The mode of inheritance is unknown.
- Causes originating in the family or relating to social class have been disproven.
- The distinction from mania may be difficult during an acute episode.
- Following a first episode, treatment is continued for 2 years. If relapse occurs, then it will be required for life.
- The family environment and the milieu in which the patient lives are important in preventing relapse.
- The prognosis has improved over the past 30 years.
- The general practitioner has a key role in proactively managing the patient, psychiatrically and physically.

References

Baxter, D. M. (1996). The mortality experience of individuals on the Salford Psychiatric Case Register. All-cause mortality. *British Journal of Psychiatry*, **168**, 772–779.

Conway, A. S., Melzer, D., and Hale, A. S. (1994). The outcome of targeting community mental health services: evidence from the West Lambeth schizophrenia cohort. *BMJ* (Clinical Research Ed), **308**(6929), 627–630.

Harvey, C. A., Pantelis, C., Taylor, J., *et al.* The Camden Schizophrenia Surveys II. (1996).

High prevalence of schizophrenia in an inner London borough and its relationship to socio-demographic factors. *British Journal of Psychiatry*, **168**, 418–426.

Kendrick, T., Sibbald, B., Burns, T., and Freeling, P. (1991). Role of general practitioners in care of long term mentally ill patients. *BMJ* (Clinical Research Ed), **302** (6775), 508–510.

Kendrick, T., Burns, T., Freeling, P., and Sibbald, B. (1994). Provision of care to general practice patients with disabling long-term mental illness: a survey in 16 practices. *British Journal of General Practice*, **44**(384), 301–305.

Marshall, M., and Rathbone, J. (2006). Early intervention for psychosis. *Cochrane Database of Systematic Reviews*, 4, CD004718.

Mellor, C. S. (1970). First rank symptoms of schizophrenia. *British Journal of Psychiatry*, **117**, 15–23.

Melzer, D., Hale, A. S., Malik, S. J., Hogman, G. A., and Wood S. (1991). Community care for patients with schizophrenia one year after hospital discharge. *BMJ* (Clinical Research Ed.), **303** (6809), 1023–1026.

Moore, T. H., Zammit, S., Lingford-Hughes, A., *et al.* (2007). Cannabis use and the risk of psychotic or affective mental health outcomes: a systematic review. *Lancet*, **390** (9584), 319–328.

Tandon, R., Belmaker, R. H., Gattaz, W. F., *et al.* (2008). World Psychiatric Association Pharmacopsychiatry Section statement on comparative effectiveness of antipsychotics in the treatment of schizophrenia. *Schizophrenia Research*, **100** (1–3), 20–38.

Valmaggia, L. R., McCrone, P., Knapp, M., *et al.* (2009). Economic impact of early intervention in people at high risk of psychosis. *Psychological Medicine*, **39**, 1617–1626.

Suggested reading for patients and carers

Reveley, A. (2006). *Your Guide to Schizophrenia.* (Royal Society of Medicine). London: Hodder Arnold.

Fuller Torrey, E. (2006). *Surviving Schizophrenia – A Manual for Families, Patients and Providers,* 5th edn. New York: Harper Collins.

Useful addresses

Shine, 38 Blessington St., Dublin 7, Ireland. Tel: 01-8601620 or 1890621631. Email: infosirl.ie.

Rethink (formerly The National Schizophrenia Fellowship), 89 Albert Embankment, London, SE1 7TP. UK. Tel: 0207 8403188. Email: advice@rethink.org.

Useful websites for patients and carers

www.shineonline.ie (this is the website of Shine, formerly Schizophrenia Ireland).

http://www.rcpsych.ac.uk/mentalhealthinfoforall/problems/schizphrenia (this website at the Royal College of Psychiatrists provides excellent information for patients and carers).

Personality disorder

Learning objectives

Approaches to assessing personality
The complexity of managing personality disorder
Recent guidelines in treating antisocial and borderline personality disorder
Other behavioural disorders and their management

Personality disorder (PD) is defined as an enduring pattern of perceiving, thinking about and relating to the environment and oneself that causes difficulties in a variety of social and interpersonal contexts. In other words the problems of interaction and of personal perspectives are present in a variety of social and personal settings. It is important that general practitioners recognize PD as it has an impact on the presentation, response to treatment and outcome of comorbid disorders. It causes a burden of suffering for family members and friends. PD currently results in the utilization of resources due, for example, to the repeated episodes of self-harm or substance misuse that characterize this group. Moreover there are resource implications in other health and non-health settings since many people with medically unexplained symptoms have personality disorder; and many come into contact with the criminal justice system.

After a protracted lull, interest in PD was given a large boost by the publication of a document detailing government policy in relation to the treatment of those with this condition (National Institute for Mental Health in England 2003). It recommended that treatment be delivered by specially trained multidisciplinary teams dedicated to this group and funding has been made available to pilot this development. It also recognized that some services would need to be delivered within a forensic setting. More recently the NICE guidelines for antisocial and borderline PD (2007 and 2009) provide useful clarity on when therapy and medication should be used. Commissioning guidance clarifies the roles of primary care, specialist mental health services and the criminal justice system in a stepped care approach. Training is advocated for most specialist mental health workers dealing with personality disorder. NICE Guidelines focus exclusively on the categories of antisocial and borderline that are associated with violence or that make heavy demands on the psychiatric services (see p. 130).

The diagnosis of personality disorder is one which should be made with caution since it often alienates service providers such as psychiatrists and psychologists. Conjuring up images of difficult, dependent or at times violent people, it has a stigmatizing effect, even in the presence of axis 1 disorders such as anxiety or depressive disorders. For this reason it is essential that the diagnosis is made only when the doctor is certain that the traits are of lifelong duration and lead to significant social as well as personal suffering. In primary care it may be more useful to describe traits and associated problems rather than attempting to identify a single category since there is considerable overlap between the various categories. This is illustrated by vignette 1 below.

Case 1

Mr. X was a 23-year-old man referred to mental health services by the probation service. He had started cutting himself superficially and was avoiding leaving his room. He had recently been given a community sentence for assault and, although in the past had used heroin for several years, was now binge drinking from time to time. He was attending a group for alcohol training as a part of his sentence and lived with his parents for the first time in several years.

He was hard to engage in conversation, looking away, shuffling his feet and answering in monosyllables. He showed little empathy for his victim or his family and was unable to see the point in life at all. He had no motivation to engage in training or get a job and saw alcohol as temporary relief to boredom. However, on closer questioning it became clear that he was fearful of going out into the town centre because of the way people looked at him. He believed that they thought he was a 'low life' and had previously responded by being aggressive with people, occasionally violently. He would join other groups of young men and gain kudos for minor acts of vandalism or aggression to strangers. Recently, however, he had disengaged from these groups and felt less confident about this way of displaying strength.

He was felt to have elements of both avoidant and antisocial personality disorders. However, the overall formulation emphasized his past problems with attachment and trauma. His mother had left home when he was 8 and his brothers had encouraged him in criminal acts from an early age. His father was an alcoholic and he had problems of attachment. The recent changes to his outlook suggested the possibility of a more positive evolution and following a joint meeting with the criminal justice team he was offered a mentor and provided with cognitive behavioural therapy to deal with his anger and avoidance behaviour. Over months his drinking bouts declined, he joined a fishing group associated with the mental health service and was provided with supportive housing by a housing association.

Comment

This case illustrates the difficulty of pinning down an exact diagnosis. Often it is more useful to describe those elements of personality problems (i.e. the criteria within each diagnosis, such as feelings of emptiness) rather than making an exact psychiatric diagnosis. It also illustrates the fact that past trauma and abandonment are often a prelude to personality disorder, particularly borderline and antisocial types. The right therapy is rarely clear-cut and in this situation social support based on his immediate needs, such as housing, and his interests, such as fishing, appeared to be an effective start to this process.

Categories of personality disorder

The nosological status and the categories of personality disorders vary across continents and even sometimes between individual psychiatrists. The explanation lies in the derivation of these from subjective clinical opinion. Ideally this should be a starting point from which to attempt to prove their validity (existence) rather than assuming them to be immutable. So vague have been the descriptions of these categories that the level of agreement between psychiatrists in clinically diagnosing personality disorders is only around 30%. In the USA the problem of definition has been partially overcome by using rigorous criteria to facilitate accuracy of diagnosis although the level of agreement between clinicians in clinical practice still remains low.

In ICD-10 there were 10 categories of PD with two others added subsequently (personality change following a catastrophic experience and organic personality disorder). The American system of classification (DSM-IV) names 11 categories. The categories have been the subject of much criticism, with many claiming that these are arbitrary epithets rather than scientifically validated disorders based on true clustering of traits and behaviours. Even where clustering is proven, the philosophical and clinical value of labelling by cluster rather than detailing the actual thoughts and behaviours is contested.

DSM describes a number of additional categories that are not included in the European system of classification. Schizotypal personality disorder is regarded among European psychiatrists as a variant of schizophrenia and classified in that section of ICD-10. However, American psychiatrists view it as a personality disorder since such people appear to others as distinctly odd and strange. They often demonstrate magical thinking and have great difficulty describing their interpersonal problems as their speech is often metaphorical and circumstantial, requiring interpretation. They may claim clairvoyance and describe illusions and derealization.

Narcissistic personality disorder is also included in DSM-IV but not in the European classification. Persons with this disorder view themselves as unique and appear self-important. They see themselves as cleverer than others and may appear self-absorbed. Special treatment is expected and they often present as boastful. European psychiatrists, treating a person with these features, would probably make a diagnosis of histrionic personality disorder.

Passive-aggressive personality disorder is also not classified in ICD-10 but in DSM is classified as a category for further study. It is characterized by covert obstructiveness and stubbornness to mask underlying aggression. Depressive personality disorder is also incorporated as a category for further study and is characterized by persistent pessimism, gloom and unhappiness. The content of conversation is negative and dreary and there is little joy in the person's demeanour.

In an attempt to overcome the unwieldy classification of its 11 categories, DSM has grouped them into three clusters – cluster A, also called the odd or eccentric type (paranoid, schizoid or schizotypal categories), cluster B, also called the dramatic, emotional or erratic type (borderline, histrionic, narcissistic or antisocial categories) and cluster C, also referred to as the anxious or fearful group (obsessional or anankastic, dependent or asthenic and avoidant categories). It is cluster B disorders which attract the most attention due to the considerable distress and harm to selves and others. These disorders are also associated with difficult childhoods and trauma. For this reason they are also commonly associated with psychiatric comorbidity. This potential shared aetiology adds weight to arguments about classification.

The principal categories identified in European psychiatry are as summarized below. However, it is highly likely that changes will be made to some or all of these categories when ICD-11 and DSM-V are published in the next few years.

Obsessional or anankastic personality disorder

This refers to the predominating traits of punctiliousness, order, punctuality, perfectionism and rigidity. Lack of spontaneity, a dislike of surprises and sometimes indecisiveness are also found. Such people thrive in areas that require order and regulation but because of inflexibility they often alienate others. Occasionally, obsessive compulsive neurosis may supervene. See Case 2 below.

Case 2

Mr X was 35 when admitted to hospital following an overdose. For 6 months previously he had been feeling depressed since beginning his new job. He was a successful businessman and had rapidly progressed up the management ladder to become one of the directors of his firm. He was 'head hunted' 9 months earlier for a post in the public relations and marketing side of his firm. He reluctantly accepted the post with persuasion from his wife. His hesitation stemmed from his introspective and reserved manner. He had few friends, preferring to spend his time at home rather than socializing. He had no hobbies except watching television – he rarely read and showed no interest in sport or in the arts. He was meticulous and organized and found the flexibility of having to travel at short notice difficult to cope with. His wife was ambitious for him and felt that his drive and high standards suited him to his new post. His first overdose occurred after he had been bought a set of golf clubs by his firm so that he could make local business contacts. On admission after the overdose he had initial insomnia, impaired concentration and marked suicidal ideation. His symptoms improved within 2 days without any pharmacological treatment and this continued during his 2 week stay. Throughout this time he engaged well with staff and showed no signs of low mood, sleep disturbance or impaired concentration. His appetite was good. He was advised that he was unsuited to his present post and he decided to ask for a change. This was procured and he maintained his improvement at the time of writing.

Comment

Mr X had an obsessional (anankastic) personality which had been of initial benefit to his career, resulting in him being sought out for promotion. His reserve and limited diversions as evidenced by his hobbies and inflexibility made him unsuited to the specific demands of his new position. Being emotionally inhibited and having an ambitious spouse he felt unable to confide and chose to persist in his unhappy state. Finally, unable to tolerate the stress of his predicament he overdosed. Changing his job to one which suited his personality resulted in an improvement in his well-being. Diagnostically there was some initial uncertainty about the mental state (axis 1) diagnosis – the possibility of a depressive illness was considered but ruled out in view of his spontaneous improvement and staff reports. The axis 1 diagnosis was therefore an adjustment reaction, and the axis 2 diagnosis a personality disorder of obsessional type.

Passive-dependent or asthenic personality disorder

Shyness, worrying, inability to make decisions, emotional dependence and low self-esteem characterize this group. Social anxiety and withdrawal are common.

Histrionic or hysterical personality disorder

This refers to those who are shallow, flirtatious, self-centred, attention-seeking, dramatic and childish in behaviour. Unfortunately this label is frequently applied without adequate evidence and it is also used as a term of disapproval (Thompson and Goldberg 1987). There is no relationship with the condition known as conversion or dissociative disorder (formerly hysteria) and the association is phonetic not clinical. These people not uncommonly find work in the media and entertainment.

Paranoid personality disorder
Paranoid personalities are those who are suspicious of the motives of others, have difficulty trusting and in consequence make few close relationships. They respond poorly to justified criticism and are sensitive to the extent that they easily take umbrage. This may lead to difficulties with friends and colleagues. Paranoid psychosis may occasionally supervene when the suspicion becomes psychotic in intensity.

Schizoid personality disorder
This is associated with coldness, a desire to be alone and to shun people, few relationships and often an interest in the eccentric. There is no definite evidence of a relationship to schizophrenia although earlier work suggested this association. It is probable that the features were a manifestation of early illness rather than of persistent personality type. It is also different from schizotypal disorder (see Chapter 8).

Cyclothymic personality disorder
These personalities are those who are subject to swings of mood from depression to happiness. The swings are generally not related to circumstances and are not severe enough to require hospitalization. Duration is usually a few days. Recent work suggests that this does not belong to the personality disorder category but is a subclinical form of bipolar disorder. Treatment with lithium salts has been tried with some success (Akiskal *et al.* 1977), but this study needs replication.

Antisocial personality disorder
This is associated with antisocial behaviour, impulsivity, emotional coldness and an absence of guilt. Alcohol abuse is sometimes associated. Unsurprisingly a significant proportion of people in contact with the criminal justice system have this disorder. Some individuals do well in management if impulsivity is controlled.

Anxious personality disorder
The anxious personality is tense, self-conscious and avoids relationships unless there is the certainty of acceptance. It is also called the avoidant personality by some. It may be difficult to distinguish from chronic generalized anxiety and from long-standing phobias although these latter conditions will have a clear onset whereas the traits of anxious personality disorder are not situation-specific and will be present since childhood.

Emotionally unstable personality disorder
This is divided by ICD-10 into two subgroups; the impulsive and the borderline types. DSM only identifies borderline type and this is increasingly becoming the main term used.

The impulsive personality is characterized by poor emotional control, unpredictable moods and argumentative behaviour. Forward planning is absent and decisions are often made which are subsequently regretted. A number of other terms were used clinically including 'immature', but now have no place in clinical practice.

Borderline personality disorder is a frequently used descriptor that has a vast body of associated research; the view of some is that it is a type of either sociopathic or hysterical personality whilst others hold that it is a variant of schizophrenia. This disorder is associated with chronic feelings of boredom, intense relationships which alternate between over-idealization and hostility, impulsiveness and emotional instability. Gender identity problems and body image distortions are associated with eating disorders in this group. Depressed mood and self-harm are also frequently reported. Occasionally brief psychotic episodes may occur. However, since this is a diagnosis made almost exclusively in young women and prospective studies show that it is an unstable diagnosis, many are sceptical of its validity (Tyrer 2002). Sexual abuse appears to be a frequently associated antecedent and is considered of aetiological significance.

Case 3

Ms X is a 22-year-old woman living in supported accommodation, having become homeless at around the age of 18 when she left foster care. She had a baby girl aged 1 who was in care because of Ms X's inability to look after her. Ms X was the eldest of three children and her mother left the family home when she was 4. She had little contact with her thereafter. Her father attempted to bring up the children but he was unable to manage Ms X's behaviour and began to beat her. At 12 she was taken into care. She has since reported that her uncle sexually abused her. She came to the attention of her GP because of low mood and threats of self-harm. She began cutting herself after the birth of her baby and was referred to the psychiatric services. She also had a social worker with whom she had a very poor relationship. A diagnosis of borderline personality disorder was made and she was referred for psycho-therapy in relation to the sexual abuse but was unable to tolerate this and the cutting increased. She also began to abuse alcohol. Therapy was discontinued. She defaulted from the outpatient clinic but about 6 months later represented with an overdose and a history of ongoing rapid mood fluctuations. By then she was in a serious relationship but her partner was violent to her and she ended it. She presented regularly to the accident department in an intoxicated state, cutting herself or threatening self-harm. She agreed to attend for dialectical behaviour therapy (DBT), a type of cognitive therapy used for those who self-harm (see below – Treatment). Her cutting and threats of self-harm diminished and her moods stabilized somewhat. She was not on any medication although she constantly requested this.

Comment

The young woman has been diagnosed with borderline personality disorder and her history illustrates the role of abuse (physical and sexual) in its aetiology. She was difficult to engage in treatment as is common in this group and found therapy regarding the abuse overwhelming. She was appropriately referred for DBT and was responding slowly to this intervention.

Personality change following a catastrophic experience

It is well recognized that periods of extreme stress, such as being in a serious accident or following a severe psychiatric or medical illness, can effect a change in personality that persists even after the primary illness has been successfully treated. In order to make the diagnosis, the features must persist for more than 2 years, with no prior history of personality disorder, and it presents either as persistent withdrawal, lack of interest and lack of trust in people or with dependence and making excessive demands on others.

Organic personality disorder

This diagnosis is made when there is permanent personality change following brain injury, usually head injury or secondary to alcoholic brain damage. Commonly the frontal lobe is affected, leading to disinhibition.

Dangerous and severe personality disorder

In England and Wales those deemed to have 'dangerous, severe personality disorder' (DSPD) can be subject to a compulsory treatment order with detention in a unit specializing in the treatment of this condition. The aim is to reduce the threat of violence posed to the public by this group. They present from three sources – those leaving secure hospitals, some leaving prison and some people in the community. However, the DSPD programme continues to provoke controversy and draws criticism from civil rights groups as well as psychiatrists, who point out that this legislation is penalizing those who have yet to commit a crime. In addition, as the prediction of future violence is unreliable, many more are likely to be incarcerated than are predicted by the home office. DSPD has no clinical status in psychiatry and is an epithet drawn up by government in the context of the criminal justice system. It is likely that it consists mainly of a small group with severe antisocial personality disorder.

Personality assessment

Personality assessment in general practice is useful for the following reasons:

- personality disorder can complicate treatment of other conditions
- personality traits or disorder may be the dominant problem and even if not treatable an explanation can be helpful
- significant personality disorder may underlie presenting problems such as chronic depression or anxiety
- the aim is as much to elicit problematic traits as to make a diagnosis.

Clinical methods

The clinical assessment of personality might include the following:

(1) enquiry about specific personality traits related to one or more specific personality disorders (e.g. emotional lability/impulsivity/anger)
(2) enquiry as to whether these features are of recent onset or whether they have been present since the teens
(3) ascertain whether these traits cause interpersonal problems
(4) obtain collateral information from those who know the patient well, ideally for a long time.

First, the general practitioner must attempt to *separate lifelong traits from current symptoms*, e.g. the apathetic, quiet patient with a depressive illness will give the impression of having a passive-dependent personality unless the doctor makes specific enquiries about the patient's usual behaviour. The assessor should begin by a simple statement such as 'I'm trying to find out what sort of person you have been throughout your adult life. I know you may be different now because of your problems, but I want you to remember how you were before you became ill'. The traits and behaviour which the GP assesses must therefore be persistent over a number of years.

Second, the doctor must be aware of the common *sources of bias*. It is well recognized that male doctors may diagnose attractive women as having hysterical personality disorder, especially if they are distressed. Similarly men are sometimes labelled as psychopathic on inadequate grounds. Social class also contributes to bias, with personality disorder being diagnosed more frequently in lower socio-economic groups.

Third, *a single abnormal trait does not constitute a personality disorder*. The prosaic adage that 'nobody is perfect' should be borne in mind before the patient is labelled as being personality disordered. Thus a patient who describes himself as always being tidy and conscientious may not necessarily have a personality disorder unless other abnormal traits are also present. The threshold for this diagnosis should be high and unless the trait is causing problems to those who come into contact with the patient such labelling should be withheld. Even then it needs to be done in a supportive way.

Fourth, information about personality is often best obtained from *informants*, who have known the patient for a long time. This is especially true when dealing with somebody who may be alcohol-dependent, depressed or psychotic. Because of either deliberate obfuscation or lack of insight these patients are unreliable making independent information essential.

Fifth, personality disorder does not protect against psychiatric illness. A person with a sociopathic personality disorder may become clinically depressed and require treatment for this. 'Either/or' thinking may lead to treatable disorders being neglected and subsumed under an all-embracing rubric of personality disorder. It is thus important to attempt to assess for other conditions even when the doctor is certain that PD is present.

There are a number of attributes that should alert the doctor to the possibility of a personality disorder. These include frequent changes of job and an inability to sustain long-term relationships, resulting in multiple partners. Excessive dependence on others for help with day–to-day decisions may lead to self-referral to multiple counsellors or frequent utilization of voluntary-sector services. Repeated episodes of self-harm, petty criminality and substance abuse also point to this diagnosis. Further indicators include decompensatation into anxiety or depression during transition periods, whether this involves emotional change, such as bereavement, or physical changes, such as moving house or being promoted at work. A history of sexual abuse in childhood is a known risk factor for personality disorder as is a history of disruptive behaviour in childhood. Finally patients whom GPs see as 'difficult' or 'heartsink' (see below) may have a personality disorder diagnosis (see below). Those with personality disorder overlap significantly with patients who have medically unexplained symptoms.

Interview schedules

Many structured interview schedules have been developed for measuring abnormalities of personality. Amongst the earliest was the Rorschach ink blot test, which used the patient's interpretation of ink blots to develop a comprehensive understanding of the psychodynamics of the patient's personality. This is not widely used today since there was no standardization of the test. Still used is the Minnesota Multiphasic Personality Inventory (Buros 1972) but its use is limited by the time it takes to administer and by the interpretation of scores; it may also be contaminated by current psychiatric disorder. The Eysenck Personality Inventory (Eysenck and Eysenck 1969), favoured because it is easily administered, has been widely used in general medical research. It describes the patient's personality on dimensions which are labelled neurotic, introversion–extraversion and psychotic. The dimensional concept is difficult to grasp and there is also concern about the particular dimensions chosen. The scores in each dimension have been shown to be unreliable and to change as intercurrent illness changes. More recent schedules have overcome the problems of older ones which made no attempt to distinguish between symptoms of illness and enduring traits of personality and which obtained information from the subject only. These include the Standardized Assessment of Personality (Mann *et al.* 1981) and the Personality Assessment Schedule (Tyrer and Alexander 1979). They consist of a series of questions about individual traits of personality and information is collected from informants only in the former and from both subject and informant in the latter. These schedules have considerably enhanced research in this area. The Standardised Assessment of Personality Abbreviated Scale (SAPAS) (Moran *et al.* 2003) has also been developed and this includes self-complete questions which are not generally demeaning, can be completed quickly and can be used to open up discussions. It should be combined with a clinical assessment of personality also as it is a screening rather than a diagnostic instrument.

The commonly measured and useful traits associated with personality disorder are listed in Table 9.1.

There is no simple or rapid technique for assessing personality and even with schedules such as those described above the interview is lengthy and is only as reliable as the information obtained. Questions with 'hidden' meanings such as those used in popular magazines have more commercial than scientific appeal. Thus clinical assessment remains for the present the only viable method available to the general practitioner.

Table 9.1. Traits relevant for assessment in personality disorder

General anxiousness

Conscientiousness

Rigidity

Impulsivity

Anger/aggression

Dependence on others

Indecisiveness

Suspiciousness/jealousy

Sensitivity to criticism

Lack of interest in relationships

Excessive introspection

Negativity

Exuberance

Differential diagnosis

Personality disorder can be difficult to distinguish from a range of other conditions.

Many of those with personality disorder also have co-occurring symptoms such as anxiety and depression, as well as PTSD and substance misuse. In some instances these emotional states are an inherent part of the personality. Typically the person with anxious personality will describe excessive anxiety in response to stressful events that passes quickly. The person with antisocial or borderline personality disorder often describes shifts in mood in the context of life's ups and downs. These do not warrant specific treatment with antidepressants or anxiolytics but require support measures. However, when they present for the first time a diagnosis of depressive episode or generalized anxiety may erroneously be made.

The relationship between borderline personality disorder and PTSD is more complex and is a classic differential conundrum, with repeated abuse and/or domestic violence resulting in both emotional lability and avoidance. Some commentators prefer the concept of 'complex trauma' for this group. Bipolar disorder is another important differential diagnosis in those with borderline personality disorder. Mood changes in rapid cycling bipolar can be similar in intensity, but, unlike the rapid fluctuations seen in personality disorder, they are generally not precipitated by stressors in those with bipolar disorder.

The distinction between paranoid psychosis and paranoid personality disorder can also be difficult to make and it can be even more problematic to identify the superimposition of psychosis on a pre-existing paranoid personality disorder.

Formulation of the diagnosis

In considering an intervention what is more important than the actual personality disorder category are the basic traits and behaviours that give rise to problems. This evaluation may require several consultations. Certain aspects need to be considered:

- comorbidity is common, e.g. PTSD
- a number of symptoms (e.g. anxiety, flashbacks, paranoia) can be present and require intervention
- past histories of abuse-witnessing or being a victim of domestic violence may require intervention
- self-harming behaviours (substance misuse, physical harm, risk-taking) are important components of the formulation
- insight into thinking patterns, behaviours and culpability may be variable.

Some practitioners find it useful to work with individuals mapping out past experiences, current thinking and positive and negative behaviours in order to help individuals understand the origins of current symptoms and responses, thus assisting them in taking some responsibility for change.

Epidemiology

Studies in general practice have consistently shown that about 5% of patients with psychiatric morbidity have personality disorder diagnosed clinically by their general practitioner as the primary diagnosis. When assessment is made using an interview schedule this rises to around 26% (Patience *et al.* 1995) and most of these patients will also have an additional diagnosis, e.g. passive-dependent personality disorder and generalized anxiety disorder. Among attend-ees in primary care for all reasons Moran *et al.* (2000) identified 27% as having personality disorder although those diagnosed by the research psychiatrist generally were not the same as those so diagnosed by the general practitioner. In general, personality disorder is higher in urban than rural general practices because of the attraction of the anonymous city for those who are chaotic and disturbed. Personality disorder is slightly more common in men than women and the obsessional, sociopathic and passive-dependent types are the most common.

Personality disorder is present in about 10% of the general adult population and is most frequent in those under 45. Antisocial PD is found in about 2% of the general population while borderline is present in around 0.7%.

The sex distribution varies with category (borderline more common in women, antisocial more common in men) while PD overall is diagnosed more frequently in white than in non-white populations although it is unclear whether this represents a true epidemiological difference or reflects diagnostic bias. Comorbid substance abuse is common, as are social exclusion, relationship problems and employment difficulties.

The 'difficult patient' and the general practitioner

The patient with a personality disorder rarely presents directly for help with this, and more usually presents when a crisis or some intercurrent physical illness/problem supervenes. Treatment of the presenting problem is called for first. This may involve crisis intervention, pharmacotherapy and containment or a combination of these. However, the patient will often pose additional problems that require special consideration. Some studies (Schafer and Nowlis 1998) have found that patients identified as 'difficult' by family practitioners had unrecognized personality disorder when compared to control patients and that dependent rather than antisocial or borderline type predominated in this group.

The term 'heartsink' has been commonly used in general practice to refer to the GP's feeling of 'dysphoria' at the prospect of seeing difficult patients. O'Dowd categorizes such patients as 'dependent clingers', 'entitled demanders', 'manipulative help rejectors' and 'self-destructive deniers' (O'Dowd 1988). 'Heartsink' patients are associated with frequent attend-ance and difficult GP–patient relationships and a number of studies have identified an association between these factors and psychological morbidity, including depression (Smits *et al.* 2008; Dowrick *et al.* 2000) and personality disorder (Pare and Rosenbluth 1999; Gross *et al.* 2002).

Non-adherence to treatment is a frequent difficulty and adherence issues should be discussed in an open way while giving the patient responsibility for decision-making where possible. For those engaged in counselling or cognitive therapy non-adherence may take the form of cancelling appointments at short notice or failing to complete assignments. There may of course be alternative explanations, other than personality disorder, for resistance to treatment. The explanations proffered by the patient may be genuine, as for example when confronting an issue raised during counselling that may be too painful at the time. In the event of persistent non-adherence, treatment must be suspended as damage can be done by unwanted therapy.

Coercion is another problem frequently associated with personality disorder. This may be overt, as when the patient asks for extra time off work even though there is no indication for it, or more subtle, as when the doctor gets drawn into subterfuge, e.g. a patient constantly complains about aspects of her marriage but yet refuses to discuss this openly with her spouse. A more serious example would be a request to the doctor to contact a partner ostensibly about another matter and then to discretely raise the problem. The GMC, Irish Medical Council and Defence Union guidance on confidentiality, openness and ethical conduct is now well understood, but doctors still need to maintain their guard against unethical requests.

Patients may also visit different doctors and give contradictory accounts of previous treatments. A common problem is 'playing off' the consultant against the general practitioner and when in doubt this should be clarified, on the spot if necessary; e.g. a patient whom a psychiatrist was seeing for an eating disorder and alcohol abuse asked permission to drink in order to stimulate her appetite. Permission was withheld. The following day she went to her general practitioner with this request also and failed to mention that she had discussed it only the previous day. He promptly contacted the psychiatrist to clarify respective positions and to ensure consistency in the advice given.

Blaming the doctor is a frequent and powerful technique used by the difficult patient. The patient who does not have a request for admission to hospital or for medication acceded to may threaten self-harm or may lay the blame for any consequences at the doctor's feet. Such threats must not be dismissed since patients do harm themselves when angry. The risks of these threats must be assessed taking into account the patient's past history, their family support and the danger of reinforcing the patient's maladaptive behaviour. When in doubt the advice of a colleague or specialist should be sought and documented and at times that of the defence organization also.

Flattery is frequently used to win the approval of another and words of gratitude are appreciated by the doctor no less than anybody else. Practitioners need to beware that this may preface a dramatic fall in popularity. Constant expressions of indebtedness need to be treated warily since they may indicate that the patient feels a special affinity with the doctor over and above the usual doctor–patient relationship. In some forms of therapy, especially the 'talking therapies', it may dupe the doctor into believing that the patient is being helped whereas no progress is in fact being made. The doctor who has been propitiated may also find it difficult to be objective about the patient and may become over-involved.

Dictating terms, such as wanting to be seen at special times or demanding certain treatments, etc., will often be exhibited by patients who are demanding in their personal lives also. It is common practice to acquiesce to such demands initially since they often seem reasonable but the doctor must be aware that other inadmissible requests may follow. This may cause considerable friction and at its most extreme the patient may accuse the doctor of refusing treatment. Such a modus operandi is clinically and therapeutically crippling to the doctor and the patient may have to be confronted about this.

Frequent visits or telephone calls are difficult to deal with. Obviously when these are requested to control panic attacks or to deal with the actively suicidal person they must be followed up with appropriate emergency intervention. However, when they are for routine inquiries they should be curtailed. One of the authors (PC) recently took over the care of a patient from a retiring colleague. She had previously been seen every 2 weeks although the patient's condition was stable. Attempts to increase the gap between appointments were met with regular telephone calls complaining of anxiety or of insomnia. The fact that the patient was using these to keep in contact with the doctor was discussed with her and an agreement was reached that telephone calls would only be transferred if there was an urgent problem.

Those contacts which are to dispel various medically unexplained physical symptoms (MUS) are more difficult since there is the inevitable fear that there is an organic basis for the symptom. Rather than refuse to attend when the 'emergency' presents, the doctor should afterwards draw up a 'contract' with the patient regarding this behaviour (see Chapter 12). For instance the patient may agree to desist from such emergency calls in return for a regular agreed appointment with the doctor to explore personal difficulties. The patient's family may need to be involved in reaching this decision also since they are sometimes the instigators of such requests. It is tempting also to arrange yet another physical investigation so as to 'do' something even though there are inadequate grounds or it has been done previously. The temptation should be resisted since it may reinforce the illness behaviour and the patient should be advised that the matter will be discussed in less compelling circumstances – the doctor may then if necessary give the patient a specific appointment for further discussion. This is another situation when discussion with a colleague to agree a non-interventionist approach can be useful and this should be clearly documented.

Treatment
General measures
Many of those with PD will be treated by the generic psychiatric services, not specifically for personality disorder per se but for comorbid disorders, such as substance misuse or depressive illness, or for associated problematic behaviours such as self-harm, poor problem-solving abilities or deficits in social skills. Others will be treated for childhood traumas that may have had an aetiological role in the behaviour such as physical or sexual abuse or other parental problems. The range of therapies varies from dialectical behaviour therapy (DBT) for self-harm, to problem-solving and anger management. Other interventions include generic coun-selling, solution-focused therapy or psychodynamic psychotherapy. However, impediments to successful outcome remain and include lack of motivation, poor insight and unreliability. The tendency for some patients to become over-dependent on the therapist or to see themselves as passive agents in the process also militates against successful treatment. NICE guidance advises strongly against the use of brief therapy in the absence of a package of specialist care. The new IAPT services may provide treatment for comorbid anxiety and depression if the personality issues are not over-riding. Constraints in relation to time and to skills are also a problem. A diagnosis of PD has at times excluded patients from treatment due to therapeutic nihilism but rather than refusing intervention the focus should be on setting limits and containing behaviour as described above (The 'difficult patient' and the general practitioner).

Practitioners can provide information on self-help reading material to patients who require help with social skills and self-confidence. Many centres, both lay and medical, now run social skills groups and the doctor would do well to have details of those run locally.

Practitioners can help some patients who are shy and lacking confidence by assigning simple tasks for the patient such as rehearsing answering the door or the telephone. The patient can be advised to write what he will say and then to record it on tape for the next visit when constructive criticism and advice about the next stage will be provided. Suggestions about voice pitch, speed, etc., and demonstrations by the doctor himself take little time and are often useful in bolstering self-confidence. Information about posture, eye contact and body language can be incorporated into other sessions. Encouraging a positive self-image requires a different strategy. Discussion should concentrate only on the patients' positive attributes and listing these will focus attention on them. People with low self-esteem often fail to meet their own practical needs, have an exaggerated tendency to put others before themselves and are often taken advantage of. They should be encouraged to say 'no' to the undue demands thrust upon them and to regularly reward themselves with treats. Assertive training courses are also often available in the local community as well as from the psychiatric services.

Drugs have little part to play in the management of personality disorder although they may have for comorbid conditions. There is a suggestion that lithium is helpful in aggressive behaviour but this remains to be evaluated more fully. Lithium has been more successfully used in cyclothymia. Antiepileptic drugs such as phenytoin and carbamazepine have also been used but their value is yet to be established. Many patients with personality disorder request and are prescribed drugs, especially benzodiazepines, to help cope with the problems of living which they face. This should be discouraged since the risk of dependence is all too obvious in those with long-standing disturbance. Some of the benzodiazepines also have a propensity to release aggression and in those with antisocial personalities may worsen the problem. Antidepressants should only be used with comorbid depression and avoided in those with mood lability alone.

Specific guidelines and interventions

More specific guidelines have emanated from NICE on the treatment of antisocial PD and of borderline PD, suggesting that there are now a range of treatments available and that the prognosis may be more hopeful than in the past although a number of barriers still exist, particularly with regard to the scope for interventions in primary care. Dialectical behaviour therapy (DBT) is perhaps the most promising evidence-based therapy – possibly because it addresses head on the nurturing of more normative emotional responses to conflict and stressors.

1 Antisocial personality disorder

In the context of primary care, the NICE guidelines on antisocial personality disorder (2009) recommend that evaluation of a current violence risk should be accompanied by referral to the secondary care personality disorder services or to a forensic psychiatry team. The guidelines also recognize the limited evidence base for treating antisocial personality disorder and outline the four areas at which interventions will be targeted:

- interventions specifically targeting the personality disorder
- interventions targeting associated behaviours such as aggression, impulsivity
- treatment of comorbid disorders such as anxiety, substance misuse
- management of offending behaviour.

In addition it is important to consider the safety of children or other dependants in the care of these people.

While the guidelines are silent on the role of the general practitioner in managing comorbid conditions, they do caution on the possibility of non-adherence to treatment and on the risk of interaction between medications and alcohol or illicit substances.

However, for the first time, there is an emphasis on prevention by identifying children with conduct disorder who may be at risk of developing personality disorder over time.

2 Borderline personality disorder

The guidelines (NICE 2007) relating to borderline personality disorder do not comment on the role of the general practitioner. However, of relevance to them is the fact that many present with fluctuations in mood that lead to prescriptions of antidepressants resulting in polypharmacy. For example, a 6 year prospective study found that 40% of patients with BPD had at some point been prescribed three or more drugs, concurrently. The guidelines caution against the use of polypharmacy and advise pharmacological treatments only in crisis. They also recommend that medication not be used for individual behaviours or symptoms and caution against prescribing so as to simply 'do something'.

Organization of care

The resurgence of interest in PD has been accompanied by guidance and debate about how best to organize care for this diverse group of individuals. It has mainly centred on those with 'cluster b' diagnoses such as borderline PD and antisocial PD.

Two new concepts have been introduced in the UK – stepped care and PD specialism.

1. Stepped care simply suggests that there is a tiering of intensity of care and that all levels of health service will need to have some input. Primary care is included as step one and probably most people with PD are seen solely by primary care – although mostly not explicitly for PD. As problems become more severe care might involve community mental health teams, acute inpatient and long-term secure and medium-secure 'hospitals' for those with dangerous and severe psychopathic personality disorder. It is recognized that the criminal justice system is also an area for care of PD. Contact with probation and prison programmes amounts to an early step in treatment, integrating simple and sometimes more complex psychological programmes for 'resettlement' – reducing reoffending, rather than improved health being the primary goal.

2. Specialism, the second concept, adds another diversion and further complexity to the debate. Some commentators favour specialist teams for specific groups – either for those newly diagnosed or for those with more extended and complex PD. Others favour PD 'services' which might or might not carry 'case loads', but would provide a range of other services including:

- consultation – advise only
- consultation – see and liaise
- training
- provision of dialectical behaviour therapy (DBT).

Provision of DBT requires a dedicated team of therapists and many argue that it should be separate from the overall individual coordinating care.

Stepped care reaffirms the role of the generalist in care for PD, but this is still a relatively evidence-free zone. We have given some guidance on how to deal with individuals and it is to be hoped that specialist PD services, if they are developed further, are mandated to support primary care as well as mental health teams.

Furthermore it is clear to clinicians in primary care that individuals deemed to be at step one – in primary care – are virtually never easy to manage and have complexities which are generated by comorbidity (physical and mental), difficult family situations (with children and other dependants potentially at risk) and social exclusion (homelessness, unemployment, isolation, etc.).

Implications of the diagnosis

The relevance of personality disorder to the general practitioner lies not so much in the treatment of this condition, which is time-consuming, intense and best carried out in specialist settings, but in the effect personality has on the outcome of concomitant psychiatric disorder and on response to treatment for physical conditions. Psychiatric illnesses have a poorer prognosis when premorbid personality is abnormal and response to medication is adversely affected by abnormal personality. Not only is there more contact with the psychiatric services but there are more frequent visits to the general practitioner, symptoms are slower to resolve and functioning more impaired in the long term (Tyrer 1988). It is apparent that assessing personality is of more than esoteric interest and that it has important prognostic implications.

Formal assessment of personality may become standard practice for the family doctor, who may be in a good position to provide accurate information since in most cases he will be familiar with the patient prior to the onset of illness and over a period of several years. It would benefit the patient and those involved in treatment, whether specialist or generalist, if this information could be formulated concisely. Perhaps the most important note to end on is the need to maintain optimism. New treatments are more effective and there is emerging evidence that many traits diminish over time.

Impulse and habit disorders

There are a group of patients with impulsive behaviour and habit disorders, characterized by failure to resist an impulse that is usually ego-syntonic but often harmful. There is increasing tension prior to committing the impulsive act, with a sense of pleasure or gratification once it has been completed. These disorders are variously viewed as personality disorders or as mental state diagnoses or as overlapping into both groups.

Intermittent explosive disorder

As the name suggests, this disorder consists of intermittent bursts of aggression that are out of proportion to any precipitating social stress and triggered by minor conflict. Individuals or their relatives usually describe the episodes as 'spells' or 'attacks'. Associated with the violent outbursts are feelings of tension and, relief after the episode followed by remorse. Many describe racing thoughts and an energy surge during the event followed by lowering of mood and decreased energy. Most have a lifetime comorbidity for a mood disorder, including bipolar disorder. In general, the age of onset is in adolescence and men predominate by a 4:1 ratio, although some women describe similar symptoms premenstrually. In view of the favourable response to mood stabilizers many believe that it may be linked to bipolar disorder. There is little research on this disorder.

Pathological gambling

The essential feature of pathological gambling (PG) is a chronic and progressive failure to resist impulses to gamble, with the behaviour leading to much damage to personal and family life. Efforts to stop or resist gambling generally fail, and the behaviour shows some resemblances to an addiction. Deprived of the opportunity to gamble, the person becomes restlessness and irritable and over time there is an increase in the size and frequency of the stake required to achieve the desired level of excitement. In pathological states the gambling will persist even in the face of mounting debts, marital breakup or other legal problems. Some gamblers steal to maintain their habit. PG is a serious problem and may be associated with other addictions, particularly alcohol and tobacco, but there may also be disturbed eating, sleeping, sexual and relationship problems, as well as impaired function at work. Some present with depression or following an overdose.

PG is not rare. A review of over 120 studies gave a lifetime prevalence of 1.6% (Schaffer *et al.* 1999) and surveys of prison populations show that around 10% of prisoners are pathological gamblers. PG is most obvious among men and among those who indulge in horse and dog racing, with which dramatic losses soon become apparent. Women prefer bingo and football pools but morbid patterns are less obvious because losses are smaller and spread over longer periods of time. The internet provides a new forum for gambling.

The condition tends to begin in adolescence for males and late in life for females. It waxes and wanes but is often chronic. The aetiology is unknown and theories abound. There are suggestions that gambling will at least temporarily help people switch out of negative internal mood states such as feelings of loneliness or other forms of dysphoria. The obvious self-destructive nature of the behaviour has provoked much analytical speculation, but there is little scientific study on the problem. There may also be social pressures including early exposure to gambling. Learning theorists point out that the usual sequence of repeated gambling losses with occasional random wins provides a pattern of intermittent reinforcement, the most potent schedule for conditioning. In this respect a big win is thought to be particularly hazardous, and the financial reinforcement of winning prolongs the habit. Personality disorder, mania and childhood ADHD are considered risk factors also.

Various treatment approaches are offered, encompassing most known types of psychotherapy. Counselling and support for the family may also be helpful. Both psychodynamic psychotherapy and aversive behavioural therapy have been attempted, but neither claims much success. Most gamblers find the notion of complete abstinence abhorrent, but a few may accept the wisdom of a moratorium for a few months. Among the more severe cases there is usually a disturbed appreciation of the value of money, and in these instances it is wisest for all the family income to be paid into an account over which only the spouse has sole control. Gamblers Anonymous uses the Alcoholics Anonymous model and is the first step for many. There is a little optimism on the pharmacological front, with preliminary studies suggesting a role for naltrexone, either as monotherapy or in combination with an SSRI. Also, lithium and valproate have been used with some success. Clearly, this will be a fruitful area for research in the future. In general non-pharmacological treatments appear to be somewhat more effective than pharmacological interventions (naltrexone, mood stabilizers and SSRIs) but cognitive therapy seems to be no more efficacious than less expensive alternatives such as brief interventions (Leung and Cottler 2009). Recent work suggests that cognitive behaviour therapy may be helpful along with a 12-step group programme.

Trichotillomania

Trichotillomania is defined as the irresistible urge to pull one's hair. This is often associated with subsequent rituals, such as mouthing the hair afterwards, or even ingesting it (trichophagy). Most subjects report a state of tension before pulling their hair out. The hair-pulling is not described as painful, but subjects report tingling and pruritis in the affected areas. As well as the scalp, the eyebrows, eyelashes, beard and pubic hair may be involved. Hair pulling tends to occur during states of relaxation – while sitting down watching television, reading, listening to music, etc.

The aetiology of the disorder is not understood and some regard it as being driven by a desire to self-mutilate, others as arising from impaired early relationships and others believe it to be biologically determined, reflecting inappropriately released motor activity. The repetitive nature of the hair-pulling suggests a link to OCD.

The disorder is not uncommon in general practice and presents most commonly to dermatologists before the seeking of any psychiatric help. Behavioural strategies appear to be the most useful. Drugs such as cloimipramine or an SSRI may also be helpful in view of the possible link to OCD. While both behaviour therapy and drug treatment may offer some relief in the short term, little is known about relapse rates or long-term outcome, but a recent longitudinal study found a poor prognosis even with psychiatric treatment.

Adult attention deficit hyperactivity disorder

Attention deficit hyperactivity disorder (ADHD) is one of the most common psychiatric disorders of childhood. The belief that it is attenuated with increasing age and disappears in adulthood has been shown to be incorrect and studies now show that 25% still always meet the criteria in early adulthood, with the proportion falling to 8% by the late 20s, while 60% have at least one disabling symptom as adults. Complications such as antisocial personality disorder, found in up to one-third, and substance misuse in 16% indicate that its ramifications are significant. While studies of this condition in adults are few in number they suggest that 0.5–1% of the young adult population has this disorder. Many psychiatrists still have little experience in managing this disorder in adults, with a consequent deficit of services for this patient group.

This disorder is incorporated into this chapter since personality disorder is a common complication of severe, untreated ADHD.

There is no evidence that environmental factors such as parental attitudes, deprivation, toxins or pre- or perinatal complications are responsible for ADHD. Some studies demonstrate the importance of genetic factors, with monozygotic twins showing a 50% concordance for the disorder, and adoption studies show an increased concordance for ADHD in the biological rather than the adoptive families of child sufferers. In addition imaging studies such as MRI have found abnormalities in the corpus callosum and caudate nucleus although these require replication. Blood flow studies have also pointed to abnormalities in the prefrontal cortex, an area concerned with attention processes.

In relation to the core features of the disorder, these include hyperactivity, poor ability to maintain attention and poor impulse control. Three broad groups are described – the inattentive form, the hyperactive-impulsive form or the more common combined type. To make the diagnosis the features must be present even before school age, should be pervasive rather than sporadic and should give rise to significant impairment. Harbingers of antisocial personality disorder include aggression and absence of guilt for suffering inflicted and deliberate cruelty. Substance abuse may supervene and depressive illness and anxiety are frequent comorbid conditions. Although personality disorder is a challenge to treat, it does modify as middle age is approached and there is some evidence that anger management and cognitive therapy can be of assistance in attenuating the abnormal behaviour.

ADHD is a chronic and often severe psychiatric disorder. When it continues into adult life it can have serious consequences for employment, relationships and general emotional well-being. Since impulsivity is one of the features of ADHD the condition is often associated with a poor work record and multiple jobs. Hyperactivity also reduces the ability to attend meetings and engage in concentrated work for long periods. The domineering and noisy behaviour of many sufferers lead to poor peer relationships and rejection both in childhood and adulthood. As a result long-term, stable relationships are difficult. Aggression may be associated with violent crime and imprisonment. Many develop depressive and anxiety disorders and substance misuse is a complicating problem.

The pharmacological treatment is usually with methylamphetamine and other psychostimulants although licensing laws vary in different jurisdictions. However, since alcohol and personality problems are complications of ADHD, the use of psychostimulants is not always recommended because of the risk of abuse and interaction with other agents. Alternative pharmacological treatments include clonidine and tricyclic antidepressants. Psychological treatments are required both for the patient and for family members. Cognitive behaviour therapy can be used to establish a reward and punishment system for behaviour and to help the young adult accept their disorder and to take responsibility for their actions. Studying techniques can assist in optimizing concentration. When complications such as alcohol abuse arise these should be treated in the usual way. Diagnosis and response to treatment can both be aided by use of an ADHD scale.

The earlier the disorder is recognized and treated the better the prognosis since this will reduce the adverse effects on relationships and the attention difficulties that are related to poor academic performance. The inattentive subtype has the best prognosis. Adverse effects such as personality disorder, impaired relationships and substance abuse are more persistent and may continue into middle life.

Summary

- When assessing personality it is essential to separate symptoms of current disorder from persistent traits of personality.
- Informants are necessary to obtain objective information about personality.
- Personality disorder frequently co-exists with psychiatric illness.
- Guidelines for treating the most serious personality disorders (antisocial and borderline) have been issued.
- Treatments are mainly psychological in nature.
- Specialist teams for the treatment of some of those with personality disorder are recommended in these guidelines.
- The importance of personality lies in the effect it has on the outcome of psychiatric disorders – the presence of an abnormal personality adversely affects prognosis.
- Personality disorder is a stigmatizing diagnosis that should be made with caution.
- Related conditions such as pathological gambling are difficult to treat.
- Adult attention hyperactivity disorder has recently been recognized as a condition that in some persists into adulthood.

References

Akiskal, H. S., Djenderedjian, A. H., Rosenthal, R. H., and Khani, M. K. (1977). Cyclothymic disorder: validating criteria for inclusion in the bipolar affective group.

American Journal of Psychiatry, **134**, 1227–1233.

Buros, O. K. (1972). *The Seventh Mental Measurements Yearbook.* Highland Park, NJ: Gryphon Press.

Crews, C., Batal, H., Elasy, T., *et al.* (1998). Primary care for those with severe and persistent mental illness. *Western Journal of Medicine*, **169**, 245–250.

Dowrick, C. F., Bellon, J. A., and Gomez, M. J. (2000). GP frequent attendance in Liverpool and Granada: the impact of depressive symptoms, *British Journal of General Practice*, **50**(454), 361–365.

Eysenck, H. J., and Eysenck, S. B. G. (1969). *Manual of the Eysenck Personality Questionnaire (EPQ).* London: University of London Press.

Gross, R., Olfson, M., Gameroff, M., *et al.* (2002). Borderline personality disorder in primary care, *Archives of Internal Medicine*, **162**(1), 53–60.

Leung, K. S., and Cottler, L. B. (2009). Treatment of pathological gambling. *Current Opinion in Psychiatry*, **22**(1), 69–74.

Mann, A. H., Jenkins. R., Cutting, J. C., and Cowen, P. J. (1981). The development and use of a standardized assessment of abnormal personality. *Psychological Medicine*, **11**, 839–847.

Moran, P. A., Jenkins, R., Tylee, A., *et al.* (2000). The prevalence of personality disorder among UK primary care attendees. *Acta Psychiatrica Scandinavica*, **102**, 52–57.

Moran, P., Leese, M., Lee, T., *et al.* (2003) Standardised Assessment of Personality – Abbreviated Scale (SAPAS): preliminary validation of a brief screen for personality disorder. *British Journal of Psychiatry*, **183**, 228–232.

National Institute for Mental Health in England. (2003). Personality disorder: no longer a diagnosis of exclusion. Policy implementation guidance for the development of services for people with personality disorder.

Nice Clinical Guideline 77 (2007). *Borderline Personality Disorder. Treatment,*

Management and Prevention. London: National Institute of Clinical Excellence.

Nice Clinical Guideline 77 (2009). *Antisocial Personality Disorder. Treatment, Management and Prevention.* London: National Institute of Clinical Excellence.

O'Dowd, T. C. (1988). Five years of heartsink patients in general practice. *British Medical Journal*, **297**, 528–530.

Osborn, D. P. J. (2000). Participation in screening for cardiovascular risk by people with schizophrenia or similar mental illnesses: cross-sectional study in general practice. *BMJ*, **326**, 1122–1123.

Pare, M. F., and Rosenbluth, M. (1999) Personality disorders in primary care. *Primary Care–Clinics in Office Practice*, **26** (2), 243–278.

Patience, D. A., McGuire, R. J., Scott, A. I. F., and Freeman, C. P. L. (1995). The Edinburgh Primary Care Depression Study: personality disorder and outcome. *British Journal of Psychiatry*, **167**, 324–330.

Schafer, S., and Nowlis, D. P. (1998). Personality disorders among difficult patients. *Archives of Family Medicine*, 7(2), 126–129.

Shaffer, H. J., Hall, M., and Bilt, J. (1999). Estimating the prevalence of disordered gambling behaviour in the United States and Canada: a research synthesis. *American Journal of Public Health*, **89**, 1368–1376.

Smits, F., Wittkampf, K. A., Schene, A. H., *et al.* (2008). Interventions on frequent attenders in primary care: a systematic literature review, *Scandinavian Journal of Primary Health Care*, **26**(2), 111–116.

Thompson, D. J., and Goldberg, D. (1987). Hysterical personality disorder. The process of diagnosis in clinical and experimental settings. *British Journal of Psychiatry*, **150**, 241–245.

Tyrer, P. (ed.) (1988). *Personality Disorders: Diagnosis, Course and Management.* London: Wright.

Tyrer, P. (2002). Practice guidelines for the treatment of borderline personality disorder: a bridge too far. *Journal of Personality Disorder*, **16**, 113–118.

Tyrer, P., and Alexander, J. (1979). Classification of personality disorder. *British Journal of Psychiatry*, **135**, 163–167.

Suggested reading for patients

Davies, W. (2000). *Overcoming Anger and Irritability*. London: Robinson.

Friedel, R. O. (2004). *Borderline Personality Disorder Demystified: The essential Guide to Understanding and Living with BPD*. New York: Marlowe & Company.

Useful websites for patients

http://www.rcpsych.ac.uk/mentalhealthinfoforall/problems/personalitydisorders/pd.aspx

http://www.personalitydisorder.org.uk/about/

Substance misuse

Learning objectives

Defining alcohol dependence syndrome
Screening in primary care
Brief interventions in primary care
The role of the general practitioner in the management of benzodiazepine dependence
Shared care between general practitioners and the addiction services in the treatment of opiate addiction
Harm minimization, detoxification and outcome
Addiction to other legal and illegal substances

Alcohol

In the past alcohol services run by psychiatrists were primarily for those who were physically dependent and needed inpatient detoxification and follow-up. General practitioners, on the other hand, have always had contact with individuals at all stages of dependence, and until relatively recently would also independently prescribe for home detoxification, give advice and treat complications with little specialist support and without the safety of protocols supported by local governance arrangements.

In recent years the focus has shifted away from exclusively treating those with established alcohol dependence towards a two-stage strategy involving (1) the early identification of at-risk drinkers and (2) delivering interventions that will stall the transition to dependence. There has been assumed some urgency due to the spiralling problem of alcohol-related problems, especially in young people. Moreover, the early identification and provision of treatment to this group is more than a pious aspiration as there is increasing evidence that brief interventions, ideal for delivery in a primary care setting, have a positive impact on harmful drinking. There has also been a renaissance of GPs being involved in home detoxification, but supported by specialists and the wider primary care team. The Royal College of GPs has now developed a Certificate in Alcohol Treatment which focuses on recognition and management of hazardous drinkers. A number of PCT commissioners are developing contacts for practices to become more involved in both the management of hazardous drinking and detoxification.

Definitions and terminology

One approach is to define alcohol misuse by the quantity consumed and various professional bodies and organizations have specified that consumption of 21 or more units per week (a unit being half a pint of beer or a glass of wine) for men and of 14 or more units for women constitutes at-risk drinking. This has the advantage of being intuitively simple but has the disadvantage of excluding those who develop difficulties with a lower intake and/or those who are unaffected by larger quantities. When discussing alcohol misuse in a clinical setting it is easy to become diverted into a debate about what constitutes alcoholism when dealing with an alcohol misuser. The term 'alcoholic' conjures up the notion of destitutes on skid row and in the early stages of dealing with the problem its use is likely to impair the process of encouraging abstinence.

The alcohol dependence syndrome, described by Edwards and Gross (1976), avoids use of the term 'alcoholic' and it outlines the features of that disorder and includes:

(1) the predominance of drinking over other activities

(2) the development of tolerance

(3) narrowing of the drink repertoire such that the pattern of consumption is unrelated to external events; in the normal drinker there is a variability in the amount consumed, e.g. at a weekend or at a social function more is ingested than usual; this variability is lacking in the person dependent on alcohol

(4) withdrawal symptoms occur and they are relieved by further alcohol

(5) a period of abstinence is followed by rapid reinstatement of dependence if drinking is resumed

(6) there is tolerance to the effects, necessitating a heavier consumption to produce the same effects.

Hazardous or at-risk use of alcohol is defined as a pattern of drinking that increases the risk of harmful consequences to the user. It is sometimes used to loosely cover those who have experienced mild as opposed to serious harm from alcohol.

Harmful use of alcohol is more serious and is defined as drinking that causes damage, physical or psychological, to the user, but without dependence.

Binge drinking has several definitions but one definition is drinking more than double the daily recommended benchmark on the person's heaviest day, i.e. 8 units for a man and 6 for a woman.

Screening and assessment

Screening large populations such as those attending accident departments, inpatients in general hospitals and attendees in primary care represents the first stage in assisting those who may be hazardous users, harmful users or even dependent on alcohol. A number of screening questionnaires have been developed for this purpose.

Questionnaires

Questionnaires that screen for alcohol misuse have some value but are dependent on the truthfulness of the subject and others are more demanding since they require recognition of alcohol problems for their diagnostic value.

For general practice screening the CAGE questionnaire (Mayfield *et al.*, 1974) is very useful since it consists of just four questions:

Have you ever felt you should Cut down on your drinking?
Have people Annoyed you by criticizing your drinking?

Have you ever felt bad or Guilty about your drinking?
Have you ever had a drink first thing in the morning to steady your nerves or get rid of a hangover (Eye-opener)?

Two or more positive answers points to the possibility of alcohol dependence and to the need for further evaluation.

Another questionnaire, the Alcohol Use Disorders Identification Test (AUDIT) (Babor *et al.* 1992), is a 10-item self-completed questionnaire designed for use in primary care. It examines the frequency of alcohol consumption, alcohol-related problems and dependence symptoms. Each question is scored from 0 to 4 with a possible total sore of 40. A score of 8 or more indicates hazardous drinking. It takes about 3 minutes to complete.

Others that have been used are the Fast Alcohol Screening Test (FAST) (Hodgson *et al.* 2002, a four-question test, and the Paddington Alcohol Test (PAT) (Patton and Touquet 2002), a three-question test. Neither was developed specifically for use in primary care although they compare favourably with the AUDIT. The MAST (Selzer 1971), is a 22-item scale but as it takes longer to complete than the other two it is less commonly used in general practice.

Laboratory markers

Chemical markers elevated in those drinking to excess include gamma-glutamyltransferase (GTT) (over 45 IU/l) and mean cell volume (MCV) (over 98 fl). Newer tests such as carbohydrate-deficient transferrin (CDT) and aspartate aminotransferase are also available.

Recent studies suggest that in primary care at least, laboratory markers are less sensitive and specific in diagnosing alcohol misuse and that evaluation using a screening questionnaire should be introduced (Aertgeerts *et al.* 2001; Coulton *et al.* 2006). In addition the use of questionnaires has been shown to be more cost-efficient. However, laboratory indicators should raise the index of suspicion when they are abnormal and lead to other investigations including, where possible, obtaining collateral information on alcohol use.

Clinical indicators of possible alcohol misuse

It is advisable to have a high index of suspicion of alcohol misuse when certain physical, emotional and behavioural conditions prevail (see Table 10.1).

Case 1

Mrs X, a 35-year-old woman, was referred with a recent history of depression. In addition she suffered occasional panic attacks but her general practitioner's main worry was her gross neglect of herself and her house. Prior to this she was a self-employed and successful beautician. She still socialized and met friends regularly for meals but her home had become dirty and she would often lie in bed until noon. Her husband was a businessman and she claimed he was supportive, although this was not felt to be the case by her general practitioner. There were no children as the marriage had not been consummated. They had sought help for this but her husband had refused to attend after the first appointment and she had 'reassured' him since then that the problem was hers. There was no definite family history of psychiatric illness but Mrs X thought that a brother may have had a drink problem in the past. She said she drank socially and her husband was also a moderate drinker. Her mother was killed in an accident when she was 14. She had a very poor relationship with her parents and she was not close to her siblings. At presentation she complained of constant tiredness, feeling slow in the mornings, waking 2 hours earlier than usual and crying frequently. Suicidal ideas were absent. Attempts to explore her relationship with her husband were always intercepted by comments such as 'He basically cares' or 'He doesn't believe in all of this', etc., and requests to interview him were always blocked by her. Similarly, questions about her mother's death and her response to it were dealt with in a superficial manner. Antidepressants were prescribed in view of the symptom pattern and the deterioration in self-care and she claimed some improvement but the panic attacks continued. In addition she was noted to be tremulous at some interviews but she attributed it to rushing for the appointments. Two months after commencing treatment her husband contacted her psychiatrist to say that his wife was having visual hallucinations. He admitted that she had been drinking heavily for several months, often beginning at 9 a.m. He also spoke of his own reluctance to admit the problem. Mrs X was admitted to hospital and diagnosed as suffering from delirium tremens. She had visual hallucinations of mice and for several days was agitated. She was treated in the usual manner with high-dose benzodiazepines and vitamins and made a full recovery. At follow-up 3 weeks later she was free from depression and panics but refused further counselling for her drink problem or her marital difficulties. She also refused disulfiram for prophylaxis. Antidepressants were discontinued on admission.

Comment

This lady illustrates several interesting points. First, the discrepancy between the severity of depression and her self-neglect was striking. Her failure to show a full response to antide-pressants in therapeutic doses along with the persisting panic attacks is a frequent finding in those whose primary problem is alcohol misuse. She admitted that before her appointments with me she would not drink – hence the tremulousness at interview. Her husband's failure to admit the problem was a reflection of the severe marital difficulties which this couple experienced. Her excessive drinking was probably due to these and to other unresolved conflicts from her past. In view of these persisting difficulties and her failure to continue in therapy, the prognosis was considered to be poor. If, at initial interview, she had admitted the alcohol problem antidepressants would not have been prescribed. She exhibited some of the indicators of alcohol misuse outlined in Table 10.1.

Table 10.1. Indicators of possible alcohol misuse

- Pancreatitis
- Gastritis
- Unexplained peripheral neuropathy
- Tremors, especially in the morning
- High mean cell volume
- Abnormal liver function tests
- Panic attacks not responding to treatment and occurring during periods of relative abstinence
- Depression which is resistant to treatment
- Relationship violence or anger
- General deterioration in self-care and social functioning for which there is no obvious explanation
- Monday morning absenteeism
- Frequent dismissal from jobs
- Repeated drunk driving offences

Epidemiology

Community studies from England (Drummond *et al.* 2005) show that overall 26% (38% men and 16% women) have alcohol use disorders that include hazardous or harmful drinking and dependence. The figure for dependence alone is 3.6% (6% men and 2% women), and 23% (32% men and 15% women) engage in hazardous drinking. One-third of presentations to accident departments in Britain and Ireland are alcohol-related, and at peak times 70% of admissions to the accident departments are alcohol-related.

Figures based on hospital admission figures are known to be inadequate since many with alcohol dependence do not receive treatment at all. Nevertheless, admissions for alcohol problems constitute 10% of all psychiatric admissions in England and Wales and a much higher proportion in Scotland, Ireland and mainland Europe. Attempts at calculating the prevalence of alcoholism on the basis of the numbers with cirrhosis of the liver annually shows that France has the highest prevalence, with England and Wales having relatively low rates. It is agreed that the selection bias inherent in this approach makes it no longer acceptable and it has been abandoned. Indirect evidence for the escalating problem of alcohol misuse comes from the rising numbers of convictions for drunkenness offences and for drunken driving convictions.

There is evidence that 20% of those presenting to the GPs drink to excess yet 98% of these are not recognized (Kaner *et al.* 1999) while a WHO study found that the rates of alcohol dependence and harmful use of alcohol among general practice attendees were 2.2% and 1.4% respectively (Kisley *et al.* 1995), with men predominating.

Types of alcohol dependence – older classification

Older classifications of alcoholism relied on patterns of drinking and the name of Jellinek is particularly associated with this approach; thus those who had a craving for alcohol were believed to be separate from those who drank in binges or from those who drank to relieve psychological distress. However, over the years it has been shown that there is little justification for retaining these subdivisions since individual patients are not true to type and present with different patterns at different times in their drinking careers. Even the simple classification of alcoholics into primary and secondary, according to whether the alcohol misuse is secondary to some other psychological condition such as depression, or not, is felt to be of little help in terms of treatment and outcome.

Aetiology

The debate about aetiology centres on two arguments – one the illness theory, the other the social learning theory. Until the middle of the century alcoholics were generally regarded as weak, lacking in moral fibre or in some way degenerate. The work of Jellinek was instrumental in reversing this and in promulgating the view of alcohol dependence as an illness. This became the dominant theory in the 1950s and 60s and is still accepted by many, most notably Alcoholics Anonymous. Regarding alcoholism as a disease serves the purpose of encouraging more humane treatments and stimulating research into this disorder. However, the counter argument is that alcohol misuse does not possess the properties of the disease, i.e. a known cause, course, symptom pattern and response to treatment. Indeed there is some evidence that in the early stages of excessive drinking the process may be reversed by simple counselling. Moreover, since active treatment is generally no more successful than simple advice and since a proportion eventually return to social drinking it can be argued that there is no consistent pattern observable.

With our increased understanding of learning theory and social theory other causes for alcoholism are now suggested. The social model is generally the one favoured by the medical profession, who argue that whilst the disease model served a useful humanitarian purpose, it has robbed the patient of responsibility for controlling his drinking and changing his lifestyle.

The search for the cause amongst those adhering to the disease model centred initially upon the genetic inheritance of alcoholism. There is some evidence from adoptive studies that the sons of alcoholics are more than twice as likely to become alcoholic as the general population and that children adopted into alcoholic families are not at increased risk. Work from the United States points to a genetic link with unipolar depression. In addition the concordance is higher for monozygotic than for dizygotic twins and heritability is higher for men than for women. It is likely that the inheritance is polygenic. A different approach to causation has focused on a supposed abnormality in alcohol dehydrogenase but the findings are so far unproven.

Social learning theory is based upon the acceptability of heavy drinking in our culture and on the ready availability of alcohol at relatively low prices. The evidence for this is the observation that during prohibition admission rates for alcohol-related problems declined considerably (even though criminal activity increased). The work of Ledermann, a French demographer, has also lent some weight to this argument by his demonstration of a logarithmic relationship between the average consumption and the numbers of problem drinkers in a community. His methodology has received much criticism but his hypothesis is intuitively attractive and also suggests a means whereby the problem may be controlled, i.e. reducing the per capita consumption by formal controls such as stricter licensing laws, heavier taxes on alcohol and a host of other legal restraints.

The role of personality in determining who becomes alcoholic has received some consideration also. The view that there was a particular personality type who became alcoholic has now been disproven, although there is no doubt that those with antisocial personality disorder are more at risk of developing substance misuse including alcohol dependence than other groups. Also at risk are those who as children had conduct disorders or attention deficit hyperactivity disorder (ADHD).

In recent years the rate of alcohol misuse and dependence amongst women has increased considerably. It is uncertain whether this represents a real increase in its prevalence in women or just an increased willingness to admit the problem. There is no doubt, however, that women are more vulnerable to both the medical and psychiatric complications of alcohol misuse than their male counterparts. Opinions have varied as to the factors underlying heavy drinking in women and the focus has been on the changing role of women in society, although much is inconclusive.

One way of bringing together these diverse models is to think of the early stages as influenced by personality traits, social context and other psychiatric conditions, and the later stages, when the brain has been permanently altered or damaged, as more of an illness.

It is apparent that the search for a single cause for alcohol misuse and dependence is naive. Moreover it must be remembered that many people possess the at-risk characteristics described above but do not become problem drinkers. Our understanding is therefore incomplete.

Prevention and brief interventions

There is evidence from a number of studies that brief interventions delivered in primary care are effective in reducing alcohol consumption and subsequent alcohol-related harm (Bertholet *et al.* 2005). These are only useful in those who are harmfully or hazardously using alcohol. They are not effective when dependence is present. There is great variability in the intensity and content of these interventions.

Patient information leaflets detailing the medical and psychological effects of alcohol as well as outlining treatment options and providing useful telephone numbers may be provided. Face-to-face interviews, two or three, lasting no longer than 10 minutes each are commonly used. Delivered by a trained nurse or counsellor, the acronym FRAMES identifies the core components of the interventions:

F – **Feedback** on the health risks, physical and psychological, to the patient
R – **Responsibility** for effecting change should be delegated to the patient
A – **Advice** on behavioural change
M – a **Menu** of treatment options
E – the session should be conducted in an **Empathic** manner
S – **Self-efficacy** and optimism that the chosen goals can be achieved.

For the general practitioner who does not have access to such a service (or who has not been commissioned to provide it), simple advice on limiting alcohol intake should be offered to all those who may be heavy or problem drinkers. Research suggests that this advice is frequently taken on board and that such people do not progress to alcohol dependence.

These brief interventions may be combined with motivational interviewing in order to deal with the ambivalence that some have to changing their habits. Motivational interviewing has evolved out of the realization that readiness for change is a key component in therapy, especially for substance misuse disorders. It is a form of semi-directive counselling in which the therapist aims to assist the person in considering the possibility of change. This is done be exploring the risks and problems associated with the behaviour while also identifying the disparity between what the patient does and what she/he hopes to achieve. Envisaging a better future may stimulate this motivation. The key elements are outlined below:

(1) Empathize with the patient and outline your understanding of his/her perspective

(2) Explore the discrepancy between how the person wants their life to be and how it now is

(3) Accept reluctance to change as natural rather than abnormal

(4) Accept the person's autonomy while allowing them to move towards change at their own pace

(5) Avoid confrontation or argument.

Motivational interviewing requires training, but is increasingly used by primary care practitioners for a range of health promotion and disease modification goals.

Detoxification

For those dependent on alcohol more active treatments than those outlined above should be used and detoxification should be offered, although there is little point in forcing treatment upon the unwilling patient, notwithstanding the understandable pressure that families may sometimes apply in order to bring this about. Whereas in the past GPs were often involved in the compulsory admission of a person for treatment of alcohol dependence, this is no longer possible in Ireland or Britain under the various mental health legislations that have been enacted. However, if there is a possibility of a severe mental illness then it may be possible to admit such a person compulsorily for assessment (see Chapter 23). Often it is a relative who first seeks treatment for a family member, who may be both insightless and reluctant. A few interviews with the patient aimed at giving insight into the problem and into the effect this is having on his family and health may sometimes motivate the otherwise uninterested patient. In addition, the possibility of separation or of job loss may also galvanize an alcohol misuser into seeking treatment.

The preferred location of detoxification depends on a variety of factors as well as an understanding of local service provision, which is highly variable.

1. Home detoxification (GP or specialist)
    (a) Good support from friends and family
    (b) No history of fits on withdrawal
2. Emergency detoxification in inpatient setting
    (a) Delirium tremens
    (b) Tremor and tachycardia
3. Specialist inpatient/residential detoxification
    (a) Lack of social support
    (b) Poor record of adhering to detoxification
    (c) History of fits and head injury.

Many patients, especially those seen in general practice and having their first detoxification, may request that it take place at home, and this may be provided by GPs or community-based alcohol services. While some GPs used to provide home detoxification routinely, it is now advisable to ensure that systems are in place for risk assessment, and daily monitoring. Support from specialist teams can be helpful, and because workload is not inconsiderable, GPs in Britain are requesting contacts to provide this service. For those who are highly motivated and who have the support of their family this may be possible. Typically a patient would be commenced on chlordiazepoxide or alprazolam in divided doses sufficient to relieve withdrawal symptoms. Chlordiazepoxide may be used in doses of up to 50 mg q.d.s. and alprazolam up to 1 mg q.i.d. in hospital patients, but among general practice patients much lower doses may be used if the level of dependence is only moderate. Reduction is titrated against the patient's symptomatology and in general detoxification should be complete in about 2 weeks. There is some evidence to suggest that alprazolam is a more rapid detoxifying agent. Several studies have shown that carbamazepine in doses up to 800 mg per day is as effective as benzodiazepines although it is much less frequently used. Multivitamin supplements, orally or intravenously, are also prescribed to minimize the risk of Wernicke's encephalopathy or Korsakoff's psychosis. There is generally no requirement to prescribe a hypnotic since the benzodiazepines used for detoxification will aid sleep. If symptomatic relief of the withdrawal syndrome cannot be brought about without recourse to the full doses detailed above, the patient should be hospitalized.

In addition some of those who are alcohol-dependent lack the motivation necessary to allow such a scheme of management by their general practitioner and default from the treatment plan. Admission to a supportive inpatient environment is required in these circumstances. The treatment regime is similar to that used for home detoxification with the exception that the dose of benzodiazepines may be higher. Occasionally an α_2 agonist, clonidine, is used in combination with a benzodiazepine. Hemineverin is seldom used now due to the risk of misuse. Whichever drug is used, care should be taken to discontinue it before discharge from hospital.

Rehabilitation

Rehabilitation is a long-term goal and means focusing on and achieving social goals such as secure housing, employment and sustainable relationships as well as preventing harm to others. There is less evidence to guide this and services are highly variable, with services increasingly commissioned from voluntary sector organizations in both the UK and Ireland.

Specialist units focus on the patient's alcohol-centred lifestyle and encourage changes to this. Self-awareness is considered an important component and the role of alcohol in aiding the patient in dealing with problems such as anxiety, shyness, etc., is identified and corrective measures introduced. Unfortunately the results from these are disappointing and suggest that the financial and training input into these has not proved as efficacious as common sense would have suggested. It has been suggested that there may be special groups of alcoholics, e.g. those recently diagnosed, who derive benefit from such intensive therapy. However, although this has intuitive appeal, it remains to be proven scientifically. Some specialist centres who carefully select patients for their programmes claim long-term success.

Rehabilitation is also likely to require successful management of underlying psychiatric disorders such as depression, anxiety, PTSD, OCD and personality disorder, which may be revealed after abstinence has been achieved.

Relapse prevention – pharmacological interventions

Disulfiram and citrated calcium carbimide are drugs which inhibit the metabolism of acetaldehyde. The build-up of acetaldehyde causes nausea when alcohol is consumed with it and many patients value this prop to sobriety, at least in the immediate period following detoxification. Disulfiram implants have also been used but their efficacy is uncertain.

Acamprosate calcium facilitates the maintenance of abstinence by stimulating transmission of GABA, an inhibitory neurotransmitter involved in substance dependence. It reduces craving the usual dose is 666 mg TID but lower doses should be used in those under 60 kg. Liver function should be checked prior to prescription since severe liver failure is a contraindication. It is not useful in the management of detoxification and is recommended in conjunction with counselling, treatment being for about 1 year.

Supportive organizations

Alcoholics Anonymous, together with its sister organization Al-Anon, provides help and support for alcoholics and their families. These groups are based on an illness model and also have a very strong spiritual overlay. The approach is one of self-disclosure, which to many is unacceptable. Because of its anonymity there are no data available on its efficacy. For some patients, however, it provides support and guidance which are invaluable.

Many also attend other local organizations, many voluntary or charitable, that provide help to those who are alcohol-dependent. Some also attend alcohol counsellors for continuing support, especially at difficult periods in life when there is a temptation to drink again.

Controlled drinking

Up to 15% of those dependent on alcohol return to social drinking following a period of abstinence. The realization of this formed the basis for the retraining of alcoholics in their drinking habits which became fashionable in the 1970s (Clark 1976). This consists of video-taped recordings, using simulated bar-rooms, of the patient in this setting. Aspects of his drinking behaviour are noted and fed back to him. These include taking bigger gulps, continually keeping his glass in hand and any other behaviours which could potentially be relearnt. Agreeing daily limits, keeping a diary of consumption, identifying triggers to overdrinking and developing strategies for saying 'No' are also included.

Follow-up studies have demonstrated the value of controlled drinking and it is no longer dismissed out of hand. Whilst it would be a foolhardy doctor who recommends that an alcoholic returned to social drinking, it is likely that in the future the specialist services will be able to assist the GP in identifying the special group for whom this may be possible. Also the possibility of controlled drinking is likely to attract more patients into treatment, particularly those who are not yet dependent but having problems with control.

Alcohol dependence in specific groups

Many offenders, particularly revolving-door criminals with repeated minor offences, have alcohol problems. Some will respond to programmes provided by the criminal justice system and others require detoxification when entering prison. Probation sentences now include Alcohol Treatment Orders which require adherence to programmes.

For the homeless person who has long-standing alcohol dependence the GP will need to work closely with social care, mental health services, half-way houses and hostels following detoxification. Although this group represents less than 5% of the total presenting for treatment, it represents the greatest treatment and humanitarian challenge. Although many present to casualty departments they frequently default from follow-up treatment. For many controlled drinking or abstinence is emotionally impossible and the GP's role is more focused on physical care and liaison with specialist services to support housing.

There has also been a slow but steady rise in the development of primary-care-based teams, with substance misuse and mental health specialists providing care for homeless individuals and more recently focusing on offenders.

Psychiatric complications of alcohol misuse

1 Depression

Alcohol misuse is associated with feelings of gloom, despondency and dysphoria. The relationship between alcohol misuse and depressed mood is a complex one. First, the mood change tends to be transient and may be a direct consequence of the central effects of alcohol. In addition, many heavy drinkers have family, financial and marital problems making them unhappy and which can even constitute depressive illness. The GP confronted with the person who misuses alcohol and who complains of depression should withhold antidepressant treatment for at least 1 month following detoxification or significant reduction in consumption as the symptoms tend to subside over time (Liappas *et al.* 2002). In the small group who do not improve (less than 10%) (Brown and Schuckit 1988) antidepressant medication may be required, provided the patient is now abstinent since there may be untoward interactions between alcohol and antidepressants. In general women are more prone to depressive illness following detoxification than are men and indeed a pre-existing depressive disorder is often present. If the individual has a strong history of recurrent depression then the prescription of an antidepressant sooner after abstinence has been achieved may be justified. However, the risk of interactions between alcohol and the anti-depressant is considerable and the patient should be advised of this. Moreover, the use of alcohol may lead to a recurrence of the depressive symptoms, rendering the antidepressant ineffective.

2 Anxiety disorders

Panic attacks frequently occur during periods of relative abstinence. These usually subside when prolonged abstinence has been established. However, social phobias often manifest themselves following detoxification and this is usually a manifestation of a pre-existing social phobia for which alcohol may have been used to bring about relief. The treatment of the social anxiety is along the lines described in Chapter 6. As yet joined pathways allowing for seamless transition from alcohol services to psychological therapy have not been developed.

3 Other substances

Many of those who are dependent on alcohol also abuse other drugs in addition to alcohol; in particular benzodiazepines or chlormethiazole prescribed to relieve withdrawal symptoms are common drugs of misuse. It is thus advisable to be circumspect when prescribing to those with a history of dependence and anxiolytic medication should never be prescribed on a long-term basis.

4 Marital and sexual problems

These are a common accompaniment to alcohol misuse. The violence, poverty and unem-ployment which are associated with alcoholism are common sources of conflict. Unless the patient becomes abstinent there is little point in pursuing marital therapy since any attempts at resolving the conflicts will be sabotaged during periods of drinking. Sexual difficulties, especially impotence, are common complications since alcohol increases the desire but reduces the ability to perform sexually. As with marital disharmony, unless abstinence from alcohol is achieved treatment of the sexual problem is doomed to failure.

5 Pathological jealousy and psychosis

Alcohol misuse is commonly associated with morbid jealousy (referred to as the Othello syndrome). This often improves after cessation of drinking but a minority become deluded about their spouse's infidelity and require treatment, which may include antipsychotic medication. Occasionally auditory hallucinations (referred to as alcoholic hallucinosis) occur in the context of clear consciousness and must be distinguished from the hallucina-tions of delirium tremens. These occur at times of either relative abstinence or relative increase in alcohol intake and although improvement occurs once abstinence is established some turn out to have schizophrenia.

6 Delirium tremens

Delirium tremens is the acute confusional state which occurs during withdrawal from alcohol. It lasts up to 4 days and is accompanied by agitation, visual hallucinations and intense fear. It has a mortality of about 15% due to the electrolyte disturbances which accompany the condition. Emergency treatment with tranquillizers, correction of the electrolyte imbalance and intravenous vitamin supplements are essential although care must be taken to administer saline rather than glucose solutions if Korsakoff's syndrome is not to develop.

7 Brain damage

Brain damage is a common complication of alcoholism and may range from the mild vermian atrophy which occurs early in the history to the more severe amnestic syndrome, often eponymously called Korsakoff's psychosis, and caused by thiamine deficiency. Haemorrhagic lesions in the mammillary bodies, in the thalamus and hypothalamus have been found at post-mortem examination. Korsakoff's psychosis is associated with confabulation, a profound impairment of recent memory, disorientation in time, apathy and impairment of perceptual and conceptual function. It is sometimes preceded by Wernicke's encephalopathy – a condition characterized by nystagmus, peripheral neuropathy, ataxia and confusion. More generalized impairment of intellect may occur and presents with similar symptoms to those occurring in dementia from any other cause. CT scans show generalized atrophy. Wernicke's syndrome is treated with intravenous thiamine whilst it is prescribed orally in the treatment of Korsakoff's syndrome. Sometimes more focal changes occur such as frontal lobe damage, cerebellar degeneration, temporal lobe lesions and a host of other rarer abnormalities.

8 Personality deterioration

This is frequently described in alcoholics, who often appear to become coarse and aggressive. The debate about whether this is the cause or the result of excessive drinking has aroused much controversy. Whilst it is recognized that personality deterioration can occur both due to the social consequences and due to frontal lobe damage, recent work on personality suggests that psychopathy is a common prodrome of alcohol misuse and tends to be the cause rather than the effect of this.

9 Suicide

Suicide is a common outcome, particularly in chronic, middle-aged men who are alcohol-dependent. It tends to be associated with concurrent depressive symptoms and is often precipitated by interpersonal loss or conflict. Long-term studies have demonstrated that between 7 and 21% die by suicide while a recent study (Flensborg-Madsen et al. 2009) found that having a substance misuse disorder increased the risk of suicide more than three-fold even when the presence of psychiatric illness was controlled for, while in a group without any psychiatric disorder apart from misuse of alcohol the risk was increased more than nine-fold. Thus, of itself alcohol misuse is a risk factor for suicide independently of other psychiatric disorders. Moreover, among the deliberate self-harm population (see Chapter 11) alcohol misuse has been shown to be a major problem, with up to 50% of men showing evidence of dependence. In addition alcohol is frequently taken prior to such an attempt. Even in the general population alcohol has been implicated as a significant factor associated with suicide due to its destabilizing effect on mood (Goldberg et al. 2001).

   Both the physical complications and the psychological disabilities associated with alcohol misuse are more prevalent in women than men. Whether this is because women are more vulnerable or because they tend to be secret drinkers and are therefore more chronic has yet to be clarified. It is essential to be alert to the distress of the alcohol-dependent person, particularly at times of conflict, if suicide and attempts at self-harm are to be avoided.

Outcome

Little is known about the effects of intervention at the GP level upon alcoholism. However, heavy drinkers who are counselled to cut down their intake have been shown to respond positively to this. The effects of inpatient treatment for alcohol dependence have been studied extensively but unfortunately it seems to have little impact on outcome when compared with simple advice. Although some centres such as Hazelden in Minnesota have demonstrated the effectiveness of intensive counselling, as patients are specially selected on the basis of their motivation, family support and personality these findings may not be generalizable. The confrontational method used in 'Minnesota Model' residential centres is not suitable for all patients and increasingly treatment is based on cognitive behavioural models. Overall, between a third and a half of those treated continue to have a drinking problem when followed up for several years, and up to 15% have been shown to return to social drinking. Prognosis is best in those with good premorbid personalities and in those who have stable families for support. Untreated, alcoholics have a high mortality and morbidity. Although there is little research available on this group, one study in 1953 showed that 50% continue with their problem until death, roughly one-quarter moderate it or become abstinent and the remaining quarter become worse.

Other considerations in prevention

Apart from the preventive approaches of screening and brief interventions described above, more broadly based population measures have also been attempted. The compulsion 'to do something' whenever a major problem is identified is as evident in relation to alcoholism as to any of the other problems of our modern times. Simple answers to complex problems have been suggested and the question of education about alcohol and its complications is one such simple solution which has been suggested and tried. Unfortunately the evidence so far (and it is extensive) is that whilst education increases people's knowledge about alcohol it does not affect attitude or behaviour. A number of studies have examined the effects of education programmes on teenagers, recidivist drunken drivers and groups recruited through advertisements. They confirm the relative ineffectiveness of education programmes in bringing about behavioural change.

Attempts to identify problem drinkers in the workplace are promising but are still in their infancy in Britain and Ireland. The approach is to recognize and provide help for those who may have emotional problems from any cause. Efforts to identify problem drinkers per se have proved less successful than a more general and holistic approach to occupational medicine.

A different approach to prevention stems from the observations of Ledermann, outlined above, of an association between the national per capita alcohol consumption and the prevalence of alcoholism. Although this hypothesis has been criticized, its application lies in reducing the mean consumption by increasing taxation on alcohol. Other approaches to influencing the per capita consumption include tighter control of the conditions under which alcohol is sold and licensing restrictions. This strategy has to be balanced against the economic effects of such measures that may make it prohibitive and some would view them as Draconian and an infringement of civil liberties. The optimum balance between the opposing philosophies of social libertarianism and prohibition has not been identified.

Other substances

Older text books emphasized the distinction between drugs that were associated with misuse but that did not cause physical symptoms on withdrawal and those that did. This distinction

Table 10.2. Drugs of abuse and dependence

Drugs of dependence	Drugs of abuse	Uncertain dependence
Alcohol	Cannabis	Nicotine
Benzodiazepine	Cocaine	Methaqualone
Opiates	LSD	Glutethimide
Barbiturates	Amphetamines	
Chlormethiazole	Mescaline	
Minor analgesics		

rested on the absence of tolerance and on psychological symptoms only on discontinuation (see Table 10.2). However, the recent editions of DSM and ICD do not make this distinction to the same extent and most substances are now regarded as causing psychological, behavioural and physical dependence, although this view is not without its critics. For example, cocaine and cannabis, in the past thought not to be associated with a physical withdrawal reaction, are now listed as among those that display this response. Caffeine is also now regarded as a substance that can produce physical dependence.

The value of this distinction is that it indicates the speed with which these substances can be discontinued. Those which produce physical dependence, such as opiates and benzodiazepines, must not be stopped abruptly, whilst those associated primarily with psychological dependence may be, although craving and other psychological symptoms such as depression and agitation may ensue. For most practitioners the most common substance misuse problems are those of alcohol and benzodiazepines.

According to NHS data one in ten adults has used one or more illicit substances in the past year and about 25% of those with psychiatric illness seen in primary care have a second diagnosis of substance misuse (also referred to as dual diagnosis or comorbidity) although rates vary (Strathdee *et al.* 2002). Among adults in the USA the lifetime prevalence for abuse of illegal substances is 6.2%, with an excess in males. Clinically there is a suggestion of a link with personality disorder but this has not been adequately investigated.

Benzodiazepines

The popularity of the benzodiazepines lay in the fact that for the first time in the early 1960s there appeared on the market very powerful and effective anxiolytics which had none of the apparent drawbacks of their antecedents, the barbiturates. Time has once again become the great leveller and since the first caution that these drugs may also be drugs of dependence, the number of cases of addiction spiralled. The extent of the problem is unclear although estimates can be made from prescribing analysis. About half of regular users are believed to suffer withdrawal symptoms and these are identical to the classical symptoms of anxiety – hence their continuing prescription in times past since such symptoms were attributed to a recrudescence of the anxiety state which they were being used to treat.

Symptoms of withdrawal

The typical withdrawal reaction consists of two clusters of symptoms (Table 10.3) corresponding approximately to classic symptoms of anxiety and a more serious group of perceptual,

Table 10.3. Symptoms of benzodiazepine withdrawal

Restlessness	Hyperacusis
Impaired concentration	Hypersensitivity to touch
Tremor	Hallucinations
Insomnia	Delusions, especially paranoid
Anxiety	Depersonalization
Palpitations	Dizziness fits
Nausea	

physical and sometimes psychotic symptoms (Petrusson and Lader 1981). These generally occur within 3 days of discontinuing the drug and are more acute following withdrawal from short-acting than long-acting medication, believed to be due to the attenuating effect of the active metabolites of the latter. Symptoms last for a varying period from a few days to several weeks or rarely months.

Some work has focused also on the type of person likely to develop withdrawal symptoms and whilst there is no consistent pattern, those with passive-dependent personalities have been shown to feature more than others. The explanation for this may lie in the greater tendency of this group to become chronic users of these drugs or may be associated with a greater awareness and tendency to complain of withdrawal symptoms. Another feature is the history of dependence on other substances, especially alcohol, which characterizes these patients.

Management

A number of options are available to the general practitioner who is treating a patient wishing to discontinue benzodiazepines. The patient must be told at the outset, however, that some symptoms may occur but that these will be minimized by the judicious use of adjunct treatments and reduction regimes. In all cases it is essential not to discontinue the benzodiazepine abruptly and it is common practice to change from a short-acting to the equivalent dose of a long-acting drug, usually diazepam, either before or during the period of withdrawal. Thereafter gradual reduction, with or without adjunctive treatments, is the main approach. A reduction plan should if possible be agreed with the patient, and although flexibility is sometimes required this should be the exception. Scripts should be converted to 2 mg tablets both to reduce resale value and to illustrate the volume of consumption. A liquid preparation of diazepam can be used for reducing the final two milligrams (5 ml is equivalent to 2 mg). The dose should be reduced by one-quarter to one-tenth of the daily dose every 2 weeks but if dependence is on therapeutic doses of benzodiazepines, a reduction of 2–2.5 mg every 2 weeks should be possible. The duration of detoxification may vary from a few weeks to several months.

Several ancillary approaches are available to the doctor although it is not essential to use these and most have a limited evidence base. An excellent review by Lader et al. (2009) is recommended and some are listed below.

Tricyclic antidepressants

The tricyclic antidepressants, because of their effect on symptoms of anxiety, have found widespread use in benzodiazepine detoxification. It is important to realize that many patients receiving benzodiazepines will in fact have an undiagnosed depressive illness, presenting as anxiety, and will require suitable treatment for this once detoxification has been completed. Thus, using these antidepressants during detoxification will serve a dual purpose for many patients. Where depression is judged to be present the duration of antidepressant treatment will be as usual for depression (see Chapter 7). If depression is not diagnosed and antidepressants are being used solely to modify the withdrawal syndrome they can be discontinued once withdrawal has been completed.

Beta-blockers

Since beta-blockers are established as having an effect on the physical symptoms of anxiety, these may be used to diminish peripheral withdrawal symptoms. The dosage will vary with the degree of symptomatology and is generally in the range used for the treatment of anxiety. They will be used until the benzodiazepines have been withdrawn totally and are then discontinued themselves.

Carbamazepine

A recent Cochrane review (Denis *et al.* 2006) found some evidence from a small number of trials that this may have adjunctive properties but was unable to recommend its routine use in withdrawal.

Major tranquillizers

Major tranquillizers will assist in reducing symptoms but the drawback of drowsiness generally precludes their use.

Other drugs

Clonidine, an α_2 agonist, normally used as an antihypertensive, has been successfully used in opiate and alcohol withdrawal. It may have a use in benzodiazepine withdrawal but this has yet to be evaluated. Buspirone, a non-benzodiazepine tranquillizer, is not thought to be of benefit in withdrawal.

Psychological techniques

Cognitive therapy especially to prevent relapse has been shown to be beneficial while simple relaxation techniques are useful either alone or combined with the above approaches, especially during the discontinuation phase.

Self-help groups

Self-help groups are promoted by many and although these do not necessarily help in controlling symptoms their benefit lies in the comfort patients find from meeting others with similar problems and in stimulating motivation when this is flagging. As with all self-help groups, the danger of becoming 'stuck' and not moving out of the group to resume normal functioning and the tendency to use the group as an opportunity to endlessly 'discuss' the problem rather than as a stepping stone must be emphasized.

Case 2

Mr X was a 30–year-old married man who was referred for benzodiazepine withdrawal having been prescribed a short-acting preparation 3 years previously after his wife had a miscarriage late in pregnancy. This was the first pregnancy in the marriage and they were very excited about the prospect of parenthood. His wife miscarried at 22 weeks and Mr X was extremely upset. He arranged a religious burial ceremony for the baby and within a week began to have panic attacks. He went to his GP complaining of anxiety, depression, insomnia and anorexia and was prescribed a short-acting benzodiazepine. He continued to take this for about 2 years but on hearing of the risk of dependence tried without success to discontinue it himself. In the intervening 2 years he felt gloomy and had stopped going out initially because of lack of interest but subsequently due to panic attacks. When seen at the clinic a diagnosis of benzodiazepine dependence and of depressive illness was made and he was commenced on a tricyclic antidepressant. He began to obtain some symptomatic relief from his depression after 3 weeks of treatment at a dose of 100 mg nocte. At this point the first reduction in the benzodiazepine was made whilst increasing the antidepressant to 150 mg. Subsequently he underwent monthly reductions in benzodiazepine until he could no longer tolerate further changes in dosage. At this point he was changed to diazepam, a long-acting benzodiazepine, and reduction continued thereafter until it was discontinued. At no time did the patient require admission to hospital and overall the reduction occurred over a 6 month period. Subsequently antidepressants were continued for a further 9 months.

Comment

This gentleman had a depressive illness and his symptoms of anxiety were part of this condition, which had gone unnoticed and untreated for some time. It is common for patients to cope with the initial reductions in benzodiazepines, probably because they are highly motivated at the outset and later experience more difficulty. Changing to a long-acting drug is associated with fewer withdrawal symptoms because of the cumulative effects of the active metabolites. There is also more flexibility of dosage. In this gentleman's case the withdrawal symptoms were also reduced by the sedative properties of the antidepressant he was receiving.

Prevention

(1) The cautious use of benzodiazepines hardly needs reiterating and the advice at present is that they should not be prescribed on a regular basis for longer than 4 weeks. Also long-acting drugs are to be preferred to short-acting ones and flexible rather than regular dosage is recommended.

(2) The accurate diagnosis and treatment of depression, especially when anxiety is to the fore, will reduce the inappropriate prescribing of these substances.

(3) As outlined in Chapter 6 there are many techniques available to the practitioner in dealing with anxiety. Using this broad range of treatments is to be commended.

(4) Except in circumstances where insomnia or short-term anxiety is a source of great distress problems of living should not be 'treated' with drugs and a willingness to accept the limitations of medicine in dealing with understandable human suffering is a philosophical stance which has become a medical necessity in view of the iatrogenic problems associated with benzodiazepine over-prescribing. If circumstances demand intervention then this must be short-term.

Opiates

Many general practitioners have little contact with opiate addicts but those working in the inner cities will be frequently confronted with this problem and the attendant legal and medical difficulties. In addition general practitioners are increasingly involved in the ongoing management of opiate addicts in collaboration with specialists in substance misuse.

The epidemiology of this problem is unknown since there are difficulties inherent in measuring its prevalence, not least being the reluctance of patients to admit the dependence. In an attempt to overcome this uncertainty the Home Office made compulsory the notification of opiate abusers to the Addicts Index in Britain. No such law exists in Ireland. There are estimated to be over 250 000 drug addicts in Britain, most using opiates (mainly heroin) and crack cocaine, and more than 181 000 are in contact with the drug treatment services. Among the 15-year-old age group, 1% are estimated to be chronic users. The fashion in opiates changes periodically and although heroin remains constantly the substance of first choice for most addicts, methadone, pethidine and DF118 have been variously sought after. Some are also now abusing buprenorphine, an opiate substitute increasingly used in treatment. Many people will also use other drugs either alone or with opiates and so combination with hallucinogens, cocaine and others is commonplace.

Social and demographic features

Opiate dependence is largely found in those under 26 and there is an excess of men. Many have histories of non-drug-related offences even prior to the addiction and further offences continue in an effort to steal drugs from pharmacies, etc. Other offences such as shoplifting and prostitution are common as the addict attempts to finance the spiralling debt which invariably ensues. Up to 50% are diagnosed with antisocial personality disorder although this behaviour may be the result of the lifestyle associated with addiction rather than an inherent personality disorder. Addicts tend to congregate in the poorer non-residential areas of large towns and cities. Many are unemployed and have few close, lasting relationships outside the drug culture. All social classes are represented.

Presentation

Frequently the addict first presents as a result of pressure from the courts. Opiate addicts should be assessed initially by a service for substance misuse: the doctor who attempts to detoxify or otherwise treat an opiate user may rapidly attract patients who wish to have their habit facilitated. Addicts also often present at times of crisis for themselves, including weekends or when money or supplies are not available. In such circumstances it is tempting to prescribe on humanitarian grounds. Again, this is ill-advised and may be dangerous since the patient will often exaggerate his need and death may follow from overdose.

Those who have been prescribed long-term opiates for genuine painful conditions may also misuse their drugs at times (see Case 3). Many are not aware of the addiction until withdrawal is attempted whilst others have a well-developed preference. Cautious prescribing, with supervision from a family member and the doctor, can be continued if there has been no gap in medical prescribing while awaiting specialist assessment.

Case 3

Mr X was referred by his family practitioner because he was demanding increasing amounts of opiates for back pain. He had been involved in a road accident 3 years earlier and having had to have his vertebrae fused continued to complain of pain. His wife was taught while in hospital to administer the opiate injections and thereafter he attended his GP, who prescribed these drugs under the instruction of his orthopaedic consultant. His GP felt that he was deceiving him about the severity of his back pain and having confronted him he admitted this. Mr X was admitted for detoxification and this was successfully carried out using clonidine. Throughout his stay in hospital he remained repentant and motivated and although he still described some back pain agreed that it was not constant nor did it interfere with his day-to-day activities as he had suggested. His reason for taking opiates was for euphoria. Prior to discharge he was referred back to his consultant for further consideration of his analgesic requirements.

Comment

Cases such as this are difficult since the doctor is totally dependent on the accuracy of the patient's history when making decisions about treatment. The iatrogenic addict is often not recognized and the patient who complains of constant pain despite 'successful' prior treatment should alert the prescribing doctor to the possibility of opiate abuse.

Detoxification

Detoxification is most easily carried out in inpatient treatment units but in some circumstances, where the patient has a stable family for support, it may be done as an outpatient. A larger number of drug treatment centres now exist in Britain although they are much scarcer in Ireland. These centres have community drug prevention teams attached in order to support the primary care services in the detection, early intervention and maintenance treatments that have evolved.

Detoxification is most commonly done by substituting methadone for the other opiates which the patient has been using. Care must be taken lest the doctor unwittingly overdoses the patient since most substance misusers do not generally have an accurate record of their opiate consumption and may exaggerate it for the purpose of procurement. It is best to titrate upwards as withdrawal symptoms appear rather than the reverse. The dose is then decreased at a rate which is also titrated against symptoms, the objective being to minimize these. In general short-acting substances such as heroin produce short but intense discontinuation symptoms whilst longer-acting opiates lead to a less severe but more prolonged withdrawal phase.

However, when an opiate antagonist such as naloxone or naltrexone is used the reaction can be severe. For this reason they are seldom used except in the maintenance phase.

Using methadone for detoxification the process takes about 2–3 weeks. Buprenorphine can also be used especially if rapid detoxification is required and there are fewer side effects than with clonidine or lofexidine, both α_2-adrenergic agonists, which may also be used. Occasionally buprenorphine and clonidine are used in combination.

Following detoxification from heroin the opioid antagonist naltrexone can be used to maintain abstinence since it blocks the agonistic effects of opiates, especially euphoria, making continuing abuse less likely and ultimately leading to extinction of the behaviour due to the absence of any psychological rewards. The initial dose is 25 mg increasing to 50 mg the following day. However, it can cause severe withdrawal symptoms if the patient is still physically dependent and should only be instituted when detoxification is fully completed. A period of 7–10 days opiate-free, confirmed by urinalysis, is required. If there is a risk of occult abuse a naloxone challenge test should be performed. However, there is no mechanism to compel the person to comply with this treatment so high levels of motivation are required.

Maintenance and harm minimization

In order to maintain abstinence the prescribing of buprenorphine, methadone and/or needle exchange is the usual first step in treatment. Decisions about dosage are made by the specialist services or by general practitioners in shared care schemes. In order to reduce the risk of selling-on abuse daily prescriptions are recommended, while take-home prescriptions are only used after trust and stability are established. Supervised consumption at pharmacies is normal.

Buprenorphine, a partial μ-opioid agonist and κ-opioid antagonist, is also used for maintenance. However, it may also be misused for recreational purposes and adverse events including cutaneous complications may develop after injection. Strict controls are recommended so as to reduce the potential for misuse including the registration of those who prescribe it as well as daily supervised consumption (Ho *et al.* 2009).

There are ethical concerns about some aspects of harm reduction. These include the use of injectable heroin for those who will not or cannot be maintained on methadone, with the related requirement for the provision of injection rooms.

Alongside maintenance, attention should be paid to supporting a change in lifestyle and development of relationships and employment. Many patients describe missing the ritual of searching and of injecting more than the drug effect and will often describe a void in their life. Counselling can be directed towards satisfying recreation, finding a job if possible and towards building a trusting relationship with the therapist (GP, psychiatrist or counsellor), since the former addict will be especially vulnerable at times of crisis.

For some, for long periods, complete abstinence from heroin cannot be achieved despite maintenance medication. Flexibility, with occasional lapses (positive urine samples), is probably preferable to zero-tolerance policies, as long as maintenance medication is collected regularly. There is ongoing debate about harm-reduction policies in relation to the need for gradual reductions in replacement regimes. Our view is that social stability and inclusion are the primary goal and that once these have been at least partially achieved goals in methadone reduction should be encouraged.

Shared care

Increasingly general practitioners work collaboratively with the specialist addiction services to treat this challenging group of patients. In the UK general practitioners with the necessary qualifications are advised to participate in these schemes and this development has been made possible by initiatives from the Royal College of General Practitioners such as the Certificate in the Management of Drug Misuse (parts I and II). The shared care model involves the general practitioner in prescribing various alternatives to heroin or other opiates, the main substitutes being methadone and buprenorphine. Initial assessment including a urine sample and full history is required in collaboration with specialist service. Those with the part II certificate can provide tier 3 interventions at a special interest level. The principles of management are outlined in Department of Health Guidelines (2007).

The doctor–patient relationship

This is perhaps more compromised than with any other group of patients. Trust is often lacking since the addict may be attending to obtain drugs rather than to gain advice whilst the doctor may find himself questioning his patient's motives. Distrust is also a function of past abuse and attachment problems which many patients have experienced. The doctor may also have to refuse medication which would bring symptomatic relief – a practice which is alien to the caring doctor. Not surprisingly, many find this difficult and adopt a permissive approach to prescribing.

Safeguarding children

Increasing attention is now being paid to ensuring that children (and other dependants) of people with substance misuse problems are given the highest attention. Health visitors, school nurses and social services often need to be involved. Balancing the needs of children to be looked after by their biological parents against stability requires regular information-sharing and liaison between the various organizations involved.

Pregnancy

Addiction to opiates in the neonate is an increasing problem and about three-quarters of all infants born to addicted mothers experience a neonatal abstinence syndrome (NAS). The mortality among newborn infants acutely withdrawing from opiates is much higher than among adults, where it is almost never fatal. In addition there is a risk of miscarriage when withdrawal occurs earlier in pregnancy. Maintaining the pregnant woman on methadone may be the least hazardous and if a reduction is required it should be carried out slowly and with monitoring of fetal movements, and preferably in the second trimester when it is least hazardous. During the third trimester doses may need to be increased due to changes in its metabolism at that time. However, there is conflicting evidence as to whether the severity and duration of the NAS is correlated with the dose of methadone used by the mother so there is little to guide the clinician as to the safest dose (Lim *et al.* 2009). However, it seems that the stability which methadone brings to the pregnant woman, especially as it reduces the risk of acute maternal withdrawal, which is associated with fetal death, offsets the complication of NAS. Methadone maintenance is not a contraindication to breastfeeding. There is emerging evidence regarding the possible use of buprenorphine in pregnancy.

Outcome

The physical consequences of opiate addiction stem probably from the use of contaminated materials and dirty needles. These include thrombophlebitis, hepatitis, muscle contractures, finger gangrene and AIDS. Thrombophlebitis may result in veins becoming permanently damaged. Veins should be examined not just in the antecubital fossa, but also in the arms and forearms, the ankles, neck and fingers. The social consequences include poverty, repeated crime both petty and serious, prostitution (homosexual and heterosexual) and loss of family and friends. Opiate addiction is not associated with any particular psychiatric syndrome although depression is often described during detoxification. This may not require treatment and improves spontaneously. However, as with alcohol, PTSD, anxiety, depression and personality disorder can be revealed after stabilization.

Recent studies from general practice point to the acceptability of providing methadone maintenance treatment in primary care. A study in Britain shows that the frequency of heroin use was reduced from a mean of 3.02 episodes per day to a mean of 0.22 episodes per day, confirmed by urinalysis. Mean numbers of convictions and cautions were reduced by 62% for all crime. HIV risk-taking behaviour, social functioning, and physical and psychological well-being all showed significant improvements (Keen *et al.* 2003). While this study is positive in its findings, the patients are likely to be among the more stable addicts as those with poor motivation and continuing abuse remain under the care of the specialist services.

The feasibility of abstinence post-detoxification has been highlighted recently, with 23% of those who entered inpatient treatment with the goal of abstinence remaining drug-free at 2–3 years follow-up, while 50% reported recent opiate abuse and 57% were on maintenance methadone (Smyth *et al.* 2005). Abstinence was associated with having completed the course of detoxification and with the absence of a family history of substance misuse. Abstinence rates of 22–86% have been found across a range of studies, with voluntary participation in a detoxification programme showing the strongest association with being drug-free post-treatment (Kornor and Waal 2005).

Suicidal behaviour is common among those who misuse opiates, with up to 50% having a history of deliberate self-harm (Tremeau *et al.* 2008) although the risk factors are no different from those of other diagnostic groups and these include a past or positive family history of suicidal behaviour, impulsivity and aggression. Suicide is also a consequence and a recent 20 year follow-up study of hospitalized opiate addicts treated either for self-poisoning or admitted for detoxification confirmed this (Bjornaas *et al.* 2008). The mortality rate from all causes was higher than in the general population and 37.8% of the index sample had died, 11.4% in accidents, 7.1% by suicide, 2.9% by other violent means, while the remainder had variously died of cancer, cardiovascular disease and other unnamed illnesses.

Amphetamines and related substances

Amphetamine was discovered in 1887 and was marketed in the 1930s as an over-the-counter treatment for nasal congestion. Within a few years reports of abuse began to appear. Amphetamine sulphate, the most common preparation, is easily synthesized in home laboratories although a stronger version, methylamphetamine ('ice'), is also available and its effects are said to last much longer. Amphetamines are often used on their own but they may also be abused in conjunction with opiates and while they are associated with some physiological changes such as fatigue, headaches, muscle cramps, profuse sweating and insatiable hunger when withdrawn, the main discontinuation symptoms are emotional in nature. These consist of profound craving for the drug, severe depression, often suicidal in intensity, especially associated with methylamphetamine abuse, lethargy, nightmares and either agitation or psychomotor retardation. For the patient's safety hospitalization is advised during this period. Symptoms begin within a few hours of discontinuation, peak within 2 days and resolve within a week usually.

In the early 1960s most abusers were women who had been prescribed these drugs for obesity or depression. Today, they are mainly men and are similar to opiate addicts – in fact amphetamine abuse now seldom occurs in isolation and amphetamines are often abused to counteract the dysphoria many opiate addicts experience in the aftermath of a 'buzz'.

The immediate effects of amphetamines are to reduce fatigability, decrease hunger, improve concentration and heighten awareness in association with an intense feeling of bodily pleasure. In some users an amphetamine psychosis can occur with paranoid delusions, hallucinations in multiple modalities, and thought disorder. Consciousness is clear and in the acute phase is indistinguishable from schizophrenia. However, when the symptoms are chronic, amphetamine psychosis lacks the affective flattening and poverty of speech characteristic of chronic schizophrenia. It is uncertain whether amphetamine psychosis occurs in those who are predisposed to schizophrenia or whether it is sporadic. The treatment is as for any acute psychosis and if chronic symptoms supervene maintenance treatment will be necessary as for schizophrenia. Occasionally high-dose amphetamines may produce life-threatening cerebrovascular accidents and focal neurological signs.

Methylene dioxymethamphetamine (MDMA) or 'Ecstasy' is a party drug, used socially, which rapidly induces energy, alertness and euphoria. Adverse effects include severe headache, tension in the jaw and teeth-grinding, panic attacks and elevated blood pressure. After use irritability, depression and insomnia are commonly described and then fade after 2–3 hours. Occasionally hallucinations and paranoid ideation may occur and paranoid psychosis has been described with high doses, as have abnormalities of gait and nystagmus. Seizures, renal failure and cardiovascular accident have also been documented. Malignant hyperpyrexia with disseminated intravascular coagulation can also result from dehydration but rapid rehydration can cause circulatory overload and death. Occasionally MDMA may be combined with fluoxetine to enhance its effects, believed to result from a massive release of central serotonin. Although not physically addictive, it can induce psychological dependence. Treatment is symptomatic and most users presenting to the medical services do so for control of psychotic symptoms or for the treatment of acute dehydration.

Khat (pronounced COT) is derived from a plant of the same name and can be bought from greengrocers in East London, where it is imported from the Horn of Africa. Nowadays, it is chewed or made into a tea and used by immigrants from Somalia, the Yemen and Ethiopia. Its active ingredients, cathinone and cathine, are stimulating and are class C drugs under the Misuse of Drugs Act. In other countries it is more strictly controlled by law. Similar in effect to amphetamines, it increases alertness and reduces appetite. It also induces a feeling of calmness but regular use results in insomnia, anxiety and anorexia. Chewing the leaves results in intense thirst and produces a strong aroma. It may lead to irritability and even violence and it may lead to psychological dependence along with depression on discontinuation.

Cocaine

The acute effects of cocaine are generally similar to amphetamines but tactile hallucinations, referred to as formication, are common. Cocaine acts as a stimulant and because it produces a sudden feeling of euphoria (a 'rush' or 'flush') it may be used repetitively. 'Crack' is an extremely potent form of cocaine that can induce intense craving after only a few experiments. With both forms of cocaine, usually smoked or snorted, paranoid delusions and episodes of psychosis are frequent, occurring in up to 50% of abusers. The risk of violence or homicide associated with cocaine has led to its legal recognition as a class A drug (under the Misuse of Drugs Act, 1971) along with opiates. Sometimes visual and tactile hallucinations may be described also, although less commonly than delusions. A special form of tactile hallucination, referred to as formication, or a sensation of insects crawling beneath the skin, is also a feature of cocaine abuse. The psychosis may persist and resemble a schizophreniform illness.

Notification of cocaine abusers to the Home Office, in Britain, was mandatory but the Addicts Index has been replaced by data collated from drug treatment centres. In 2009 there were over 3000 cocaine addicts receiving treatment. As with amphetamines, cocaine with-drawal is not associated with a physical withdrawal syndrome but it can produce a profound depression, termed a 'crash'. This is usually short-lived and terminates in less than a day although when the abuse is severe the withdrawal may be prolonged for several days. Inpatient care during withdrawal is not mandatory since these drugs may be discontinued without physical withdrawal symptoms but it is advisable in view of the associated depression. Moreover, cocaine is frequently abused alongside opiates and opiate detoxification may need to be carried out concurrently. With long-term snorting, cocaine users are subject to ulceration of the nasal mucosa. No one treatment has been shown to be effective in reducing the withdrawal symptoms although dopamine agonists such as bromocriptine have been tested with varying results. Management of acute psychotic episodes is as for any psychotic episode.

Hallucinogens

Lysergic acid diethylamide (LSD) is the most popular of this group of drugs and is a class A controlled drug. It is usually taken by mouth and the first effects are felt 30–90 minutes after ingestion. These include dilated pupils, sweating, increased heart rate and high blood pressure. Perceptual disturbances including vivid visual hallucinations, heightened senses of colour and auditory changes are common. Sensory inputs are blended (synaesthesiae) so that sounds may be seen and colours felt! Thought processes are distorted and thinking becomes illogical and with a magical quality to it. During the peak of the experience there may be a loss of personal identity which some regard as a quasi-religious experience whilst others become terrified with a feeling of impending insanity and loss of control. Vivid recollections of the past and delirium are sometimes present and distractability is marked. The acute symptoms fade in about 6 hours but residual symptoms, e.g. distractability, persist for up to 24 hours. When these symptoms induce fear and panic in the patient they are referred to as 'bad trips'. These may present to the general practitioner and treatment is as for any acute psychosis. They require prompt treatment since bizarre accidents can ensue. 'Flashbacks' are another adverse feature of LSD abuse and can occur for up to 1 year after the last episode of abuse. These too should be treated with major tranquillizers. Occasionally a psychosis, schizophrenic in type, may supervene and a 'psychedelic syndrome' with inert and passive behaviour has been described in chronic users. Psilocybine is the active ingredient in 'magic mushrooms' and has effects similar to those of LSD. It is an occasional drug of abuse.

Solvents

These include glues, petrol, nail varnish remover, etc., and their abuse is confined to children and teenagers. Most strikingly, these usually come from poor and emotionally deprived back-grounds. The general action of solvents is as a central nervous system depressant. Tolerance develops although the withdrawal symptoms are mild. The initial effects, occurring after a few minutes and lasting for up to a few hours, resemble alcohol intoxication with euphoria followed by depression. Occasional psychotic episodes have been reported. With prolonged inhalation cardiac arrhythmias and loss of consciousness may occur. Chronic abusers may develop hepatic or renal damage and aplastic anaemia has been reported. Delirium or irreversible dementia may develop with persistent use and the associated behavioural disturbance may require symptomatic control with major tranquillizers. Benzodiazepines should be avoided since they may further increase the risk of respiratory depression. Solvents may be discontinued without a physical withdrawal syndrome but there is some evidence that solvent abusers frequently progress to alcohol abuse. Long-term management should centre on the family pathology rather than the solvent abuse in isolation.

Cannabis

This is a class B controlled drug, having had its criminal status upgraded in early 2009. Within minutes of smoking the subject is relaxed and experiences perceptual distortions, which are not as severe as with the hallucinogens. Sexual arousal occurs and energy increases. Heavy use can cause cannabis intoxication with a heightened awareness of colour, sound and detail. Time also appears slow and there may be feelings of detachment and out-of-body experiences. Skills such as driving and using machinery are impaired for up to 12 hours after smoking. Either elation or depression can occur in those subject to mood swings. Expectation and ambience is also thought to contribute. Psychotic reactions have been described although much less commonly than with hallucinogens or the other 'hard' drugs. There is dispute about the aetiological role of cannabis in long-term psychosis but the work of Arseneault et al. (2004) identifies an aetiological role for cannabis in conjunction with other factors in causing schizophrenia. Moreover, they argue that at a population level the incidence could be reduced by 8% if cannabis use was eliminated. A systematic review of the relevant literature (Moore et al. 2007) concluded that there is now sufficient evidence to warn young people that using cannabis could increase the risk of developing psychosis later in life.

The role of cannabis in causing an 'amotivational' syndrome characterized by self-neglect and apathy is in dispute. Cannabis detoxification does not require inpatient treatment and is unlikely to occupy much of the practitioner's time since use of cannabis is generally sporadic and recreational. Acute psychotic episodes require sedation in the usual way and the use of cannabis by those with a pre-existing psychosis considerably destabilizes their condition and may require additional medication to re-establish control of the illness (see dual diagnosis below).

Nicotine

Nicotine is the most common drug of abuse and cigarette smoking produces pharmacological and psychological dependence. Unlike other substances nicotine intoxication has not been described. There is no doubt that craving occurs and this coupled with the relaxing effects of nicotine make stopping difficult. Social factors contribute to smoking initiation and to its maintenance by encouraging the use of cigarettes in some environments. Moreover, those whose parents or siblings smoke are more likely to do so themselves since they act as role models. Claims have been variously made for the success of hypnotherapy. Chewing gum impregnated with nicotine, transdermal nicotine (patches) and group and cognitive therapy are standard treatments available within the NHS.

Hemineverin

This drug is occasionally abused, especially by alcoholics for whom it may have been prescribed during detoxification. It produces a physical withdrawal syndrome and should be gradually reduced in those who are dependent. This may be avoided by cautious prescribing and it should not be given for longer than 10 days. Its former popularity in alcohol detoxification has waned considerably in recent years and with its declining use, the problem of dependence should decline also.

Barbiturates

Once common, barbiturate dependence is now rare and confined mainly to established opiate addicts. These drugs should not be suddenly discontinued because of the risk of fits. The addict should be prescribed a long-acting barbiturate, e.g. phenobarbitone 50 mg t.i.d., and this is then decreased, usually under anticonvulsant cover over a period of a few weeks. Ideally this should be carried out in an inpatient setting. If fits supervene they should be controlled in the usual way with a short-acting barbiturate or with diazepam intravenously.

Other drugs of abuse are analgesics such as paracetamol. This is associated with mild feelings of pleasure, peptic ulceration, anaemia and in severe cases analgesic nephropathy. Withdrawal headaches combined with denial of the problem make this difficult to detect and treat.

Laboratory investigations

The presence of drugs in the body may be detected by either urine or blood analysis. Techniques involving saliva and hair sampling are not widely available and are still in their infancy. The usefulness of a particular test depends on being aware of the drawbacks of the method as well as the metabolism of the drug.

A negative finding does not exclude the possibility that illicit drugs have been taken, merely that the concentration in body fluids was not high enough or that the half-life of the drug was too short to allow detection when the sample was taken. In particular heroin and cocaine have short half-lives. The half-lives of the commonly abused drugs are shown in Table 10.4. False positive results have also been described and interpretation of results must be made in conjunction with clinical and historical information rather than as an end in itself. For example, repeated negative testing for opiates is significant in a patient claiming to be dependent and requesting methadone. In addition some drugs are metabolized before excretion in urine, thus making detection of the parent substance impossible. For example, heroin is metabolized before any urinary excretion occurs so urinary testing makes detection of the parent substance

Table 10.4. Metabolic profile of common drugs of abuse

Drug	Half-life (hours)	Unchanged drug in urine
Chlormethiazole	5	5%
Amphetamine	12	3%
Methylamphetamine	9	43%
Cocaine	1	4%
Diazepam	48	?
Heroin	0.5	0%
Morphine	3	5%
Methadone	15	4%
Codeine	3	?
LSD	3	1%
Cannabis	30	?4%

impossible. On the other hand, over 40% of methylamphetamine is excreted unchanged in urine, making urine testing particularly valuable when assessing the consumption of this drug.

When a urine sample is provided it is important to ensure that it has actually been provided by the patient since abusers of illicit drugs can substitute samples. Not only will regular sampling assist in building up a picture of the patient's drug misuse over time but the threat of spot checks can have a deterrent effect.

Dual diagnosis

Dual diagnosis is defined as the presence of a substance misuse disorder and another comorbid psychiatric condition. The latter can be a common or severe mental illness. The third element, present in some, is an underlying personality disorder, thus leading to a triple diagnosis. There is no implication as to whether the substance misuse or the psychiatric illness is primary – merely that both are present simultaneously. How common is dual diagnosis? Among those with alcohol dependence psychiatric comorbidity rates of 30% have been described while among other substance misusers a figure of 45% has been found. Alternatively among those with schizophrenia more than 50% have been shown to misuse illicit substances, thereby increasing the risk of destabilizing their illness. Further complications of comorbid substance misuse are the increased risk of violence or suicide and poorer clinical and social outcomes (Abou-Saleh 2004).

In trying to understand the mechanism by which severe mental illness can lead to substance misuse two possibilities have emerged. The self-medication model is the theory that those with significant mental illness misuse substances as a form of self-medication. This explanation may well be important for those with common mental illnesses but has not been well investigated. The alternative is that those with major mental illness are more vulnerable to the effects of such substances and is termed the supersensitivity model. This is supported by a growing body of evidence. For some individuals initial recreational drug use can lead to dependency following stressors and the development of depression.

Screening for substance misuse in those presenting to the generic psychiatric services or for major psychiatric illness in those attending the substance misuse services is essential. The same holds true for primary care although disentangling the effect of substances on symptoms is likely to be more problematic in this setting since this can only be satisfactorily achieved after a substance-free period. Tools such as the AUDIT (Babor *et al.* 1992) and the Dartmouth Assessment of Lifestyle Instrument (DALI) (Rosenberg *et al.* 1998) complement urine screens and collateral information in establishing whether substance misuse is present.

It is recommended that those with dual diagnosis be treated in the generic services using an integrated approach so as to avoid having to involve two services and for continuity of care (Department of Health 2002). This entails the delivery of both components of treatment by a single team in a single location. Alternatively, some services engage in multidisciplinary case management so as to enhance the substance misuse component although the danger of fragmentation exists. Assertive outreach, motivational interviewing, psycho-education and cognitive therapy in conjunction with pharmacotherapy have been variously incorporated into these service delivery models (Abou-Saleh 2004). Some services have established dual diagnosis teams with clinical competencies in both domains in an effort to enhance outcomes. Notwithstanding these strides, a recent systematic review failed to identify the superiority of any element of treatment over another (Cleary *et al.* 2008) and there was no difference between integrated and non-integrated models. However, in some aspects of treatment studies were limited in both methodology and numbers. Significant gaps continue to exist between service aspirations and delivery. It is particularly problematic for individuals with substance misuse and depression, anxiety, PTSD or OCD where integrated models are the exception.

Summary

- Defining alcoholism by the presence of the physical, social or psychological complications is likely to result in those with milder forms of the syndrome being missed.
- The controversy over whether it is an illness is still unresolved although both illness and social models have distinct implications for management.
- The search for a single cause is naive and current theories of causation focus largely on social and personality factors. Genetic inheritance may play a part in some but the findings are disparate.
- A number of physical illnesses and chronic psychiatric disorders, especially panic attacks and resistant depression, should alert the GP to the possibility of problem drinking. Various social and employment difficulties should also increase vigilance.
- The general practitioner is one of the most successful agents in detecting alcohol abuse and reducing hazardous drinking.
- The role of the family doctor in treatment is crucial and he has a central role in counselling the patient and in the detoxification of those who are motivated.
- Although inpatient detoxification and intensive aftercare by trained personnel has been diligently studied, few centres have shown better results than those obtained from simple advice.
- Psychological complications of alcohol such as marital and sexual dysfunction as well as depression and anxiety may need treatment when the patient is alcohol-free.
- Although abstinence is the desired goal for every alcoholic, it is possible that certain sub-groups may, with specialist retraining, return to social drinking.
- The type of alcohol misuse, i.e. whether binge or regular drinker, primary or symptomatic, does not affect the prognosis.
- Benzodiazepines are the most common drugs of dependence after alcohol.
- The patient during withdrawal can usually be treated without recourse to hospitalization.
- Benzodiazepines should not be discontinued abruptly. About 50% of long-term users suffer withdrawal symptoms. These resemble anxiety but occasionally a more severe reaction may occur.
- There is no information about the best approach to management but the addition of a tricyclic antidepressant is beneficial in some cases. Propranolol is also used to alleviate the physical withdrawal symptoms. It is best to change from a short-acting to a long-acting benzodiazepine before or during withdrawal.
- Opiate dependence is not usually managed by the general practitioner, except in collaboration with specialists, but there is an important role in early detection and in encouraging the patient to seek treatment.
- Amphetamines, cocaine and LSD are not drugs of physical dependence and they may be discontinued without fear of a physical reaction. Hospitalization may be required to counteract the psychological complications of withdrawal.

References

Abou-Saleh, M. T. (2004). Dual diagnosis: management within a psychosocial context. *Advances in Psychiatric Treatment*, **10**, 352–360.

Aertgeerts, B., Buntinx, F., Ansoms, S., and Fervey, J. (2001). Screening properties of questionnaires and laboratory tests for alcohol abuse or dependence in a general practice population. *British Journal of General Practice*, **51**(464), 206–217.

Arseneault, L., Cannon, M., Witton, J., et al. (2004). Causal association between cannabis and psychosis: examination of the evidence. *British Journal of Psychiatry*, **184**, 110–117.

Babor, T. F., de la Fuente, J. R., Saunders, J., et al. (1992). *AUDIT: The Alcohol Use Disorders Identification Test*. Geneva: World Health Organization.

Bertholet, N., Dappen, J., Wietlisbach, V., Fleming, M., and Burnand B. (2005). Reduction in alcohol consumption by brief alcohol intervention in primary care: systematic review and meta-analysis. *Archives of Internal Medicine*, **165**, 986–995.

Bjornaas, M. A., Bekken, A. S., Ojlert, A., et al. (2008). A 20 year prospective study of mortality and causes of death among hospitalised opioid addicts in Oslo. *BMC Central Psychiatry*, **13**(8), 8.

Brown, S. A., and Schuckit, M. A. (1988). Changes in depression among abstinent alcoholics. *Journal of Studies in Alcohol*, **49**, 412–417.

Clark, W. B. (1976). Loss of control, heavy drinking and drinking problems in a longitudinal study. *Journal of Studies on Alcoholism*, **37**, 1256–1290.

Cleary, M., Hunt, G. E., Matheson, S. L., et al. (2008). Psychosical interventions for people with both severe mental illness and substance misuse. *Cochrane Database of Systematic Reviews*, **1**, CD001008. DOI: 10.1002/14651858.CD001088.pub2.

Coulton, S., Drummond, C., James, D., et al. (2006). Opportunistic screening for alcohol use disorders in primary care: comparative study. *British Medical Journal*, **332**, 511–517.

Denis, C., Fatseas, M., Lavie, E., et al. (2006). Pharmacological interventions for benzodiazepine mono-dependence management in out-patient settings. *Cochrane Database of Systematic Reviews*, **3**, CD005194. DOI: 10.1002/14651858. CD005194.pub2.

Department of Health. (2002). *Mental Health Policy Implementation Guide: Dual Diagnosis Good Practice Guide*. London: Department of Health.

Department of Health (England) and the devolved administrations. (2007). *Drug Misuse and Dependence: UK Guidelines on Clinical Management*. London: Department of Health (England), the Scottish Government, Welsh Assembly Government and Northern Ireland Executive.

Drummond, D. C., Oyefeso, A., Phillips, T., et al. (2005). *National Alcohol Research Project: The 2004 national alcohol needs assessment of England*. London: Department of Health.

Edwards, G., and Gross, M. M. (1976). Alcohol dependence: provisional description of a clinical syndrome. *British Medical Journal*, **1**, 1058–1061.

Flensborg-Madsen, T., Knop, Mortensen, E., et al. (2009). Alcohol use disorders increase the risk of completed suicide – irrespective of other psychiatric disorders. A longitudinal cohort study. *Psychiatry Research*, **167**(1–2), 123–130.

Goldberg, K. F., Singer, T. M., and Garno, J. L. (2001). Suicidality and substance abuse in affective disorders. *Journal of Clinical Psychiatry*, **62**(suppl 25), 35–43.

Ho, R. C. M., Chen, K. Y., Broekman, B., et al. (2009). Buprenorphine prescription, misuse and service provision: a global perspective. *Advances in Psychiatric Treatment*, **15**, 354–363.

Hodgson, R., Alwyn, T., John, B., Thom, B., and Smith, A. (2002). The FAST alcohol screening test. *Alcohol and Alcoholism*, **37**(1), 61–66.

Kaner, E., Heather, N., McAvoy, B., et al. (1999) Interventions for excessive alcohol consumption in primary health care:

attitudes and practices of English general practitioners. *Alcohol*, **34**, 559–566.

Keen, J., Oliver, P., Rowse, G., and Mathers, N. (2003). Does methadone maintenance treatment based on the new national guidelines work in a primary care setting. *British Journal of General Practice*, **53**(491), 461–467.

Kisley, S. R., Gater, R., and Goldberg, D. P. (1995). Results from the Manchester Centre. In Ustun, T. B., and Sartorius, N. (eds.), *Mental Illness in General Health Care*. Chichester: Wiley.

Kornor, H., and Waal H. (2005). From opioid maintenance to abstinence: a literature review. *Drug and Alcohol Review*, **24**(3), 267–274.

Lader, M., Tylee, A., and Donoghue, J. (2009). Withdrawing benzodiazepines in primary care. *CNS Drugs*, **23**(1), 19–34.

Liappas, J., Paparriqopoulos, T., Tzavellas, E., *et al.* (2002). Impact of alcohol detoxification on anxiety and depressive symptoms. *Drug and Alcohol Dependence*, **68**(2), 215–220.

Lim, S., Prasad, M. R., Samules, P., *et al.* (2009). High-dose methadone in pregnant women and its effect on duration of neonatal abstinence syndrome. *American Journal of Obstetrics and Gynaecology*, **1**(70), e1–e5.

Mayfield, G. D., McLeod, G., and Hall, P. (1974). The CAGE questionnaire: validation of a new alcoholism screening instrument. *American Journal of Psychiatry*, **131**, 1121–1123.

Moore, T. H., Zammit, S., Lingford-Hughes, A., *et al.* (2007). Cannabis use and the risk of psychotic or affective mental health outcomes: a systematic review. *Lancet*, **390** (9584), 319–328.

Patton, R., and Touquet, R. (2002). The Paddington alcohol test. *British Journal of General Practice*, **52**(474), 59.

Petrusson, H., and Lader, M. H. (1981). Withdrawal from long-term benzodiazepine treatment. *British Medical Journal*, **282**, 643–646.

Rosenberg, S. D., Drake, R. E., Wolford, G. L., *et al.* (1998). Dartmouth Assessment of Lifestyle Instrument (DALI): a substance use disorder screen for people with severe mental illness. *American Journal of Psychiatry*, **155**, 232–238.

Selzer, M. L. (1971). The Michigan alcoholism screening test. *American Journal of Psychiatry*, **127**, 1653–1658.

Smyth, B. P., Barry, J., Lane, A., *et al.* (2005). In-patient treatment of opiate dependence: medium-term follow-up. *British Journal of Psychiatry*, **187**, 360–365.

Strathdee, G., Manning, V., and Best, D. (2002) *Dual Diagnosis in a Primary Care Group (PCG)*. London: Department of Health.

Tremeau, F., Darreye, A., Staner, L., *et al.* (2008). Suicidality in opioid–dependent subjects. *American Journal of Addiction*, **17**(3), 187–194.

Further reading

Crome, I., and Chambers, P., with Frisher, M., Bloor, R., and Roberts, D. (2009). The relationship between dual diagnosis: substance misuse and dealing with mental health issues. Social Care Institute for Excellence (SCIE) Research briefing 30. Available online.

Useful website for general practitioners

www.nta.nhs.uk/areas/clinical_guidance/ clinical_guidelines/docs/ clinical_guidelines_2007.pdf

Suggested reading for patients

Jay, J., and Jay, D. (2008). *Love First: A Family's Guide to Intervention,* 2nd edn. Minnesota: Hazelden Publishing.

Baylissa Frederick, V. (2009). *Benzo-wise: A Recovery Companion.* Iowa: Campanile Publishing LLC.

Pryor, W. (2004). *The Survival of the Coolest.* Clear Books: London (this memoir deals with heroin and alcohol addiction)

Useful websites for patients

www.rcpsych.ac.uk/mentalhealthinfo/problems/ alcoholanddrugs.aspx

www.addictionrecoveryguide.org

Useful addresses

Alcoholics Anonymous, General Service Office, PO Box 1, 10 Toft Green, York, YO1 7NJ, UK.

Alcoholics Anonymous, General Service Office, Unit 2, Block C, Santry Business Park, Swords Road, Dublin 9, Ireland.

Al-Anon, 61 Great Dover St., London, SE1 4YF, UK. Tel: 02074030888. Email: enquiries@al-anonuk.org.uk.

Al-Anon Information Centre, 5 Capel Street, Dublin 1, Ireland. Tel:: +353 1 8732699. Email: info@al-anon-ireland.org.

Local Council on Alcoholism,
.... (please fill in address and telephone number here)

Alcoholics Anonymous,
.... (please fill in your local branch number here)

Narcotics Anonymous, UK Service Office, 202 City Road, London, EC1V 2PH, UK. Tel: 020 7251 4007. Email: ukso@ukna.org or parentsandcarers.chair@ukna.org.

Narcotics Anonymous Ireland, Irish Regional Service Committee, 29 Bride St., Dublin 8, Ireland. Tel: +353 1 6728000 (information line only). Email: info@na-ireland.org.

Adfam, 25 Corsham Street, London, N1 6DR, UK. Tel: 02075537640.

National Drug Treatment Centre, Trinity Court, 30 Pearse Street, Dublin 2, Ireland. Tel: +353 1 6488600. Email: info@dtcb.ie.

....
....

(please fill in your local Narcotics Anonymous telephone number here)

Suicidal and self-harming behaviour

Learning objectives

Understanding deliberate self-harm
A typology of suicide; ideation and assessment of risk
The general practitioner and prevention
Antidepressants and suicide
Psychiatric and sociological aspects of suicide
The overlap between self-harm and suicide
Common pitfalls when assessing suicide risk

Until the 1960s it was thought that every act of self-harm was a failed suicide attempt. This attitude was challenged by the emerging clinical impression that many 'suicide attempts' were not prompted by a desire to extinguish life but by other motivations such as the desire to escape from problems, the non-verbal communication of distress, to relieve unbearable emotions through pain and the wish to control situations and sometimes to manipulate others. The term parasuicide was coined to describe this behaviour, whose motivation is heterogeneous. The definition of parasuicide is that it is any non-fatal act in which an individual deliberately causes self-injury or ingests a substance in excess of any prescribed or generally therapeutic or safe quantity. This definition includes experimental drug use since the ingestion of these substances is either not prescribed or if prescribed, as with opiates, is taken in excess. The inclusion of this latter category is, however, open to criticism as being over-inclusive since drug misusers may be motivated by purely recreational factors; however, it is not unhelpful to consider ingestion of any substance in quantities known to be potentially unsafe as a form of self-harm; and indeed there is a significant overlap in the underlying aetiology and diagnostic spectrum of the two groups. The concept of parasuicide, which makes no assumptions about motivation, has found almost universal approval for both its pragmatism and its usefulness in clinical practice and research. Increasingly the term deliberate self-harm (DSH) is replacing parasuicide, at least for the present. DSH will therefore be used in this chapter and includes self-injury and suicide attempts. As with parasuicide DSH carries no implication for what might be motivating the act of self-harm. For primary care clinicians DSH becomes important in a number of scenarios:

- routine assessment of risk of self-harm
- presentation of threats to self-harm at or during routine surgery or emergency settings

- follow-up of individuals who have recently self-harmed
- sharing care for individuals with ongoing attempts and risk of self-harm

Epidemiology

DSH predominates in women, in those under 35 and in the divorced, single or separated. The association with unemployment and low socio-economic class is well-recognized although the reason for this is not understood. The episode generally occurs in the context of a family or personal crisis and for many it represents a common behaviour pattern.

Many of those who self-harm are treated by their general practitioner in preference to attending hospital and official figures based on hospital records are thought to underestimate the number by up to 30%. A further source of attrition is the number who self-discharge before evaluation has taken place in the emergency department – this results in a further loss of about 12% of episodes. It is difficult to be precise about the prevalence since it varies from country to country and centre to centre. In England rates have varied between 285 and 460/100 000 for men and between 342 and 587/100 000 for women (Hawton *et al.* 2007), with rates being highest in women under the age of 25 and among men in the 25–34 age group while they are lowest in both sexes among those over the age of 55. The female excess is slightly reversed in those over the age of 55 (Hawton *et al.* 2007). Rates show an inverse relationship with social class and they vary with marital status, with the divorced being most at risk. In Ireland the national male and female rates of DSH in 2007 are 162 and 215/100 000 respectively (National Suicide Research Foundation 2008), with almost half being under the age of 30 and 87% under 50. Other socio-demographic associations are similar to those in Britain.

This behaviour is estimated to account for about 100 000 hospital admissions each year in England and Wales and in Ireland for over 11 000 attendances to accident departments annually. Similar to suicide, a seasonal variation has also been observed for DSH with a peak in late spring/early summer and a trough in late December/January among women, possibly related to the sense of purpose which is associated with the traditional role of women at Christmas.

Repetition is reported in about 15% annually and this is especially associated with male gender, personality disorder and low socio-economic class. The risk of repetition is highest in the immediate period following the index episode and a clustering of episodes is often observed. Over a year 1% will die by suicide, especially in the period immediately following an earlier self-harm episode. Attempts at predicting repetition or suicide by devising and applying scales have so far proved unsuccessful.

Methods used

Over 80% of episodes of DSH are by poisoning and the remainder consist of self-injury, usually by cutting or a combination of both. Non-opiate analgesics, minor tranquillizers and paracetamol are most often used in both Britain and Ireland. Those who self-injure are the group who most often engage in multiple episodes, presenting a difficult clinical challenge.

The most frequent clinical diagnosis among those who self-harm is of a stress reaction (adjustment disorder, Chapter 5) occurring in the context of some stressful event, often in connection with relationships. Other axis 1 diagnoses are less common but include mood and anxiety disorders as well as substance misuse with 3–10% misuing drugs and up to 22% alcohol. The role of alcohol is hardly surprising since it may be used by some as a remedy for untreated depression while for others its depressant and disinhibiting effects increase the likelihood of self-harm. Overall about 50% of those who self-harm use alcohol at the time of the act. Axis 2 diagnoses, i.e. personality disorders, most commonly borderline type, co-occur in up to 65% of subjects. Many of those who self-harm, particularly those who do so repeatedly, have a history of childhood trauma, a frequent aetiological factor in personality disorder. Some of these aspects are found in Case 1 below.

Case 1

G was a 19-year-old woman referred to the local mental health team by the family support service, because of concerns about her own mental health and the well-being of her 2-year-old child. She was engaged in a number of self-harming activities which tended to shift over time, but recently included making deep cuts to her thigh; 6 months ago she had made an attempt at hanging. She also engaged in binge drinking, had significant symptoms of bulimia and a past history of anorexia nervosa. Her mood was labile with angry outbursts and difficulty maintaining relationships. She had been sexually abused as a child by her uncle and raped once in her early teens. She had flashbacks of these events and voices telling her she was unclean. These precipitated her self-harm.

She was diagnosed as having both borderline personality disorder and PTSD. This could have been categorized as 'complex PTSD'. Her self-harming behaviour, including binge eating and excessive alcohol consumption, was seen as a maladaptive coping response in the face of intolerable psychological distress. Until recently she had managed to maintain the care of her child, but in recent weeks there had been a couple of episodes when she had been drunk as the only adult in the house.

Social services were involved and provided support with additional child care and attending a parenting group. She also attended some brief therapy for control of self-harm in order to limit the dangers from her cutting behaviour, which reduced significantly. After 6 months support aimed at stabilizing the social situation, she agreed to engage with therapy in order to address the traumas she had had in the past. Although the cutting continued for a further year on an intermittent basis it was not as deep as previously. After 9 months with support of the local alcohol team she gave up drinking. This was influenced by the development of a positive relationship with a young man she had known since her school days.

Comment

This case demonstrates the link between self-harming behaviour, psychiatric diagnoses and past trauma. The self-harming behaviour was serious, affected her parenting abilities, but was not life-threatening, apart from one attempt at hanging. Reduction in self-harming behaviour was achieved by a combination of social interventions and then later with psychotherapy; her own strengths enabled her to develop a positive sexual relationship for the first time and continue looking after her child.

Who is referred for specialist help?

General practitioners sometimes undertake the treatment of those who present after an act of self-harm. Those who self-poison are more likely to be referred for specialist help at the time of the act than those who cut themselves. Also likely to be referred are those self-harming for the first time and those without a family history of psychopathology or dysfunction. There is no convincing evidence that admission per se reduces the risk of repetition. If a depressive illness or some major mental illness is diagnosed, treatment of the underlying condition may reduce the risk of repetition, at least in the short term.

Aetiology of DSH

The aetiology of DSH is complex and can be divided into general risk factors and precipitants. The most common risk factors are social and include unemployment and social disintegration or anomie (normlessness), a term used by Durkheim (1951) in his work on suicide. Evidence for the importance of societal norms in controlling suicidal behaviour comes from the findings that it is highest in inner cities where the correlates of anomie (non-marital births, crime, unemployment and divorce) are prominent. The relationship to poverty independent of these factors remains unproven.

Other possible theories focus on the personal meaning such an act may have, and the idea of the 'cry for help' is one such hypothesis, although so far unsubstantiated. Messages other than a behavioural plea for help may also be conveyed by DSH and these may include anger, revenge or control. For example, individuals who have poor verbal, interpersonal or social skills may use this behaviour as a method of controlling or of bringing about change in their environment.

Psychological studies have examined the thought processes in DSH and found deficits in problem-solving and, in particular, identified inflexible thinking leading to impairment in generating responses to stressful situations. This cognitive understanding, while providing a theoretical model for intervention designed to prevent repetition, has so far been unsuccessful in this regard and several studies involving training in problem-solving have not had a beneficial effect in reducing DSH repetition. Biological research has investigated the role of serotonin and of noradrenaline in generating suicidal behaviour but is hampered by problems in eliminating the effects of depressive illness, itself associated with abnormalities in serotonin.

Since most episodes of self-harm are precipitated by some event, in particular those relating to interpersonal relationships, an episode of DSH which is apparently without an obvious trigger should be viewed with caution and may indicate a serious attempt at suicide warranting psychiatric inpatient treatment.

Assessment of DSH

If the patient is seen in an accident and emergency department most are assessed psychiatrically. If the patient self-discharges and presents to the family doctor later, then an assessment of the patient's suicide risk and of any potential treatment may be necessary. Assessment of DSH is also important for routine care of all mental illness. The psychiatric assessment of DSH is considered under the four headings which follow.

Assessment of suicide ideation

Suicide risk should be assessed in every patient presenting to the general practitioner with an emotional problem. Many patients will describe unfocused, fleeting thoughts in the absence of any active wish or plan to kill themselves. The patient might say 'I wish I could go to sleep and not wake up' or 'I wish I were dead' but without any further elaboration. These are referred to as passive death wishes. Nevertheless inquiry must be made about more serious

Table 11.1. Typology of suicide ideation

| Passive death wish |
| Active death wish |
| – fleeting |
| – persistent |
| – with low suicide intent |
| – with high suicide intent |
| – without plans |
| – with plans |

active death wishes which may include detailed plans to execute the act and/or avoid discovery as well as final plans about saying goodbye. GPs and patients report that assessments are not routinely carried out and this is confirmed in consultation studies.

However, it is important to bear in mind that suicidal ideation is common in the general population, varying from 2 to 15% depending on the country studied and the scientific methods used. Serious suicidal ideation, when there is strong desire for death and/or a definite plan, is much less common at less than 1%. Even serious suicidal ideation can at times be very brief, especially when occurring in the context of an interpersonal crisis. If the doctor believes that the severity of suicidal ideation poses a risk, as for instance when it is persistent and there is a definite plan that the patient may act on, referral to the accident and emergency department or the community mental health team for urgent assessment is strongly recommended. If in doubt err or the side of caution.

A typology of suicidal ideation is presented in Table 11.1 and these are not mutually exclusive so that it is possible to have fleeting suicidal ideas with high intent and so on.

Passive death wishes are thoughts of wanting to be dead but without any desire to bring this about oneself. On the other hand active death wishes are defined as wanting to take steps to achieve. However, these must be further evaluated in order to assess the degree of suicide intent, which may be high or low depending on whether there is a persistent and well-formulated plan or simply an expression of a wish to end one's life without any definite strategy. The assessment of suicide intent following a self-harm event is described below.

Assessment of suicide intent

Following an act of DSH a full assessment of the act itself must be made in order to identify those acts that are associated with high intent. This is the most pressing concern if completed suicide is to be avoided in the short term. The question 'Is the patient currently suicidal?' may be answered by considering the degree of intent at the time of the act and by assessment of the current level of intent.

Not only is the patient's account taken into consideration but inferences from the act of self-harm itself are also a guide to suicidality. The presence of a suicide note, indications of final plans, such as a will, and careful execution of the attempt alert one to a high intent to commit suicide. The medical seriousness may not be related to intent and an assessment of the patient's concept of medical lethality must be made. Violent methods are generally believed to be evidence of high intent, along with the absence of another person in the vicinity and attempts to conceal the episode.

Questions about the patient's current attitude to the episode, to living and dying and their view of the future increase the precision of the evaluation. In particular the symptom of hopelessness has been consistently found to predict high intent and must be viewed with gravity. The absence of any wish to live or of any conflict between the desire to live or die may show itself as composure when talking about suicide and is equally serious. The person with high suicide intent must be hospitalized as a life-saving measure irrespective of whether a psychiatric illness is deemed to be present or not. The role of suicide intent is illustrated in Case 2 below.

Where possible, collateral information should be sought as some who are actively suicidal may conceal their intentions.

Case 2

Mrs X was a 39-year-old married woman with marital problems relating to her husband's drinking and infidelity. Two weeks earlier she had been prescribed antidepressants by her general practitioner because of a depressive illness. Her symptoms consisted of early wakening, diurnal mood swing, palpitations, loss of interest and impaired concentration. She did not have any suicidal ideation at the time this medication was prescribed. On the evening of the overdose she returned home to find a note from her husband saying he had left to live with his lover. Mrs X went straight to the bathroom and took an overdose of eight paracetamol. She was alone at the time and shortly became frightened that she may have harmed herself permanently. She telephoned her mother, who arranged her admission for medical treatment. The liaison team agreed that the general practitioner had correctly diagnosed a depressive illness and that the self-harm was of low intent; they contacted her husband, who took her home and he agreed to have marriage counselling. At follow-up a week later with her GP she admitted to regretting the whole incident and although her depression remained she felt more hopeful.

Comment

In this case the suicide intent was low despite the presence of a definite depressive illness. There was a worry that this lady's impulsive behaviour was atypical and related to her pervasive despondency. Despite this concern she did not exhibit any further suicidal ideation and as the crisis which provoked it had resolved she was able to return to the care of her GP alongside relationship counselling. This case also illustrates the role of the liaison service at the acute hospital in assessing risk, making contact with the husband and GP and signposting to further care.

Assessment of psychiatric illness

Major psychiatric illness is not universal in those who self-harm. Many are acute and impulsive reactions to stressful events (adjustment disorder) while others may have depressive illness and/or substance misuse. Personality disorders also often co-occur with these axis 1 disorders or this may be the only diagnosis. Irrespective of the level of suicide intent, an attempt must be made to assess and treat any underlying illness. At the time of the assessment some patients will not exhibit any obvious symptoms but a recent history of these and/or brittleness of mood should alert the doctor to the potential for suicide. If there is doubt about the presence of psychiatric illness admission for further assessment may be indicated. If the doctor decides to treat the patient's illness himself, such as when suicide intent is low or the DSH has occurred some weeks previously, it is prudent to prescribe newer antidepressants when these are required, so as to avoid the risk of death in the event of a repeat overdose. Repeat episodes of DSH are especially common in those with border-line personality disorder (BPD) and recent NICE guidelines on their management (2007) recommend not using antidepressants as first-line treatments notwithstanding the mood fluctuations commonly described in BPD since the evidence base for their benefits in those with BPD is limited.

Assessment of social problems

By far the largest component in the assessment will be an evaluation of the social difficulties the patient is experiencing. Social problems including poor housing, unemployment, alcohol abuse and relationship problems are frequent concomitants of DSH. Social isolation is of special significance since it suggests the absence of support at times of crisis. This does not mean geographical or physical isolation but refers to loneliness and is especially significant in the elderly and infirm. The practitioner may have to involve social services and local voluntary organizations in attempting to bring about change in the patient's social environ-ment and in providing companionship to those who are lonely.

General factors associated with suicide risk

In general the closer the sociodemographic and clinical resemblance between the person who self-harms and the typical victim of suicide (see below) the graver the risk of future suicide. Thus acquainting oneself with this profile is of paramount importance. It is impor-tant to realize, however, that relying on this dictum too slavishly may result in a serious underestimation of risk in those who do not conform to this pattern (see pp. 181 and 183).

The general practitioner and prevention

Most of those who self-harm do not receive psychiatric follow-up and are returned to the care of their general practitioners. Of the approximate 30% who are referred to the psychi-atric services following assessment only about one-third keep the appointment. By contrast, however, those who are returned to their general practitioner for follow-up have a high rate of consultation, with one-third attending the week after the episode and over 50% within 1 month (Gunnell et al. 2002), although this is far short of the NICE guidelines (2004), which recommend that they be seen within 5 days of the episode. Most discuss the reason for the self-harm and report the consultation as helpful (Houston et al. 2003). This high consultation rate places general practitioners to the forefront of identifying those with major psychiatric disorders or those who might be at risk of subsequent suicidal behaviour. Whilst the repetition of DSH cannot be predicted, the possibility of developing focused psychological interventions (see below) for those at risk of repetition should be considered. In particular the high rate of consultation suggests that primary care might be a more effective outlet through which to deliver such interventions.

Interventions
Reducing repetition

Many intervention studies have examined methods to reduce the repetition of DSH. These have included task-oriented case work, behaviour therapy and insight therapy. The most successful has been dialectical behaviour therapy (Linehan *et al.* 1993) although this requires specialist training. A more accessible intervention using manualized assisted cognitive therapy (bibliotherapy based on cognitive therapy principles with an offer of up to seven sessions of face-to-face therapy) did reduce the number of repeat episodes (Evans *et al.* 1999) subsequently although this was delivered within the mental health services rather than in primary care.

An intervention aimed specifically at general practitioners was developed and evaluated (Bennewith *et al.* 2002). Those who had presented to the emergency department following DSH were sent a letter by their general practitioner and invited to attend for follow-up. The doctors were provided with an educational handout on the management of deliberate self-harm. Unsurprisingly, the study found that this made no difference to the repetition rate, probably due to the difficulty of predicting future adverse circumstances that trigger repeated self-harm in this group of patients.

Reducing suicide

The most important reason for assessing each act of DSH is to reduce the risk of completed suicide in the immediate aftermath and there is evidence that this goal can be achieved (Suokas and Lönnqvist 1991) although reduction of suicide in the long term has not been achieved due to problems in predicting rare events (Suokas *et al.* 2004).

There is no evidence that the Samaritans prevent suicide although there are humanitarian reasons for welcoming the establishment of that organization. In particular the profile of those who contact them is believed to more closely resemble the self-harm rather than the suicide population.

For individual patients the best approach in primary care is to respond in a supportive manner at times of crisis and to prescribe with circumspection. The detection and treatment of reversible causes of DSH and suicide are crucial, as is a thorough assessment of suicide risk. Advice to the effect that the patient should 'do it properly next time', as is occasionally reported, is crass, insensitive and irresponsible.

Suicide

Despite public concern, suicide is still uncommon and the individual practitioner will rarely be confronted with it. The rates worldwide have been fluctuating over the past 40 years. In England and Wales the rates decreased during the 1960s and 70s, only to increase again. In 2007 the male suicide rate in Britain was 16.8/100 000, a reduction from 21.1/100 000 in 1998. Reductions have occurred in all age groups. The female rate has been relatively unchanged for decades and in 2007 was 5/100 000. On the other hand Ireland has seen a dramatic increase in its suicide rate, due mainly to an increase in the 20–30 year age group among men. Overall the standardized male suicide rate for 2006 (the most recent year for which reliable data are available) is 23/100 000, whilst the female rate has been relatively stable over the past 15 years and stands at 4.5/100 000. This increasing rate in Ireland has been attributed to changes in Irish life, both religious and social in recent years (Kelleher 1996).

In all cultures those at particular risk are the divorced, widowed or single. Differences in social class rates have diminished and the highest rates are recorded in late spring and early summer, reflecting the peak for affective disorders. Some European studies have noted a biseasonal distribution for women, with a second peak in the autumn, although this has not been replicated in Eastern countries. There is also evidence of a 'copy-cat' effect (also called the Werther effect) for some suicides, resulting in local clusters in some instances.

Methods of suicide

Availability is the major determinant of methods of suicide and these have changed in the last 30 years. In Britain, domestic gas, which was detoxified in the 1960s, was replaced by car exhaust poisoning (carbon monoxide) until the mid 1990s. However, the introduction of catalytic converters led to a reduction in this method and hanging is now the most common method among men, whilst women continue to use more passive methods such as over-dosing. In Ireland slightly different methods are used, with men choosing hanging and drowning and women poisoning and hanging. In both Britain and Ireland antidepressants on their own are implicated in about 4% of suicides and in 2.5% in combination with other substances.

Antidepressants and suicidality

Studies examining the link between antidepressant treatment and suicidality can be very confusing. The first problem lies in the definition of suicidality. In general it refers to the totality of suicidal ideation, suicide attempts and completed suicide. Some studies consider these as a single aggregate while others separate them into three individual measures or alternatively combine some components, e.g. suicide attempts and completed suicide, into a single variable often referred to as suicidal behaviour.

Earlier concerns about the potential for at least some of the SSRIs to cause suicide have generally not been substantiated following investigation by the Food and Drugs Administration of the United States, the Medicines and Healthcare Products Regulatory Agency (MHRA) in Britain and the Irish Medicines Board along with their European counterparts. Moreover, the National Institute of Clinical Excellence (NICE) (2009) in Britain continues to recommend SSRIs as the first-line pharmacological treatment for depressive illness, in those over the age of 18. NICE also recommends that irrespective of age, those considered to be at increased risk of suicide, for any reason, should be seen every week, once antidepressants have been initiated, until the risk has subsided. Common sense dictates also that if there is a real risk of suicide the doctor should consider admitting the patient for their own safety.

The studies informing the above guideline are based on detailed and regular evaluation of the research relating to suicidality and antidepressants. For those under the age of 18 there is evidence that compared with a similar age group not taking antidepressants there is an increased risk of suicidal ideation, suicide attempts and completed suicide. The risk of suicidal ideation is believed to continue up to the age of 25 or 30, depending on the study. By contrast, among adults the risk of suicide attempts and completed suicide is significantly lower than in those not taking antidepressants (Barbui *et al.* 2009).

A large American study, carried out after the warnings were introduced, found that suicidal behaviour was highest in the month before commencing antidepressant treatment, declining thereafter (Simon *et al.* 2006) and that there was no evidence of an increase in completed suicide in the early phase of treatment. Moreover, a related study also identified suicidal behaviour in those treated in primary care with psychological therapies (Simon and Savarino 2007).

A further problem is that some SSRIs may increase the risk of self-harm while reducing suicide. A study from Finland (Tiihonen *et al.* 2006) examined the risk of suicide and attempted suicide among all hospitalized patients who were receiving antidepressants. This study was not linked to the pharmaceutical industry. A total of 15 390 high-risk patients were identified and followed up for over 3 years. It found a markedly reduced incidence of suicide and of overall mortality from physical causes (heart disease and stroke) and a markedly increased risk of DSH. Specifically examining those under the age of 20, the risk of suicide was only present with the use of paroxetine while for other antidepressive agents the risk was reduced. A further meta-analysis submitted to the MHRA also found a reduction in suicide and an increase in self-harm (Gunnell *et al.* 2005).

A problem in assessing the causal role of antidepressants in suicide is that simply assuming that when a behaviour, such as suicide, follows the use of a particular antidepressant, one must have caused the other is fallacious since this does not take account of other background factors, prior suicide attempts or the stage in the illness at which the medications are prescribed. Indeed antidepressants are frequently prescribed during a period of deteriorating symptoms with evolving suicidal ideation. Often antidepressants considered to be safer in overdose are prescribed for this group of patients, giving a false sense of security to the treating doctor. It is thus to be expected that overdosing may occur in some. Others may use a more aggressive means to ensure death so that the causal factor is the severity of depression rather than the antidepressant itself.

A further explanation is that the increase in self-harm is a reflection of the differential rate of improvement in symptoms. Since motivation and drive improve before suicidal ideation resolves, the risk of overdosing in these early days of apparent improvement is heightened. So, the person with suicidal ideation who in the untreated phase of depression lacked the drive to act on the thoughts may be able to do so during the early phase of recovery. A further possibility is that the SSRIs may induce anxiety and agitation in the early days of treatment and that this may stimulate suicidal behaviour in some. These issues remain to be resolved. All antidepressants, irrespective of the class, now carry a 'black box' warning in relation to their initial use in children and young adults.

So the current position is that antidepressants, with the exception of fluoxetine, are not licensed for use in those under the age of 18 because of the poor risk–benefit ratio with regard to all aspects of suicidality. These restrictions apply only to antidepressant usage for treating depression and are not applicable to other disorders such as OCD etc. For young adults, up to the age of 25–30, there is an increased risk of all aspects of suicidality but for suicide attempts and completed suicide the link is very weak and significant statistically (odds ratio 1.04) only when both behaviours are combined into a single measure. This is due to the small numbers. In the older age groups the risk of suicidal behaviour diminishes substantially with the treatment of depression using antidepressive agents.

All age groups, apart from those under the age of 18, show a reduction in suicidal ideation after the first few weeks of treatment once the antidepressant response occurs.

Aetiology of suicide

Two aspects to the aetiology of suicide present themselves. The first explores the reasons for the population trends in suicide throughout Europe and the second examines why individuals take their own life; in other words these theories address population versus individual trends in suicide and are discussed below.

Population studies and sociological theories

The French sociologist Emile Durkheim has contributed greatly to our understanding in this area. His theory of anomie, the loss of the force of normative values on society, is frequently used to explain the reduction in suicide at times of social cohesion, e.g. war, and the increase during periods of social disorganization, e.g. economic recession. The current trends in suicide are believed to have resulted from both the present economic decline as well as the change in traditional mores and values – both reflecting aspects of anomie. The religious dimension has been examined specifically by other workers and the roles of religious commitment confirmed as protective against suicide. Current approaches to measuring anomie focus on social fragmentation and material deprivation, although the former seems to have a greater impact than the latter (Whitley *et al.* 1999).

A further theory – the egoistic theory – views social isolation as being of significance and may explain the high suicide rate in cities, in migrants and in those who are divorced, widowed and single. The role of loneliness and isolation has been confirmed in observational studies. The third type, also described by Durkheimm, is the altruistic suicide. This is the use of suicide to achieve an ideal and examples include suicide bombers and hunger strikers. Such suicides are of little psychiatric importance as they are not associated with mental illness and prevention does not rest with the medical profession.

There are some who argue that the sociological and psychiatric explorations of the aetiology of suicide are conflicting and mutually exclusive. The authors do not subscribe to this analysis but believe the two to be complementary and that both enhance our understanding of this tragic behaviour. A sociological as well as a psychcological basis for depressive illness is well recognized by most psychiatrists (see Chapter 7) and illustrates the interaction between both forces. The absence of confidants, the role of religious beliefs, unemployment and loss of mother in childhood are aspects of anomie and egoism as described by Durkheim – such difficulties predispose to depression and also to suicide. It can be concluded that psychiatry provides clues to the cause of individual suicides, whilst sociology leads to an understanding of suicide trends in populations.

Individual trends

Recent research has confirmed the findings of decades of research of the presence of psychiatric illness, especially alcohol abuse, depressive illness and schizophrenia in most victims of suicide. On the other hand men under the age of 30 are less likely to have a psychiatric illness as compared to their older counterparts (Foster *et al.* 1999) and suicide among young people is frequently associated with substance misuse and with a diagnosis of adjustment disorder.

In addition examination of personality status has been part of recent studies and personality disorder has been shown to co-occur in over 30% of victims (Henriksson *et al.* l993), with borderline personality disorder being over-represented.

Since depressive illness is the most common diagnosis among victims of suicide preventive efforts have focused on the identification and aggressive treatment of this condition (see Chapter 7). Hopelessness and guilt are recognized risk symptoms, and those in the early stages of recovery when lassitude has lifted are also at particular risk. The relationship between depressive illness and suicidal behaviour is illustrated in Case 3 below. Among alcoholics it is the chronic middle-aged man who is at highest risk and often the final action is precipitated by the conclusion of a relationship. In contrast to this group are the young schizophrenic patients who in a period of apparent well-being kill themselves using violent methods. It is believed that the presence of insight about the nature of the illness places this group at particular risk. The impulsiveness of suicide in the group makes it difficult to predict.

The association between physical illness and suicide has been documented by many, particularly the presence of painful conditions or of cancer, and the presence of depression is believed to be the mediator. Some researchers have pointed to an increased risk of suicide among HIV-positive patients, especially in the immediate aftermath of obtaining a positive result. Others have failed to replicate this finding.

There is increasing interest in the biology of suicide and the role of serotonin in suicidal behaviour has been investigated, as has that of noradrenaline and cholesterol. The results are as yet inconclusive.

Case 3

Mr X, a 58-year-old man, was referred as an emergency after he had decided to end his life by letting his car run freewheel down a steep hill which was traversed by a concrete wall at the end. He was deterred from completing this, and applied his brakes, when he saw a boy who reminded him of his son as he neared the bottom. His car was damaged by the impact on the wall but he was physically uninjured. He was having serious financial difficulties and had become bankrupt. Debt collectors were pressing him for money. He decided that the way to resolve his situation was to end his life. On questioning he had impaired concentration so that he was unable to even read his financial documents. He had early morning wakening as well as initial insomnia and morning was the most difficult time for him. His wife was unsupportive and did not accept that he had attempted to kill himself. She constantly harangued his employees, resulting in a rapid turnover of staff. Her behaviour may have been explained by the fact that some 4 months later she was diagnosed with a frontal lobe tumour. Mr X agreed to remain in hospital and a course of antidepressants was initiated in light of the diagnosis of depressive illness. However, because of continuing suicidal ideation a course of ECT was also prescribed, leading to remission in his symptoms. This enabled him to deal with his business difficulties. He was discharged from hospital on an antidepressant and was asymptomatic at follow-up.

Comment

To the unwary his decision to end his life may have seemed the only reasonable way to deal with his difficulties since there was clear evidence of his dire financial problems and his wife was unsupportive. In this patient's case his mental state was preventing him from doing anything about his situation, e.g. going to his accountant and making the decision to declare himself bankrupt. Treating his illness facilitated this. The fear of suicide while waiting for antidepressants to work is a real one and ECT is frequently the most rapid treatment. Such patients must be prescribed antidepressants also as prophylaxis if relapse is to be avoided. This treatment should be continued for about 9 months and sometimes longer if symptoms recur on decreasing or discontinuing the medication.

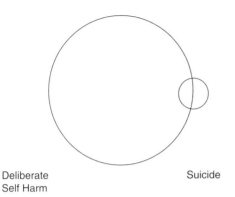

Figure 11.1. Overlap between people who attempt suicide and carry out DSH

Deliberate
Self Harm

Suicide

Relationship between DSH and suicide

In this chapter emphasis has been placed on the separation between suicide and DSH and these distinctions are evident from the epidemiological profile of each group, from the motivation and from the differing clinical status of each. However, this is an over-simplification and it is recognized that there is a small but important overlap between both populations (see Figure 11.1).

During a 1 year follow-up, roughly 1% of those who self-harm will kill themselves. Moreover, of those who die by suicide, up to 50% have had prior self-harm episodes. And while many of those who self-harm do not wish to die, many are clearly ambivalent about it and indeed some have been prevented only by the advances in resuscitation procedures. Further evidence of some overlap between suicide and DSH is the fact that almost 40% of those who subsequently kill themselves have been shown retrospectively to have attended a casualty department in the previous year for any reason, and some 15% for an episode of deliberate self-harm. In addition 5% of those who take their own lives have visited casualty in the last month of life because of a deliberate self-harm episode (Gairin *et al.* 2003). In general, the closer the resemblance sociodemographically and clinically between the person who self-harms and the profile of those dying by suicide, the graver is the risk. The prime risk factors include being male, elderly, socially isolated, physically or psychiatrically ill, hopeless and the use of violent means of self-harm. The pitfalls of adhering to these naively has already been alluded to (see also p. 183).

Prevention of suicide

Individual level

Undoubtedly doctors have a role in suicide prevention since many victims have contact with their general practitioners in the days preceding their death. While earlier studies estimated that 70% of victims had visited their family doctor in the month prior to the suicide and 40% in the week before their death the figure is now much lower and a recent study (Boer *et al.* 1996) found the corresponding figures to be 49% and 24%, respectively, particularly for those under the age of 35. Contact with psychiatrists was even lower at 12% and 6.5% for each time frame. Whilst the association between mental illness and suicide continues there is debate about whether suicide can in fact be prevented by medical means, given the rarity of the event. Some have suggested that socio-political and moral considerations are likely to make a greater impact on prevention (Wilkinson 1994).

The *adequate assessment* of individual acts of DSH is of paramount importance if suicide is not to be the short-term outcome in such patients. This has been described already (see p. 172).

The necessity to *recognize and adequately treat depressive illness* is evident since this illness has a high mortality if untreated. Recognizing it may be difficult at times, especially when the presenting symptoms are physiological rather than emotional. This is especially the case among general practice attendees. The neurotic/psychotic dichotomy, adhered to by so many, does not assist in diminishing suicide risk. The presence of even a single biological symptom, e.g. sleep disturbance, should alert the physician to make further enquiries about depressive symptomatology. Also the presence of unusual physical symptoms which do not constitute any of the commonly recognized medical syndromes along with a prior history of psychiatric disorder should arouse suspicion. Central to this is the necessity to think syndromally rather than symptomatically and failure to ask the necessary questions about the common symptom constellation found in depression may result in a woeful disregard for the fatal potential in this illness. The adequate treatment of depression necessitates the use of antidepressant drugs in therapeutic doses and subtherapeutic doses can heighten the suicide risk, especially among those with psychomotor retardation. It is clear that at the commencement of treatment due care must be taken to assess the risk of suicide and if in doubt relatives must be given charge of medication or inpatient treatment sought.

Gatekeeper training is an initiative that has been running for several years with backing from the United Nations. This targets doctors, community workers, school counsellors, general practitioners and those in a position to identify those who may be at risk of suicide. It also provides information on local resources and how these can be accessed. The most famous was in Gotland (Rutz *et al.* 1992), where family practitioners were given a 2 day training course in identifying and treating those who were suicidal. The initial results showed a reduction in suicide, for females only, and the effects were found only for the first 3 years. Other more recent studies have found positive effects but only when incorporated into a multifaceted approach to suicide prevention (Isaac *et al.* 2009).

Population level

Much debate has centred on the possibility of restricting the availability of potentially lethal substances such as paracetamol. There is a body of knowledge which holds that limiting the availability of these and similar drugs may prevent suicide at a population level. The likelihood that the overall rate would significantly diminish is in question since such attempts in relation to coal gas in Britain and Holland did not have any lasting impact. It is accepted that the methods of suicide reflect the current availability of lethal materials, e.g. firearms being the most common method in the USA, but when they are limited then potential victims may choose other available means.

It is often forgotten that many people are impulsive and resort to self-harm without a great deal of thought. This may not be related to psychiatric illness and is often determined by personality. So a person even with treated mental illness will retain their basic personality structure, which in some instances is impulsive and aggressive. Interventions to reduce impulsivity are of very limited effectiveness and so the risk of an ultimate act of suicide carried out on impulse is a possibility in some patients. It is impossible in these instances to foresee the timing of such an act.

Common pitfalls

Asking the question

There is a belief, at least among some of the public, that enquiring about suicidal thoughts will increase the risk by raising it in the consciousness of the individual. Such fears have fortunately been widely repudiated. The most direct way of assessing suicidal ideation is by such questioning although sometimes the question is not asked because it is assumed not to be present or it is not explored in any depth.

The patient may provide other clues but these are more likely to be demonstrated to those in close contact with the patient than to the physician. A common way of introducing such a line of questioning is to ask 'Do you ever feel it is difficult to just go on?' or 'Has life ever seemed hopeless?' More direct questions about the exact thoughts, 'Did you ever feel that you would be better off dead?' or 'Did you ever think you might harm yourself?', should then follow along with questions about the plans, if any, for executing this.

Failure to disclose

Patients are often reluctant to disclose suicidal ideation/intent if they are determined to carry out the act or if they fear psychiatric admission. For this reason obtaining collateral information is essential so that indirect indicators can be made known to the psychiatrist. In this regard, the patient may refuse permission to the doctor to speak with family members but when suicide intent is suspected confidentiality can be breached in the interests of patient protection.

Understandability

The doctor who knows and understands his patient may feel that there are compelling reasons why he might choose to harm himself. He may feel that in the circumstances, taking into consideration the patient's personality and the stresses to which he is exposed, nothing can or should be done. He may feel that his distress is the direct result of these burdens. It should be remembered that treatable illness can be provoked by such stresses (see Case 2 above) and to ignore warnings of suicide in such people is tantamount to negligence. Even if many of these stresses are transitory or the patient is responding to a life crisis, with support and appropriate interventions, the impact can be reduced and alternative way of dealing with the situation identified. Thus, the understandability of the reasons for depression and potential suicide is not a justification for ignoring them.

Relying on predictors

Too frequently the doctor may feel that the patient does not exhibit the features commonly associated with completed suicide. Thus, confronted with a young married woman, he may feel that her gender, marital status and age are not amongst the commonly cited risk factors. In general, the well-known risk factors are useful as general guidelines but may lull the unwary into complacency if relied upon too rigidly since they fail to take account of individual variation and personal circumstances.

Ignoring warnings

The received wisdom that those who speak about suicide will not execute it is a myth which must be dispelled. It has been shown that those who successfully harm themselves give warnings which include direct threats and indirect forewarnings such as refusing to buy new clothes, etc. These are ignored at the patient's peril. Since suicide victims have a high degree of contact with their doctors in the immediate period before the act, it behoves every doctor to be alert to these forebodings.

The family of the victim

Bereavement following suicide is frequently associated with many conflicting emotions. Feelings of guilt are the most common, with family members wondering if they could have done more to prevent the tragedy. Others feel anger and shame and articulate thoughts such as 'why did he do this to me?' These in turn may be a common source of guilt. Work in this area has shown that in all respects the duration and severity of the grief are similar to that with any death. Relatives generally find the inquest the most distressing part (Harwood *et al.* 2002) and despite their initial feelings of guilt, anger and shame welcome the support and comfort of others. There is no evidence for an increase in psychiatric illness in the family following suicide and in one study half of those interviewed felt they were better off emotionally since the suicide (Shepherd and Barraclough 1974).

When dealing with the family it is important to allow them 'space' to ventilate their true feelings. By articulating these they will eventually resolve them as with any other loss. Children are the most vulnerable family members and many will have been living in an environment which was far from satisfactory prior to the suicide. Many adults underestimate the child's capacity to understand and it is important to approach each child individually. Allowing the child time to grieve and answering his questions sympathetically is the most satisfactory approach if he too is not to carry the stigma of his parent's misfortune.

Summary

- Deliberate self-harm (parasuicide) is a behaviour with diverse motivations. The most urgent concern is that of suicide intent.
- Suicide intent is assessed by direct questioning and where it is high the patient requires hospitalization to reduce the immediate risk of suicide irrespective of whether illness is present or not.
- Hopelessness is especially associated with the future risk of suicide.
- Family and personal crises rather than psychiatric illness are the backdrop against which DSH occurs.
- Attempts at primary and secondary prevention have so far failed.
- Most of those who die by suicide suffer from psychiatric illness, of which depressive illness is the most common.
- There is debate about the role of the doctor in suicide prevention and it is argued that a combined medical and socio-political approach is best. Prediction of suicide is not possible due to its rarity
- The recognition and vigorous treatment of depressive illness is essential.

References

Barbui, C., Esposito, E., and Capriani, A. (2009). Selective serotonin re-uptake inhibitors and risk of suicide: a systematic review of observational studies. *Canadian Medical Association Journal*, **180**, 291–297.

Bennewith, O., Stocks, N., Gunnell, D., *et al.* (2002). General Practice based intervention to prevent repeat episodes of deliberate self harm: cluster randomised controlled trial. *British Medical Journal*, **324**(7348), 1254–1257.

Boer, H., Booth, N., Russell, D., Powell, R., and Briscoe, M. (1996). Antidepressant prescribing prior to suicide: role of doctors. *Psychiatric Bulletin*, **20**, 282–284.

Durkheim, E. (1951). *Suicide: a Study in Sociology* (translated by J. A. Spaulding and G. Simpson). Glencoe, IL: Free Press.

Evans, K., Tyrer, P., Catalan, J., *et al.* (1999). Manual assisted cognitive-behaviour therapy (MACT): a randomised controlled trial of a brief intervention with bibliography in the treatment of recurrent deliberate self-harm. *Psychological Medicine*, **29**(1), 19–25.

Foster, T., Gillespie, K., McClelland, R., and Patterson C. (1999). Risk factors for suicide independent of DSM-111 axis 1 diagnosis. Case-control psychological autopsy study in Northern Ireland. *British Journal of Psychiatry*, **175**, 175–179.

Gairin, L., House, A., and Owens, A. (2003). Attendance at the accident and emergency department in the year before suicide; retrospective study. *British Journal of Psychiatry*, **183**, 28–33.

Gunnell, D., Bennewith, O., Peters, T. J., *et al.* (2002). Do patients who self-harm consult their general practitioners soon after hospital discharge? A cohort study. *Social Psychiatry and Psychiatric Epidemiology*, **37**, 599–602.

Gunnell, D., Saperia, J., and Ashby, D. (2005). Selective serotonin re-uptake inhibitors (SSRIs) and suicide in adults: meta-analysis of drug company data from placebo controlled, randomized controlled trials submitted to the MHRAs safety review. *British Medical Journal*, **330**(7488), 385.

Harwood, D., Hawton, K., Hope, T., and Jacoby, R. (2002). The grief experiences and needs of bereaved relatives and friends of older people dying through suicide: a descriptive and case control study. *Journal of Affective Disorders*, **72**, 185–194.

Hawton, K., Bergen, H., Casey, D., *et al.* (2007). Self-harm in England: a tale of three cities. *Social Psychiatry and Psychiatric Epidemiology*, **42**, 513–521.

Henriksson, M. M., Aro, H. M., Marttunen, M. J., Heikkinen, M. E., *et al.* (1993). Mental disorders and co-morbidity in suicide. *American Journal of Psychiatry*, **150**, 935–940.

Houston, K., Haw, C., Townsend, E., and Hawton, K. (2003). General practitioner contact with patients before and after deliberate self-harm. *British Journal of Psychiatry*, **53**, 365–370.

Isaac, M., Elias, B., Katz, L. Y., *et al.* (2009). Gatekeeper training as a preventive intervention for suicide: a systematic review. *Canadian Journal of Psychiatry*, **54**(4), 260–268.

Kelleher, M. (1996). *Suicide and the Irish*. Dublin: Mercier Press.

Linehan, M. M., Heard, H. L., and Armstrong, H. E. (1993). Naturalistic follow-up of behavioural therapy for chronically parasuicidal borderline patients. *Archives of General Psychiatry*, **50**, 971–974.

NICE Clinical Guideline 16. (2004). *Self-harm. The Short Term Physical and Psychological Management of and Secondary Prevention of Self-Harm in Primary and Secondary Care.* London: National Institute of Clinical Excellence.

NICE Clinical Guideline 77. (2007). *Borderline Personality Disorder. Treatment, Management and Prevention.* London: National Institute of Clinical Excellence.

National Institute for Clinical Excellence (NICE). (2009). Depression: the treatment and management of depression in adults (update). Oct. 2009. http:guidance.nice.org.uk/CG90.

National Suicide Research Foundation. (2008). National Registry of Deliberate Self Harm. Annual Report 2006/2007.

Rutz, W., von Knorring, L., and Walinder J. (1992). Long term effects of an educational programme for general practitioners by the Swedish Committee for the Prevention and Treatment of Depression. *Acta psychiatrica Scandinavica*. **85**. 83–88.

Shepherd, D., and Barraclough, B. M. (1974). The aftermath of suicide. *British Medical Journal*, **2**, 600–603.

Simon, G., and Savarino, J. E. (2007). Suicide attempts among patients starting depression treatments with medications or psychotherapy. *American Journal of Psychiatry*, **164**, 1029–1034.

Simon, G., Savarino, J. E., Operskalski, B., and Wang, P. S. (2006). Suicide risk during antidepressant treatment. *American Journal of Psychiatry*, **163**, 41–47.

Suokas, J., and Lönnqvist, J. (1991). Outcome of attempted suicide and psychiatric consultation: risk factors and suicide mortality during a five-year follow-up. *Acta Psychiatrica Scandinavica*, **84**(6), 545–549.

Suokas, T., Souminen, K., Isomesta, E., *et al.* (2004). Long-term risk factors for suicide mortality after attempted suicide – findings of a 14 year follow-up study. *Acta psychiatrica Scandinavica*, **104**, 117–121.

Tiihonen, J., Lönnqvist, J., Wahlbeck, K., *et al.* (2006). Antidepressants and the risk of suicide, attempted suicide and overall mortality in a nationwide cohort. *Archives of General Psychiatry*, **63**, 1358–1367.

Whitley, E., Gunnell, D., Dorling, D., and Smith G D. (1999). Ecological study of social fragmentation, poverty and suicide. *British Medical Journal*, **309**, 860–861.

Wilkinson, G. (1994). Can suicide be prevented? Better treatment of mental illness is a more appropriate aim. *British Medical Journal*, **309**, 860–86l.

Further reading

Boer, H., Booth, N., Russell, D., Powell, R., and Briscoe, M. (1996). Antidepressant prescribing prior to suicide: role of doctors. *Psychiatric Bulletin*, **20**, 282–284.

Crawford, M. J., and Wessely, S. (2000). The management of patients following deliberate self-harm – what happens to those discharged from hospital to GP. *Primary Care Psychiatry*, **6**, 61–65.

Durkheim, F. (1975). *Suicide*. London: Routledge and Kegan Paul.

Hawton, K., and van Heeringen, K. (eds.). (1987). Assessment of suicide risk. *British Journal of Psychiatry*, **150**, 145–153.

Kreitman, N. (1989). Can suicide and parasuicide be prevented? *Journal of Royal Society of Medicine*, **82**, 648–652.

Luoma, J. B., Martin, C. E., and Pearson, J. L. (2002). Contact with mental health and primary care providers before suicide: a review of the evidence. *American Journal of Psychiatry*, **159**, 909–916.

Suggested reading for patients and families

Jamison, K. R. (1999). *Night Falls Fast. Understanding Suicide*. London: Picador.

Lucas, C., and Seiden H M. (2007). *Silent Grief: Living in the Wake of Suicide*. London: Jessica Kingsley Publishers.

Schmidt, U., and Davidson, K. (2004) *Life After Self-harm. A Guide to the Future*. Hove: Routledge.

Useful telephone numbers

The Samaritans ....
(please fill in your local number here)

Console. Living with Suicide (Ireland). 1800201890.

Survivors of Bereavement by Suicide (UK). 08445616855

Problems of the mind and body

The mind–body divide

Since Descartes the medical profession and others have systematically differentiated between problems of the mind and body. While this has been important for developments in the fields of psychology and psychiatry it is now generally recognized that there are significant disadvantages for patients and that the separation of the two is unhelpful for an integrated formulation of patients' problems and for determining the best management plans.

This chapter deals with the general issues relating to the mind–body divide and focuses on the problems of medically unexplained symptoms and the growing issue of ongoing psychological problems related to long-term physical conditions. It also covers a group of miscellaneous conditions with physical and mental health symptoms. This is indeed a wide array of diagnoses found in a variety of locations within the ICD and DSM classification systems. At one extreme we have what is seen as the physical manifestations of 'mental' problems or psychological trauma, and at the other extreme the psychological results and responses of having to bear a long-term physical condition.

But one spectrum is an over-simplification when reaching for a unified integrated approach to understanding symptoms and disease. For example, physical symptoms are virtually universal within so called psychiatric diseases. For example tiredness and the slowing down of the bodily functions are common in depression; palpitations and sweating are seen almost universally in panic disorder and hallucinations are disorders of our physical perception. Similarly psychological and emotional symptoms are common to most so-called physical illnesses, and not just as a response to them. The brain is the organ responsible for perception and pain is mediated and expressed through the brain. In itself pain is not a special sensory ability, but is perceived as a result of problems either at the end organ or throughout the sensory system of the various sensory abilities (touch, pressure, heat). Our emotional response to pain is almost immediate and the combination of our emotional response and the pain itself affects function – the end result of the illness causing the pain. This interlinking of pain, function and emotion was demonstrated by Bair *et al.* (2008).

In the past some psychiatrists and psychotherapists have gone further and argued that many physical illnesses are actually caused by emotional problems. For example, Type A personality has been linked to heart disease and was seen by some as the main cause. While this extreme position is now no longer accepted, a more nuanced one, where biological, social and psychological factors are seen as important in both aetiology and management of all conditions, has emerged. This position still allows and encourages exploration of complex interactions between the neurological, endocrine and immune systems: psychological trauma, emotions and the social environment can have a small or larger impact on the aetiology of a variety of conditions, such as psoriasis, ischaemic heart disease and hypertension. Even cancer may be affected by these complex mind and body processes.

For all these reasons and the fact that patients present with undifferentiated illnesses, disclose some symptoms but not others, and mix emotional and physical symptoms within their accounts of their illness, the general practitioner is well placed to help differentiate serious illness, which may be life-threatening, from other problems which are self-limiting. The general practitioner and others within primary care are also in a good position to work with the patients to develop management plans which take into account the physical and emotional aspects of illness. Thus, an integrated approach can encompass the physical and emotional causes and increase clarity and understanding about the nature and presentation of the condition. Perhaps most importantly a management plan can be developed which focuses on improved function and self-care for those with long-term conditions and provides timely referral and ongoing investigation for those with rarer, more complex conditions which require specialist psychiatric, psychological or physical expertise. We would argue that it is not always the role of the general practitioner to distinguish the physical or psychological aetiology of conditions as they present. Rather it may at times be as important to suggest that physical and psychological origins are possible causes of physical symptoms, and to demonstrate an expertise about the links between mind and body.

The remainder of this chapter focuses on more practical advice about how to deal with medically unexplained physical symptoms and other physical presentations which may have at least a partially psychological origin as well as support patients with long-term conditions with secondary emotional aspects.

Medically unexplained symptoms (MUS)

'Medically unexplained symptoms' (MUS) is, along with medically unexplained physical symptoms, the most recent name in a long line of nomenclature that attempts to encompass those conditions where mental health may have a great bearing on the presentation of physical symptoms. 'May' is the critical word and hence the change in nomenclature to avoid an inference that these conditions always have psychiatric origins.

Physical symptoms are ubiquitous within the general population and while most are unreported a significant proportion are brought to primary care. However, of those with medically unexplained symptoms less than 10% persist (De Waal *et al.* 2004), a small but significant proportion will go on to have explained symptoms (Carson *et al.* 2003), and more than 30% have symptoms which persist for 2 years or more (Craig *et al.* 1993).

This section describes some general issues, goes on to discuss system-wide and consultation-level strategies applicable to primary care, and finishes with a more detailed description of the complex different categories within the psychiatric classification.

The diversity of medically unexplained symptoms

Medically unexplained symptoms vary enormously across a number of dimensions:

- severity
- organ specificity
- predominance of anxiety or depression
- intent of the patient.

The severity is related to the intensity of the symptom load, frequency of attendance, the functional impairment and the length of time the individual has suffered from unexplained symptoms. At one extreme are those who have had symptoms for several years which significantly affect function and at the other those with transient symptoms during periods of stress. These specific syndromes as defined in the psychiatric classifications are described below (see pp. 195–197). Those seen in general practice can usually be managed in that setting and in most instances their investigations have often proved futile in discovering the cause of a range of physical symptoms. Their symptoms, while present, are not globally incapacitating and are likely to be deemed of mild or moderate severity.

At the milder end of the spectrum we have those presentations which are extremely common in general practice where relatively minor physical symptoms are present and there is no explained physical cause. These are generally not specifically classified as medically unexplained physical symptoms, but undoubtedly include individuals and conditions which will later go on to become significant in terms of duration, symptom load and functional impairment. Many, if not, of these symptoms will not have a predominant psychiatric origin, in the sense of being related to significant past trauma. They are more likely to be due to physiological imbalance in response to a variety of recent and current physiological or emotional stresses; or are due to diseases with a physical origin which have not yet differentiated and will often resolve before a full diagnosis is obvious or has been made. Importantly, a small proportion of such presentations go on to become physically explained and are life-threatening.

Organ specificity is another important dimension for medically unexplained symptoms. Some individuals have what are very much organ-specific problems, such as globus pharangius/hystericus, irritable bowel syndrome or pelvic pain syndrome. Each medical specialty, and indeed surgical, has their own particular syndromes for which no pathology is found.

Some people with medically unexplained symptoms, on the other hand, have symptoms which are multi-organ or multisystem. This may be due to the presence of a number of syndromes or due to a number of symptoms across a range of organs and with none of them reaching the criteria for, say, irritable bowel syndrome.

Pain and fatigue require special discussion. Chronic pain is included by some as part of the MUS spectrum and there is very good evidence that emotional state moderates the intensity and suffering from pain. Also those with a past history of trauma (both childhood abuse and witnessing dramatic events) have an increased propensity for chronic pain. Treatment with pharmacological techniques can be relatively successful. Aspects of chronic pain are also disputed. In particular when it presents as myalgic encephalomyelitis (or chronic fatigue syndrome) there is debate about the role of psychological or biological factors (see below).

Anxiety is a common accompaniment to the presentation of medically unexplained symptoms, but by no means universal. Mild to moderate health anxiety frequently accompanies the presentation of symptoms in general practice at the undifferentiated stage. Health anxiety is born from the combination of an individual's anxiety trait level and the way in which medicine is practised, encouraging individuals with symptoms to present to doctors. Those with more extreme anxiety focused on physical symptoms have been called hypochondriacs in the past. Some are severely disabled by the constant presentation of new symptoms which they believe might be a manifestation of significant illness. Some people recognize the anxiety and it is easier to provide immediate, but not necessarily long-term, reassurance to that subgroup.

The *intent* of the patient is relevant since there are some medically unexplained symptoms that are presented *deliberately* by the patient. In factitious disorder either symptoms are fabricated or injury is deliberately induced. The latter can include cutting and burning, but, in contrast to deliberate self-harm, the physical sign is readily presented to the doctor, and the patient does not admit their responsibility. The gain in factitious disorder is for care and attention and this is not usually recognized by the patient. In its most severe form it is called Munchausen syndrome, a phenomenon of multiple hospitalizations and surgical interventions for the gain of being cared for. Factitious disorder must be differentiated from malingering, where the gain is conscious although like factitious disorder the symptoms are knowingly exaggerated or fabricated. The gain in malingering may be to win a legal case, escape imprisonment, obtain disability payments or some such reward. These conditions are described in more detail below (see also p. 202).

The complex dimensions described above also encapsulate the underlying tensions amongst physicians and others regarding the aetiology and therefore the best management for these conditions. Psychiatrists and psychotherapists tend to see these conditions in terms of the patient's history, often one of past abuse, ongoing psychiatric conditions and the need for therapy. On the other hand there are those, particularly with an interest in pain and fatigue, who see these conditions as having a physical origin that is as yet unexplained. Our view is that both these perspectives have their merits and that the role in primary care is to ensure that treatable or life-threatening diagnoses are identified early, that manifest psychiatric illnesses are identified and discussed with the patient and that understandable emotional responses to distressing physical symptoms are managed positively in a primary care setting. Perhaps most importantly, functional ability for those with long-term problems should be the focus of a bio-psychosocial approach.

A systems approach to medically unexplained symptoms

Figure 12.1 depicts the system through which patients with medically unexplained symptoms flow. Very few in fact reach psychiatrists and psychologists, partly because the patients themselves are resistant, and also because expertise is limited with the NHS and other health

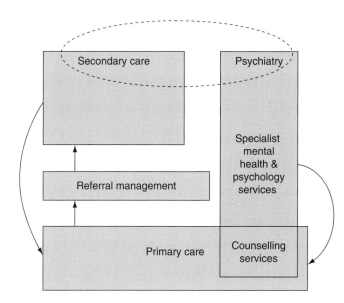

Figure 12.1. Representation of Plymouth Healthcare System. A pictorial representation of the current health care system within Plymouth

care systems. Most patients are contained within primary care, but a significant proportion reach secondary care specialties and some are managed by mental health professionals embedded within their teams.

A number of attempts have been made to calculate the financial impact of the ongoing care and investigations of people with medically unexplained symptoms. While some have estimated that up to 10% of the budget of the NHS is taken up with medically unexplained symptoms (Bermingham *et al.* 2010) this is probably an overestimate, but even if it is 3% there is significant potential for shifting budget from investigation to management, focused on improving function.

This perspective is based on the assumption that over the years we have been over-medicalizing and causing iatrogenic harm to patients with medically unexplained symptoms. As doctors we are both promoting the idea that there is likely to be a physical cause and potentially causing physical harm whenever we investigate or refer on to a medical specialist. The Plymouth Medically Unexplained Symptoms Project focused on a systems approach (NHS Evidence 2008) and made the assumption that we should be aiming to shift the balance away from referral and over-investigation towards improving the functional status of people with medically unexplained symptoms. Figure 12.2 shows diagrammatically the potential pathways for individual patients from primary care where every examination, investigation or referral to secondary care can result in increased expenditure and potential damage.

The assumption is that we need to shift the balance of the patient pathways towards the left-hand side of the diagram, reducing those referred on to secondary care.

Table 12.1 outlines the main clinical changes that would be required to achieve this shift. As well as changes to communication within the consultation with both primary and secondary care, significant system-level policies could be introduced to support these changes. These focus on positive risk management where governance for Provider Trusts and Commissioning Trusts takes responsibility for encouraging practitioners to reduce the emphasis on investigation. In addition to these system-level approaches education will be

Table 12.1. Summary of key changes required to clinical practice

Changes to primary care consultations (as a means of micro-commissioning):
Empathize and acknowledge symptoms
In MUS cases at low risk of disease, investigation and referral may not be required – clinicians can 'share risk' by discussing with patient, specialist or colleagues (and documenting)
In suspected MUS cases, when referring for investigation or specialist opinion, patient should be informed of likely 'negative' results in order to manage expectations
Inform specialists of likely MUS in referral letters (rather than feeling need to justify referral but emphasizing symptoms)
Offer and explore, but don't push, psychosocial explanation
Focus on improving functional ability
Recognize and treat comorbid anxiety and depression

Changes to specialist consultations:
In suspected MUS cases, when referring for investigation, patient should be informed of likely 'negative' results in order to manage expectations
Once low risk of disease established further investigation may not be required – clinicians can 'share risk' by discussing with patient and/or colleagues (and documenting)
Discharge to primary care once investigations are complete with clear negative results
Respond to GPs provisional MUS diagnosis and actively support it verbally to patient and in writing to GP
Offer and explore, but don't push, psychosocial explanation
Recognize and treat comorbid anxiety and depression

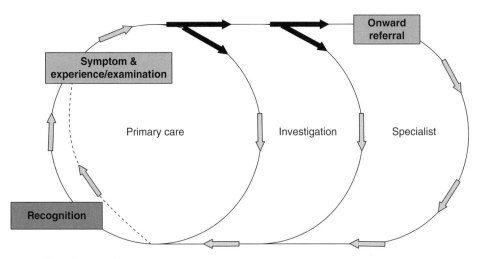

Figure 12.2. Patient pathways

required and the introduction of simple techniques to share risk amongst clinicians at local level. Many of these elements are illustrated in Case 1 below.

Case 1

Mr X was a 30-year-old man who first came to the attention of his general practitioner with a range of neurological symptoms, including dizziness, feelings of water running down inside his head, twitching of his muscles and abdominal pain. He had also been seen by a cardiologist the previous year and had reduced his work to half time, because of fears of ill health. He then presented with a further episode of pleuritic chest pain for which no cause was found. By this stage he was coming to see several of the doctors in the practice two or three times a week, as well as being followed up in several outpatient clinics.

The GPs discussed him as a critical case in a team meeting and agreed that one practitioner would take over his care to provide consistency. He was offered regular appointments which he generally took, but still came back in between with other complaints. He became increasingly angry that his symptoms were not being taken seriously and whenever the practitioners mentioned the possibility that he was anxious or depressed he resisted making the link between his stress levels and physical symptoms. Over time and ongoing communication with several specialists who were seeing him he gradually came to see that ongoing referrals were not helping him. Thereafter there was a gradual reduction in his attendance and after 6 months he went back to full-time employment in a different job. He also agreed that he had been stressed, although persisted in believing that there was a physical cause for the low-level persistent symptoms which never actually went away.

Comment

Medically unexplained symptoms such as this are not unusual in general practice. Often, however, the resolution is not as clear-cut as in this case. Management requires a combination of patience and a curiosity as to what success in treatment would look like. It often requires consistency and team working, as well as liaison with other services. Most of all it demands that GPs prioritize improved function as much as if not more than a concern to avoid missing a critical diagnosis. This form of positive risk management becomes harder in our risk averse world.

Communication within the consultation

Research into consultations with patients with medically unexplained symptoms has also led to useful perspectives. The balance of the presentation of psychological and emotional symptoms depends on the culture and specifically the culture of the medical and health service. While UK physicians have recognized that patients with medically unexplained symptoms should be treated in primary care, there is considerable international variation in the involvement of general practitioners with this group of patients. Dowrick *et al.* (2004) have shown that normalization, i.e. stressing the absence of significant disease, can exacerbate patients' perception of the problem. Furthermore, GPs are more likely than their patients to recommend investigations and somatic treatments (Ring *et al.* 2005).

Since the original research highlighting the problem in terms of cost and subsequent iatrogenic impaired dysfunction several groups have been developing models and assessing *reattribution training* for physicians. The aim of the training is to realign patients' thinking to understand that a psychological problem underlies their physical symptoms. Unfortunately the evidence for the benefits of this training in terms of patient outcomes is weak, even though it improved physician confidence. In a recent UK study Morris *et al.* (2007) actually showed increased anxiety amongst the patients and no overall benefit. Also known as the MUST trial, the reattribution intervention had four elements: feeling understood; broadening the agenda to the psychosocial; making the link between the physical symptoms and psychosocial factors and negotiating further treatment. A model developed by Fink *et al.* (2002), known as TERM (The Extended Reattribution and Management), had similar aims and emphasized the diagnosis of psychiatric disorders, the need for the GP to demonstrate expertise and follow-up for the problem. Although there are likely to be benefits to many of these strategies, it appears from qualitative evidence that it is the enforcement of a psychosocial explanation on patients which causes a negative response.

Recent research (Morris *et al.* 2010) has emphasized a broader array of positive and negative behaviours within the consultation. Clearly some of these behaviours are best introduced early in the MUS cycle for those with mild symptoms and milder functional impairment and others are more appropriate later in the cycle for those with more severe impairment and ongoing medically unexplained symptoms where the focus on function is important.

Positive consultation behaviours include (Trailblazers 2010):

- listening to the patient and eliciting ideas, concerns and expectations
- fully exploring their experience as well as their worries and family background
- understanding the impact of the symptoms on function
- fully acknowledging the patient's anxiety and suffering
- linking the patients' explanations and understanding with a bio-psychosocial model as to how the symptoms arise
- pre-empting negative referral and investigational results by explaining beforehand that they are likely to be negative (this will also enforce practitioners' sense of expertise)
- sharing uncertainty and risk both with the patient and with other colleagues in order to get medico-legal cover for a decision not to refer.

Negative consultation behaviours include:

- normalizing and dismissing symptoms without an explanation
- focusing excessively on the diagnosis rather than symptoms or function
- enforcing the idea that you think something is wrong by making referrals and investigation without explaining the likelihood of a negative result
- treating symptomatically with medications without explaining possible side effects and finding out whether the patient would want these medications
- ignoring and missing psychological cues
- enforcing psychosocial explanations when resistance is present
- showing excessive anxiety or uncertainty to the patient
- feeling the need to provide a diagnosis rather than understanding the symptoms.

A number of other approaches have been identified which may be particularly useful for those with more entrenched medically unexplained symptoms (Dowrick and Rosendal 2009). These include:

- being honest with the patient about those areas where you agree and disagree
- being stoical and not expecting rapid changes or cure
- considering whether worsening symptom load is potentially the result of an emotional communication

- considering referral for specialized psychological treatment
- offering a fixed schedule of appointments at 2 to 6 weekly intervals, avoiding on-demand consultations
- avoiding providing certificates for time off work where possible
- aiming to ensure continuity with a single physician
- agreeing contingency plans with other physicians
- attempting to co-opt a relative as a therapeutic ally
- arranging support and supervision for yourself.

Several packages of guidelines are now available to assist the general practitioner in managing this challenging group of patients (NHS IAPT Guidelines 2008; NHS Evidence 2008).

Specific syndromes

The description of medically unexplained symptoms outlined above can be seen as the primary care viewpoint. There is an alternative model of classification which is relevant in the interface between general practice and psychiatry and this is the approach used in ICD-10 and DSM-IV. It consists of diagnostic categories described in this section.

Conversion and dissociative disorder (formerly hysteria)

Hysteria was recognized by Hippocrates but came to prominence in the writings of Freud. Uninformed opinion may create the impression that the symptoms are consciously produced and that the design is to gain some tangible benefit. The essence of hysteria is that there is no conscious awareness of the link between a traumatic event and the conversion of the psychological symptoms into physical symptoms. So the symptoms are not deliberately produced.

- The question of gain is confusing for many. Primary gain refers to gain that is symbolic or internal. For example a singer whose career is floundering develops aphonia – the gain allows the person to exit their career. The gain is unconscious. Secondary gain is defined as a more tangible psychological benefit such as receiving support that might not otherwise be forthcoming or controlling the behaviour of others such as family members and so on.
- In those over the age of 35, these symptoms may actually herald a serious physical illness such as incipient multiple sclerosis; it is this concern that understandably worries many doctors.
- While the symptoms usually resolve after the triggering stressor is removed this does not always occur.

Conversion disorder

Conversion disorder is characterized by the presence of one or more neurological symptoms. These include anaesthesia, disturbance of gait including paralysis or loss of sight or speech and other neurological symptoms. These cannot be explained by known medical or neuro-logical disorders. When making the diagnosis, it is necessary to identify two elements – a trauma that triggers the symptoms and primary gain. This diagnosis is now seldom made and then only after physical illness and other psychiatric disorders such as depressive illness have been ruled out completely. In view of the restricted criteria for making the diagnosis *that must include a psychological conflict and secondary gain*, it is apparent that, of itself, the absence of an organic cause for symptoms is not a basis on which to make this diagnosis.

Conversion disorder is uncommon and the symptoms are often focused on organs which have been injured or damaged previously. There is an excess of those with conversion disorder amongst those attending neurological and ear, nose and throat clinics. It is twice as common amongst women as compared with men. It is also more common amongst those with low IQ and those with poor education.

Treatment initially consists of physiotherapy directed at the affected organ. This allows the patient a channel for symptomatic improvement. Later the conflicts leading to the symptoms need to be explored. Abreaction, that is the exploration of conflicts when the patient is relaxed using intravenous medication, is also used if symptoms do not improve rapidly. Whilst in this state, the therapist explores the possible underlying stressors that may have been kept from consciousness through the patient's defences and, while still used, the evidence base is limited to anecdote.

Dissociative disorder

Dissociative disorder, like conversion disorder, is viewed as self-defence against a traumatic event. It serves the purpose of psychologically or physically removing the person from the trauma. When well the person has a unified sense of self. While in the throes of stress this sense of self is fragmented and may manifest itself as amnesia or (controversially) as multiple personalities.

Dissociative disorder is less common than conversion disorder and amnesia is probably the most common presentation. Memory for personal identity is impaired but other aspects of memory, such as that for skills, is intact. Whilst it can occur spontaneously most patients have experienced an emotionally painful trauma. Localized amnesia is the most common. Sometimes amnesia is associated with wandering away from home and being found in another location, usually in a distressed state. This is termed a fugue state. Whilst traditional thinking focused on psychodynamic explanations such as repression, modern research emphasizes the possibility of flaws in the underlying neuroanatomical and neurotransmitter systems.

Somatoform disorders

This is a group of disorders in which the patient presents with physical symptoms in the absence of physical cause and with persistent requests for medical investigations, unlike conversion and dissociative disorder, where symptoms are not associated with distress or repeated requests for investigations. Somatoform disorders are also less dramatic than conversion or dissociative disorders. Management by individual practitioners is to limit investigations where possible and form a therapeutic alliance as described above.

The aetiology of somatoform disorders is not understood, although vulnerability factors include a family or childhood history of serious or prolonged physical illness. Precipitants to actual symptoms include physical traumas and personal stresses, and the disorders may be perpetuated by relationships in which the attention of the partner serves to meet needs such as dependence, punishment or responsibility avoidance. However, the most common perpetuating factor is the manner in which the symptoms are dealt with by the doctor. In particular numerous physical investigations are likely to reinforce the symptoms.

Somatization disorder

This is a one syndrome in the somatoform disorder group. It is characterized by the presence of physical symptoms that cannot be explained by other disorders such as depressive illness, or by any physical explanation. The focus may be on one or multiple organs, the Latter being called Briquet's syndrome. Somatization disorder usually begins before the age of 30, affects less than 1% of the population and the symptoms often involve a multiplicity of organs and numerous investigations. It has to be present for 2 years and significantly affect function. The person is often reluctant to accept psychiatric intervention and may go to great lengths to identify an organic cause, sometimes paying personally for intricate and expensive investigations.

Somatoform pain disorder

This often presents in the context of medico-legal proceedings following an accident. Typically, the person sustains soft-tissue injury and this persists long after there is any evidence of tissue damage. This may delay return to work and activities and because of insomnia be associated with other psychological symptoms such as irritability, low mood, tearfulness and reduced concentration. However, the most important facet of somatoform pain disorder is the role of behavioural factors in maintaining the pain, such as the legal process with multiple medical consultations reinforcing the sick role. It is possible that structural and chemical abnormalities in the central nervous system's modulation of pain may also play a role, although work in this area is in its infancy. Optimum management includes acceptance of the reality of the pain experience and utilizing a cognitive/behaviour approach to living with the associated discomfort. Antidepressants also have an effect on the intensity of the pain, even in the absence of depression. The prognosis varies and there are no long-term studies of outcome in this condition but anecdotal evidence that those involved in litigation, those with chronic pain and those with long-standing personality and interpersonal problems, especially dependence, have the poorest outcome.

Somatoform autonomic dysfunction

This is a description of a constellation of organ symptoms under the control of the autonomic nervous system. It is not included in DSM-IV but is retained in ICD-10 and presents with sweating, tremor and palpitations that are not due to panic.

Other related conditions

Body dysmorphic disorder

Those with body dysmorphic disorder (BDD) (formerly termed dysmorphobia) believe that a part or parts of the body, such as the nose, ears, etc., are seriously disfigured. Sometimes there may be a minor abnormality that is exaggerated but there may be none. This belief is associated with demands for cosmetic surgery, but meeting this request does not result in improvement or if there is a reduction in the preoccupation regarding one organ, it shifts to another. As a result there are repeated requests for surgery and often the patient pursues litigation as dissatisfaction is inevitable. In addition to this excessive concern there is significant avoidance of everything from reflective surfaces to socializing. Sometimes long periods are spent mirror gazing and checking the perceived abnormality, and relationships may be placed under great strain due to the continuous focus on appearance.

Deliberate self-harm is common during periods of feeling overwhelmed by the perceived abnormality. It may also manifest with anxiety symptoms such as fear of being in crowds, with the underlying problem only identified on detailed questioning. There is often a history of various forms of childhood abuse and personality disorder is a common co-occurring disorder.

Cosmetic surgeons and physicians are aware of this condition as it is found in up to 7% of their clientele and up to 12% of those attending dermatology clinics, yet it can be difficult to identify until a number of operations have taken place and the patient's displeasure becomes apparent. Therefore, when a person presents with a relatively minor blemish about which there appears to be an excessive preoccupation, BDD should be considered, along with treatment if the patient is willing.

The beliefs and preoccupations about disease and disfigurement are not of delusional intensity, but, should this occur, the condition is referred to as persistent delusional disorder (formerly called monosymptomatic delusional psychosis or MDP) and treated with major tranquillizers.

A combination of CBT and medication can lead to 50% symptom reduction in those with BDD who adhere to treatment. Unfortunately those who suffer from BDD and MDP are often hostile to doctors, since they perceive that the medical profession has no interest in them. The potential for allegations of negligence being made against doctors in these circumstances is significant.

Hypochondriasis

This differs subtly from somatization disorder in that the focus is on an illness rather than on specific symptoms. The person with hypochondriasis has an excessive preoccupation with the possibility of serious physical illness. It is thought to result from the person's inaccurate interpretation of bodily sensations. A diagnosis of hypochondriasis should not be made when the misinterpretation is due to lack of knowledge; for example, the person who misinterprets the chest pain of a panic attack as due to a heart attack. It afflicts men and women equally and up to 6% of medical outpatients are said to have hypochondriasis.

Management is often undermined by well-meaning friends who advise seeking treatment elsewhere or by alternative therapists who might make spurious diagnoses of allergies, etc. These disorders tend to be long-term conditions that impact gravely upon the patients and family members. Treatment is difficult and the doctor should avoid the pitfalls of repeated intensive investigations and of benzodiazepine prescriptions. Cognitive therapy has been used with some success in some patients. Management consists of reducing physical investigations to a minimum and assisting the person in learning to live with the symptoms.

Psychiatric manifestations of physical illness

Many physical conditions are known to be closely associated with affective and other psychiatric disturbances. These are not simply reactions to physical illness (see below) but are an inherent part of the illness itself. The psychological symptoms may even occur prior to the physical illness being diagnosed and this is especially true with carcinoma of the bronchus or of the pancreas and lymphomas, particularly Hodgkin's disease. Manic and schizophrenic presentations are much less common than depression.

There is a strong link between neurological disorders and psychological disturbances, especially depression. Following a cerebrovascular accident, depression is frequently described. This is not due solely to the physical incapacity resulting from such disorders but is related also to the site of the lesion. Right-sided infarcts in the posterior cortex are most likely to be associated with depression. Catastrophic reactions and dementia may occur also. Multiple sclerosis is associated with both depression, mania and dementia and these are related to the degree of central nervous system involvement. Contrary to the belief that such disturbances do not respond to antidepressants, there is strong evidence that pharmacological intervention can bring about a dramatic response. Parkinson's disease is also associated with a higher than expected occurrence of depression, as is Huntington's chorea and epilepsy. On occasions temporal lobe epilepsy may be confused with schizophrenia, especially when perceptual disturbances predominate. These normally subside when the epilepsy is brought under control.

Endocrine disorders such as hypoglycaemia may occasionally present with acute confusional states or with hypomania. Hyperthyroidism may be associated with anxiety, hypomania or depression in hyperthyroidism or with depression and paranoid illnesses in hypothyroidism. Mood disturbances also occur in Cushing's syndrome. Autoimmune disorders, especially systemic lupus erythematosus, are associated with a variety of psychological conditions when there is cerebral involvement. Of these depression is the most common.

Controversial diagnoses

A number of conditions have both physical and psychological components to their aetiology and/or presentation. These have also been hotly debated.

Premenstrual dysphoric disorder

Premenstrual syndrome is a general term for the physical, psychological and physiological changes that occur in the luteal phase of the menstrual cycle. Premenstrual dysphoric disorder (PMDD) is the more specific term used to describe a condition in which mood symptoms predominate. It is recognized as a psychiatric disorder in DSM-IV although this is controversial. It is estimated that 2–10% of women meet the criteria for PMDD. However, some may erroneously believe they have PMDD when in fact the premenstrual exacerbation is due to an underlying condition that is common in many psychiatric conditions such as depressive illness.

Twin studies strongly support a genetic contribution to PMDD, while others have suggested a high oestrogen to progesterone ratio. Serotonin has been found to be low in blood and platelets as well as showing decreased uptake during the luteal phase of the cycle. Other theories focus on societal and personal issues relating to womanhood.

The clinical features are a mixture of psychological and physical symptoms that occur in the premenstrual phase of most cycles and remit in the week post-menstruation. These consist of depression, hopelessness, anxiety, tension, lability of mood, irritability or anger, decreased interest in usual activities, tiredness, increased or decreased appetite, hypersomnia or insomnia, weight gain, feeling bloated, breast discomfort and feelings of being overwhelmed or out of control resulting in impairment in occupational and interpersonal functioning. Irritability is one of the most common symptoms in the condition and one that probably has most impact on others.

Many non-pharmacological treatments are of unproven efficacy but remain popular for mild symptoms and in those who do not wish to take pharmacological agents. These include aerobic exercise, reduction in caffeine intake, relaxation exercise and high-fibre and low-salt diets, the latter being useful only when symptoms due to fluid retention are prominent. There is some evidence for the benefits of cognitive therapy and of PMS support groups. If PMS impacts negatively on the family or the family response is abnormal then family therapy may be useful.

Of the pharmacological treatments oral contraceptives continue to be prescribed yet there is no evidence that psychological symptoms improve and they may even become more severe. The SSRIs are the most effective treatment for PMS (Brown *et al.* 2009) and there appears to be no difference between individual products, although the slight difference in side-effect profile suggests that citalopram and fluoxetine have fewer sexual side effects. Unlike the antidepressant response, the response in PMS occurs very rapidly. This makes the intermittent use of SSRIs, during the luteal phase only, a possibility that is more acceptable than continuous dosage to many women. Cloimipramine and venlefaxine have also been found to be effective. Antidepressants should be discontinued after about 1 year to evaluate symptom recurrence. Buspirone and alprazolam are supported by some empirical evidence and diuretics are of use if cyclical weight gain is evident, although their efficacy in other symptoms is uncertain. Pyridoxine (vitamin B6), calcium supplements and L-tryptophan may be effective. There is no evidence for the benefits of herbal remedies and evening primrose oil in spite of their popularity.

Chronic fatigue syndrome

Chronic fatigue syndrome (CFS) defies classification and three aetiological views have been expressed, viewing it as either psychiatric, physical or straddling both. The condition has attracted unprecedented interest and even the name has caused controversy, with the term myalgic encephalomyelitis (ME) implying a strong organic basis, and seen by some as a separate entity caused by CNS inflammation.

The debate has abated somewhat in recent years although there is still no consensus on the most likely cause. However, it is now recognized that it is frequently preceded by infection with EBV, Q fever or viral meningitis but not the common respiratory infections. Varicella has recently been implicated.

The prominence of fatigue and myalgia has led some to suggest that CFS is a disorder of neuromuscular function. EMG studies have confirmed abnormalities of muscle structure but function is not impaired, suggesting that the abnormalities are consequent upon disuse, a common result of the symptoms.

The suggestion that it is primarily a psychiatric disorder evokes negative reactions from some doctors and the majority of patients, although up to two-thirds of patients with CFS meet the diagnostic criteria for major depression, anxiety disorder or somatization disorder. It is likely that there is overlap in the diagnostic criteria, making the finding of a high prevalence for psychiatric disorder an artefact. Alternatively CFS may be a variant of depression but without the negative beliefs and cognitions.

CFS effects between 0.2 and 0.5% of the population and occurs equally in both sexes. Excluding those who have a clearly diagnosable organic condition, three groups emerge: those who, as well as having a clear-cut depressive illness, complain of fatigue and myalgia; those who develop the symptoms of fatigue over several months, becoming increasingly concerned at its impact on their lives, but are willing to engage in treatment; and, the most difficult to treat, those who believe strongly that their continuing symptoms are due to an external cause such as a virus, often reinforced by family, friends, alternative practitioners, internet sites or support groups.

This latter group may come to regard rest as an essential component of management based on the 'energy-bank' model. This says that each person has a limited supply of energy, which if used too quickly causes a deficit (overdraft) requiring rest to replenish it. This theory is validated for them by the fact that they suffer fatigue even after simple exercise. These patients are likely to oppose any efforts to introduce a graded exercise programme and also often subscribe to theories that allergies, yeast infections and vitamin deficiencies contribute to the illness.

CFS is diagnosed when the patient describes fatigue for more than 6 months that interferes with everyday activity by 50% or more. Generalized muscle pains, post-exertional fatigue and mental fatigue, such as poor concentration and difficulty thinking and focusing, are also prominent. Sleep, although normal in quantity, is not refreshing and headaches, painful glands and a feverish sensation (but no actual rise in temperature) are also described. Depressed mood and anxiety are often secondary to the incapacity. Routine tests are probably all that are required in the presence of a normal physical examination and typical history. Other investigations should be determined by the history and physical abnormalities since these may reinforce the patient's belief that CFS is a disease process that further tests will eventually identify. See general advice on consultations for MUS (p.194).

Poor prognosis is associated with long duration of symptoms, with exclusive physical attribution of the symptoms and with belonging to a support group. Children and adolescents have a better prognosis, while continuing medical investigations or granting early retirement worsens the outcome also. Without treatment the outcome is poor, with between 13 and 18% improving after 1 year of treatment and only 6% becoming symptom-free.

The relationship between doctor and patient is especially important in the disorder due to the anger and mistrust which these patients experience. Reassurance that the symptoms are taken seriously and not just regarded as 'all in the mind' has to be balanced against colluding with the patient's belief that the symptoms are purely of organic origin. The cornerstone of treatment is graded activity. Many will have been cautioned against activity and will describe worsening myalgia and fatigue following exercise. Activity must be gradual and balanced, and 'boom and bust' exercise, a common feature of sufferers, must be avoided, as must total inactivity. Patients must also be informed that myalgia will increase temporarily after activity begins but coupled with suitable rest periods is not damaging and is part of recovery. Antidepressants can be used when depressive illness accompanies the disorder. Analgesics have little effect on myalgia and there is no evidence that vitamins, nutritional supplements or specific dietary exclusions are helpful.

Fibromyalgia

There is also debate about the existence of this condition. Some regard it as mainly psychiatric in origin while others regard it as physical. Most cases are treated by rheumatologists. It is recognized that there is a greater than chance association between the condition and comorbid depressive illness. It is believed to be closely related to CFS (see above) except that in the latter fatigue predominates over pain while in fibromyalgia the pattern is reversed.

The aetiology is believed to be varied and theories include immunological, stress-related, hereditary and pain-signalling causes. Each has its adherents and detractors. It is more common in women and is sometimes found in association with arthritic or immunological disorders. Treatment is broad and consists of low-impact exercise, a diet that excludes alcohol and caffeine, and tricyclic antidepressants to reduce muscle pain and spasm and induce sleep. More recently the SNRI duloxetine has been used and pregabalin has recently become the first medication licensed for use specifically in fibromyalgia. It is believed to work by blocking nerve pain.

Feigned conditions

Some may be surprised to see a section on feigned disorders in this book. However, in some instances individuals consult about symptoms that on the face of it seem genuine, but the motivations are primary or secondary gain.

Factitious disorder

This is a condition in which symptoms, usually physical but at times psychiatric, are intentionally produced with the objective of assuming the patient role. It is commonly referred to as Munchausen's syndrome after the fantastic tales of adventure described by that Baron. The patient's behaviour is directed at gaining admission to hospital or having multiple physical investigations. Sometimes urine or blood may be deliberately contaminated to achieve this end or stitches may be tampered with. Symptoms are often exotic, false names may be used and there may be a history of multiple operations. So convincing is the patient that preventing yet further investigations can be very difficult. The psychodynamic causes of factitious disorder are poorly understood since it is difficult to engage these patients in therapy. Anecdotal evidence is that many patients have a history of emotional deprivation, rejection or sexual abuse in childhood and frequent hospitalizations at that time. The perception of nurses, doctors, etc. as carers rather than parents is recapitulated in the later sick role. A related but controversial diagnosis is Munchausen's syndrome by proxy (factitious disorder by proxy) in which a parent, usually a mother, harms the child in order to vicariously gain attention for herself. One of the problems with this diagnosis is that it is based on a subjective assessment by a third party as to motivation after all other possible causes for the child's signs and symptoms have been explored. This means even considering rare causes such as metabolic and dietary disorders.

Malingering

Malingering is diagnosed when symptoms are feigned for the purpose of external gain such as compensation following road traffic accidents, repatriation from combat or avoidance of imprisonment for criminal offences. It is a difficult diagnosis to make and care must be taken to obtain *objective* information concerning symptoms and functioning. It can be considered as a possible diagnosis where there is the likelihood of gain from the symptoms and where there is a discrepancy between dysfunction and symptoms.

Treatment of malingering and factitious disorder is very difficult since the sufferer has a specific treatment agenda and is commonly unwilling to engage in further emotional exploration. Often the focus is containment and avoidance of admission by alerting hospitals and colleagues to the treatment-seeking habits of these patients. There are no adequate studies of outcome in feigned disorders.

Psychiatric symptoms associated with commonly used medications

An increasing proportion of psychiatric disturbance, especially depression, is due to pre-scribed drugs. The affective disturbance covers the whole range from mild to severe psychotic depression. Those with drug-induced depression frequently have either a past or a family history of affective disorder. Antidepressants are not usually required since discontinuing the offending drug causes an improvement. If, however, symptoms persist then the treatment is as for depressive illness. Antihypertensives are amongst the most commonly cited offenders, nowadays most commonly α- and β-receptor blockers rather than reserpine and methyldopa.

Depression has been reported as a frequent complication of the use of oral contraceptives and the reported incidence has varied from 2 to 40%. This is the most common reason for discontinuation. The proposed mechanism is that high doses of oestrogen cause a deficiency of pyridoxine which in turn impairs the metabolism of 5-hydroxytryptamine, the neuro-transmitter which is believed to be responsible for depression. However, the addition of pyridoxine did not prove effective when investigated in controlled studies.

Corticosteroids have frequently been reported as causing depression and less commonly hypomania or mania. One of the difficulties is that these drugs are widely used in medicine for conditions which themselves are associated with psychiatric complications. Non-steroidal anti-inflammatory agents have also been reportedly associated with depression although this may be associated with the conditions for which they are prescribed rather than the drugs themselves.

Major tranquillizers have long been considered a possible cause of depression and there have been many reports of suicide. Although depression is recognized as a common symptom in schizophrenia, it is only in recent years that the extent of this has been fully appreciated, and much of the depression, presumed due to treatment, may be part of the illness itself. A further confounding factor is the presence of insight into the nature of the illness together with the extrapyramidal side effects which occur. Both of these may them-selves contribute to changes in mood. Other drugs such as laevodopa and cytotoxic agents, especially the vinka alkaloids, have a similar association with depression and recently the anti-acne drug isotretinoim has been implicated in causing depression and possibly suicide, although this link is complicated by the possibility that young people with severe acne may have low mood secondary to this. The patient information leaflet now contains a warning that those taking this drug should be carefully monitored for depression.

Mental health problems of those with long-term physical conditions

This section deals with patients who have ongoing or serious physical conditions for whom there are secondary psychological symptoms. While there is now less emphasis on consid-ering the pre-existing psychological factors which may have been in themselves aetiological factors for physical conditions (e.g. type A personality and heart disease), the focus is now on identifying the comorbid psychiatric conditions and offering treatment, as it is recognized that these can influence the physical outcome.

It is now well recognized that patients with many physical conditions often have co-existing depression and/or anxiety. These problems require recognition and, if appro-priate, treatments in their own right. They also have an impact on help seeking, adherence to treatment and self-care. However, there are two major barriers to providing care for such patients:

- many patients will admit to psychological symptoms, but resist the idea of a psychiatric diagnosis
- many patients with significant physical problems, such as stroke and arthritis, are elderly and have limited access to health care facilities, being partially or fully restricted to living at home.

The Quality and Outcomes Framework Document for the GP contract has, since 2006, recommended screening people with diabetes and heart disease for depression. Two questions have been demonstrated as a useful way of detecting or recognizing depression in this group of patients (Arroll *et al.* 2003).

'During the last month have you often been bothered by feeling down, depressed or hopeless?'

'During the last month have you often been bothered by having little interest or pleasure in doing things?'

However, the subsequent conversation in dealing with a positive response requires skill when consulting with those who have limited access to treatment or who resist the diagnosis. For many years practice nurses and other community nurses who have supported people with physical health conditions in community health centres or at home have utilized empathy and their lay responses to distress to support people with anxiety or depression. These nurses, with limited mental health training, are now being expected to facilitate diagnosis of depression in a group of patients who may well be resistant to hearing this.

Specific medical conditions with comorbid mental health problems

One-quarter of people with diabetes are estimated to experience depression, twice the rate in the general population (Boehm *et al.* 2004). Those with depression and diabetes also typically have poorer health outcomes since it impacts on their self-management and self-care and increases health expenditure (Simon *et al.* 2005). People whose hyperglycaemic control is poor are more likely to have more severe depression than those whose glycaemic control is good (Lustman *et al.* 2000) although the direction of this association is unclear and it may be reciprocal, with depression producing hyperglycaemia and hyperglycaemia provoking depression. However, the relationship between diabetes and depression is not straightforward and a recent study found that a psychological intervention did improve mood and diabetes-related distress but not hyperglycaemic over a 3 month follow-up period. There was a significant longitudinal correlation between 'diabetes distress' and HBA1C control (Van der Ven *et al.* 2005).

Case 2

Mr D has non-insulin-dependent diabetes and ischaemic heart disease and is now aged 57. He always thought of himself as being fit and well. Emotions had rarely registered during his life and he saw himself as a traditional 'no nonsense' type of person. Following his diagnosis with angina and later diabetes he became increasingly tired, with poor sleep and irritable at home.

He attributed this to the diabetes and angina, but after some time his wife persuaded him to visit his GP. His GP was quick to diagnose depression, but was well aware that Mr D would not accept such a diagnosis easily. Initially the GP did not press for a formal diagnosis or treatment, but after prompting by Mr D's wife he engaged in a difficult conversation about mental illness. Mr D was absolutely clear that he did not want counselling, but agreed after a few further encounters to try some antidepressants. There was little chance of any placebo effect, and indeed after 3 weeks he stopped taking his medication and declined any further trials for treatment. His life was now significantly affected by the depression, with negative thoughts about the future and increasing despondence about his ability to control both the blood sugar and his weight. He was starting to comfort eat, and one day when seeing a new practice nurse who asked him searching questions about his life and family, as well as the diabetes control, he started to see the link between emotional and physical health. He agreed to see one of the new CBT therapists in the practice, as long as he could continue to see the practice nurse. They worked together, agreeing priorities between the three of them, initially using behavioural activation approaches; later the nurse incorporated motivational interviewing supported by a psychological therapist. After 6 months hard work his diabetes was again under control, he had started gardening, had lost some weight and was beginning to feel physically more confident.

Comment

This case illustrates the interdependence of physical and mental health care conditions. It shows how many people with physical health conditions are unwilling to take on the additional stigma of a mental health diagnosis. However, by acting sensibly the GP and later particularly the practice nurse were able to engage Mr D in a treatment programme which tackled both diabetes and mental health problems together.

Chronic obstructive pulmonary disease is another illness where mental health is of considerable interest. Rates of depression are high in this group, with up to 50% suffering from depression and 67% from panic disorder. The latter is particularly critical in determining an individual's response to increasing breathlessness and the chance of an emergency admission. COPD accounts for one in eight medical admissions in the UK.

Chronic pain may be related to a known condition or be unexplained, with a significant proportion of the adult population experiencing pain and distress due to this (Gureje et al. 1998). There is a need to treat both since there is an interaction that results in increasing incapacity. Sickle cell disease is a particular example where pain can be both acute and chronic and has significant psychological consequences, causing not only anxiety and depression but a dependent lifestyle, with coping dominated by the requirement for interventions from the medical profession, particularly opiate medications. An increased emphasis on self-care can reduce distress and improve perceptions of internal control (Turk and Okifuji 2002). Rheumatoid arthritis is also associated with an increased prevalence of depression and those accessing psychological therapies early on in their illness have significantly less health care utilization (Sharpe et al. 2008).

Post-stroke depression has been estimated to effect up to 25% of patients and to have a significant influence on long-term outcome (Robinson 2003). Post-stroke depression may be partly caused by the cognitive impairment and structural changes resulting directly from the stroke, but may also be secondary to the distress of loss of function. Coronary artery bypass grafts (CABG) are also associated with higher rates of depressive illness.

Psychiatric diagnosis in those with physical illness

In all but the mildest of physical illnesses there are psychological symptoms occurring as a consequence of the symptoms and of the restriction placed upon the individual. These reactions may vary from transient distress, low mood or anxiety which improve as the physical state improves to severe depressive illness and occasionally psychotic disturbances (see Chapters 5 and 6).

These psychiatric reactions lie on a continuum, and identifying the point at which understandable unhappiness/distress ends and illness begins is extremely difficult and is bedevilled by the arbitrariness of what is understandable and what is not. As in any clinical situation the doctor attempting to distinguish one from the other will take account of such factors as the symptom cluster with which the patient presents, previous reaction to stress, past and family psychiatric history along with the degree of impairment occasioned by the psychological symptoms. See also Chapter 5. In addition, the presence of an established psychiatric illness at the onset of the physical illness must also be taken into account.

Adjustment disorders

Most studies on hospitalized patients with physical illness have confirmed that the dominant diagnosis is that of adjustment disorder (with depressed mood or with anxiety) (see Chapter 5) rather than depressive illness. Following myocardial infarction up to a quarter of patients develop significant psychological symptoms. In most patients these symptoms are transient and will have remitted within 3–4 months. When a diagnosis of carcinoma is made the symptoms are even more intense and are similar to those found in the acute phases of grief, with anger, denial, bargaining and depression being described. However, these subside over the subsequent months and most patients, while remaining sad, do not require psychotropic medication but support and, at times, counselling. All serious physical conditions, including some that are not regarded as illnesses, such as termination of pregnancy and miscarriage, can induce these feelings and understanding and sympathy are the cornerstones of treatment.

Depressive illness

All physical illnesses can potentially cause depressive illness and where it is felt the patient has moved from an adjustment disorder into depressive illness, antidepressant medication is required. There is, however, a group of medical conditions which are specifically associated with a tendency to develop depressive illness. These include:

- painful musculoskeletal disorders, especially rheumatoid arthritis
- hysterectomy
- amputation
- infectious mononucleosis
- pregnancy, miscarriage and termination of pregnancy
- carcinoma
- cardiac by-pass.

In some patients the depressive illness will antedate the physical disorder (see symptomatic depression) and those who were depressed prior to the onset of the condition have a poorer prognosis than those who become so subsequently.

Anxiety disorders

These are commonly found in people with serious or long-term physical illness as well as in those preparing for surgery or undergoing investigations for possible serious physical illness. Both anxiety symptoms and circumscribed panic attacks may occur. These are usually most appropriately diagnosed as adjustment disorders with anxiety (see Chapter 5) although occasionally the symptoms may continue independently of the illness context in which they have arisen. A specific diagnosis such as generalized anxiety disorder or panic disorder is then the more appropriate label. Whether the symptoms are persistent or circumscribed, brief or more persistent, treatment is symptomatic using short-term anxiolytics and/or cognitive/behavioural techniques.

Those who have specific fears such as agoraphobia or fear of blood or needles may find some investigations particularly difficult, including MRI scans (involving lying in the enclosed space of the scanner) or injections/phlebotomy procedures. These very circumscribed symptoms may respond to reassurance or to a single dose of an anxiolytic.

Treatment for people with long term physical conditions and comorbid mental health problems

In general the treatment for specific mental health problems is not changed by the comorbid physical condition. However, many individuals are reluctant to recognize they have a mental health diagnosis. In addition constraints on access may be caused by practitioners themselves, with practitioners more inclined to deal with physical problems, with time constraints in primary care and with a lack of training in mental health issue. The recent emphasis within the Quality Outcome Framework (QOF) on screening for depression for people with diabetes and heart disease is likely to lead to increased recognition rates and improved awareness amongst patients, GPs and practice nurses. However, the long-term outcomes resulting from this, in terms of improving access to evidence-based treatment and to improving both depression and physical disease outcomes, are less certain.

There is little consistent evidence for the effectiveness of treating depression for people with diabetes and while antidepressants and/or psychotherapy can both be used with benefit on the psychological symptoms no single treatment leading to better medical outcomes has been identified (Petrak and Herpertz 2009).

On the other hand the evidence is more positive for the scheme in heart disease. Lewin *et al.* (2002) showed that the application of NICE-approved psychological therapies (NICE 2009) improved the psychological symptomatic and functional status of those with newly diagnosed angina. A more recent uncontrolled study showed that for people with refractory angina and an increasing frequency of admissions psychological therapies reduced admissions by 40% (Moore *et al.* 2007).

In summary the evidence for specific diseases is, so far, disappointing in terms of the impact on depression and the index disease, but given the substantial morbidity and potential gains further research is required to determine the exact interventions which may be of benefit. One possibility is that the interventions tried so far have been focused on depression or anxiety as an illness rather than distress or adjustment disorder and ignore how the individual as a whole, with both physical and mental health symptoms, adapts. This is partly a function of the structure of the health service, with community-based nurses and hospital-based practitioners focusing on physical health needs and specialist mental health workers focusing on depression. The recent NICE guidance (2009) has, however, taken up this issue and a number of recommendations have been made. These include:

- a stepped care approach to management
- a focus on early recognition
- treatment with both psychological and drug treatments
- the implementation of collaborative care for those not responding to first-line treatments.

Collaborative care of those with physical and mental health disorders

Collaborative care involves specialist mental health works working alongside practitioners in primary care providing a comprehensive package of care suited to the individual. This model (Katon *et al.* 2001) emerged from the chronic disease model and has four essential elements:

- the collaborative definition of problems, in which patient-defined problems are identified alongside medical problems diagnosed by health care professionals
- a focus on specific problems where targets, goals and plans are jointly developed by the patient and professional to achieve a reasonable set of objectives, in the context of patient preference and readiness
- the creation of a range of self-management training and support services in which patients have access to services that teach the necessary skills to carry out treatment plans, guide behaviour change and promote emotional support
- the provision of active and sustained follow-up in which patients are contacted at specific intervals to monitor health status, identify possible complications and check and reinforce progress in implementing the care plan.

In addition, most collaborative care models include a 'case manager' who often has particular responsibility for delivering the care plan. In mental health services collaborative care also typically includes a consultation liaison role with a specialist mental health professional and generic primary care staff. It may also include elements of many of the other interventions described above.

Although the recommendations for collaborative care of those with depression and comorbid physical illness within the NICE guidance are strong (NICE 2009) it is unclear as to how this will be implemented in practice due to the structural problems mentioned above. In particular we need to consider how we care for the individuals who have a reluctance to accept a mental health diagnosis and for those who are isolated, particularly at home.

Guidance on the clinical encounter

Individuals with comorbid physical and psychiatric illness who are reluctant to receive a psychiatric diagnosis are often older, male or from other vulnerable groups and from ethnic minorities. A number of approaches can be taken to this problem. First, time should be taken to listen to an individual's narrative about their life and pick up on cues particularly social, but also emotional, within their concerns. These can be built on over time, particularly if doctors and nurses provide continuity of care, and can gradually allow an individual to express their distress. Second, psychological therapies do not demand the explicit recognition of a diagnosis of anxiety or depression by the patient.

It is possible to offer psychological treatment either in terms of support within a consultation by a GP or practice nurse, or alternatively by referral to a primary-care-based mental health worker – but they must also be willing to engage in treatment without explicit discussion of a diagnosis if this has been rejected conceptually by the patient. Therapeutic manoeuvres in this situation may be supportive but may also include cognitive behavioural elements or may be based on solution-focused work (see Chapter 16).

Patients with significant mental health symptoms require detailed assessment. In particular suicide risk should be addressed and their social situation and support structures explored, as well as their strengths. It is important to understand their particular social goals (e.g. reconnecting with a particular friend or family member, revisiting a favourite place), so that treatment for both their emotional distress and their physical illness can be coordinated in order to help them achieve these goals. Motivation to self-care and adherence to medication is likely to be greater if these links have been made.

Those patients who are isolated at home, often with multiple physical comorbidity, such as strokes, arthritis, heart disease and COPD, may require additional tactics. Some may, and others may not, be willing to accept the diagnosis of depression or anxiety, but most will admit to being lonely or frustrated at their inability to achieve previous functional abilities. A range of psychological approaches may be helpful and the challenge for health communities will be ensuring that high-quality therapy is available at the home. Assessments by skilled and fully qualified CBT therapists may be appropriate, with follow-up visits carried out by a support worker or CBT-trained low-intensity IAPT therapist. Alternatively community nurses can be trained in basic psychological approaches and can help implement a care plan based on CBT approaches created by an experienced practitioner, particularly if they then supervise the support worker or community nurse.

Sleep disorders

Most sleep disorders are managed by respiratory physicians or by other specialists with an interest in this group of conditions. Their relevance to general practitioners is that insomnia, in particular, may lead to a concern that the patient has a psychiatric or substance misuse disorder even though features commonly associated with these are absent. Moreover, most psychiatric illnesses can be exacerbated by insomnia, for example due to jet lag, and relapse may ensue. The ICD classification is seen in Table 12.2.

Organic – insomnia is due to some underlying diagnosis/condition, e.g. pain. Treatment is of the cause. This section outlines the common primary sleep disorders. Non-organic or primary insomnia may present with difficulty initiating or maintaining sleep. Treatment is

Table 12.2. ICD-10 classification of non-organic sleep disorders

Non-organic insomnia
Non-organic hypersomnia
Non-organic disturbance of the sleep–wake cycle
Sleepwalking (somnambulism)
Sleep terrors
Nightmares

difficult and is usually with benzodiazepines or other hypnotics. Non-specific sleep hygiene measures and light therapy can also be used.

Non-organic hypersomnia is defined as excessive daytime sleepiness or sleep attacks not due to inadequate sleep or prolonged transition to the fully aroused state on wakening. It may be familial and lifelong. Treatment is with stimulants or with the SSRIs. Kleine-Levan syndrome and narcolepsy are organic diagnoses to be ruled out. Kleine-Levan syndrome, although rare, may present to psychiatrists because of the social withdrawal, excessive eating, delusions and disorientation lasting for a few weeks and occurring cyclically during the year. Narcolepsy may also present with hypnagogic or hypnopompic hallucinations. Other features are sleep paralysis, cataplexy and sleep attacks. Stimulants may be helpful.

Non-organic disturbance of the sleep–wake cycle is a lack of synchrony between the desired and actual sleep–wake cycle. It is also called circadian rhythm sleep disorder. The patient complains of insomnia and somnolence during the usual sleep times. There are several different types but those most commonly seen in primary care are the jet lag and shift work types. Both usually improve spontaneously but this can be hastened by altering the mealtimes and sleep–wake time in the appropriate direction. Among shift workers many never adjust to the altered time schedule, especially if it is only for a few days. Treatment of jet lag is with melatonin or hypnotics. Hypnotics may also assist shift workers. Those with psychiatric conditions, even those in remission, may relapse at these times so vigilance is required.

Somnambulism is one of the parasomniac disorders (a disorder of abnormal movements, behaviours, emotions, perceptions or dreams that occur when falling asleep, waking, during deep sleep or between sleep stages). It consists of complex behaviours in the early part of the night during non-REM sleep. It involves leaving the bed and walking about, of which there is no recollection. Although minor neurological abnormalities are thought to underpin it, it may worsen at times of stress. It is more common in children than adults. Medications that suppress non-REM sleep are used in treatment – these include clonazepam in particular but other benzodiazepines may also be beneficial, as may the SSRIs and tricyclic antidepressants. Precautions against injury such as locking windows and removing obstacles should also be part of the management.

Sleep terrors are also parasomniac conditions. The person experiences terror and panic associated with intense vocalizations such as screaming and autonomic discharge. The person may get out of bed but seldom leaves the room. Memory of these occurrences is sketchy. Occasionally it may develop into a sleep-walking episode. In children it may arise from stressful family situations which need to be explored. If medication is used, diazepam is the preferred option.

Nightmare disorder occurs during REM sleep and is characterized by long, frightening dreams from which the individual awakens in a frightened state. It is a lifelong condition and often the themes recur. The content is vividly recalled. Treatment is with agents that suppress REM sleep such as tricyclic antidepressants and benzodiazepines.

Summary

- Psychiatric and physical conditions frequently overlap.
- The nature of this overlap may arise from faulty attribution of some symptoms as having a physical origin, giving rise to medically unexplained symptoms termed somatoform or conversion disorders.
- Some may knowingly exaggerate or fabricate physical symptoms for gain.

- Medications and some illnesses have a direct causal link to psychiatric symptoms, e.g. steroids and elation, stroke and depressive illness. Alternatively some physical illnesses may present primarily with psychiatric symptoms, e.g. cancer of the lung.

- Long-term physical illnesses can lead to a range of emotional problems that in some amount to full-blown psychiatric disorder requiring collaborative care between primary and secondary care services.

- Some sleep-related symptoms may appear to be manifestations of underlying psychiatric disorder but are primary disorders of sleep.

References

Arroll, B., Khin, N., and Kerse N. (2003) Screening for depression in primary care with two verbally asked questions; cross sectional study. *British Medical Journal*, **327**, 1144–1146.

Bair, M. J., Wu, J., Damush, T., *et al.* (2008). Association of depression and anxiety alone and in combination with chronic musculoskeletal pain in primary care patients. *Psychosomatic Medicine* **70**, 8, 890–897.

Bermingham, S. L., Cohen, A., Hague, J., *et al.* (2010). The cost of somatisation among the working age population in England for the year 2008–2009. *Mental Health in Family Medicine*, **7**, 71–80.

Boehm, G., Racoosin, J., Laughren, T., and Kate, R. (2004) Consensus development conference on antipsychotic drugs and obesity and diabetes: responses to consensus statement. *Diabetes Care*, **27**(8), 2088–2089.

Brown, J., O'Brien, P. M. S., Marjoribanks, J., *et al.* (2009). Selective serotonin reuptake inhibitors for premenstrual syndrome. *Cochrane Database of Systematic Reviews*, **2**, CD001396. DOI: 10.1002/14651858. CD001396.pub2.

Carson, A. J., Best, S., Postma, K., *et al.* (2003) The outcome of neurology outpatients with medically unexplained symptoms: a prospective cohort study. *Journal of Neurology Neurosurgery and Psychiatry*, **74**, 897–900.

Craig, T. K., Boardman, A. P., Mills, K., *et al.* (1993) The South London Somatisation Study I: longitudinal course and the influence of early life experiences. *British Journal of Psychiatry*, **163**, 579–588.

De Waal, M. W. M., Arnold, I. A., and Eekhof, J. A. H. (2004) Somatoform disorders in general practice: prevalence, functional impairment and comorbidity with anxiety and depressive disorders. *British Journal of Psychiatry*, **184**, 470–476.

Dowrick, C. F., Ring, A., Humphris, G. M., *et al.* (2004) Normalisation of unexplained symptoms by general practitioners a functional typology. *British Journal of General Practice*, **54**, 165–170.

Dowrick, C., and Rosendal, M. (2009). Medically unexplained symptoms. In Gask, L., Lester, H., and Kendrick, T. (eds.), *Primary Care Mental Health*. London: RCPsych Publications.

Fink, P., Rosendal, M., and Toft, T. (2002) Assessment and treatment of functional disorders in general practice: the extended reattribution and management model–an advanced educational program for nonpsychiatric doctors. *Psychosomatics*, **43**, 93–131.

Gureje, O., Von Korff, M., Simon, G., and Gater, R. (1998) Persistent Pain and Well-being: A World Health Organization Study in Primary Care. *Journal of the American Medical Association*, **280**(2), 147–151.

Katon, W., Von Korff, M., Lin, E., *et al.* (2001). Rethinking practitioner roles in chronic illness; the specialist, primary care physician and the practice nurse. *General Hospital Psychiatry*, **23**, 138–144.

Lewin, R., Furze, G., Robinson, J., *et al.* (2002). A randomised controlled trial of a self-management plan for patients with newly diagnosed angina. *British Journal of General Practice*, **52**(476), 184–201.

Lustman, P. J., Anderson, R. J., Freedland, K. E., et al. (2000). Depression and poor glycemic control: a meta-analytic review of literature. Diabetes Care, 23(7), 934–942.

Moore, R., Groves, D., Bridson, J., et al. (2007). A brief cognitive-behavioural intervention reduces hospital admissions in refractory angina patients. Journal of Pain and Symptom Management, 33(3), 310–316.

Morris, R., Dowrick, C., Salmon, P., et al. (2007) Better doctor-patient communication did not improve clinical outcome: results of a randomised controlled trial of training practices in reattribution to manage patients with medically unexplained symptoms (MUST). British Journal of Psychiatry, 191, 536–542.

Morris, R., Gask, L., and Dowrick, C. (2010). Randomised trial of reattribution on psychosocial talk between doctors and patients with medically unexplained symptoms. Psychological Medicine, 40(2), 325–353.

National Institute for Health and Clinical Excellence. (2009). Depression in adults. Clinical Guide 90. London: National Institute for Clinical Excellence.

NHS Evidence. (2008). Medically Unexplained Symptoms (MUS): a whole systems approach in Plymouth. London: NHS. http://www.library.nhs.uk/COMMISSIONING/ViewResource.aspx?resID=338646.

NHS IAPT Guidelines. (2008). IAPT Guidelines 2008. Medically unexplained symptoms positive practice guide. NHS: London.

Petrak, H., and Herpetz, S. (2009). Treatment of depression in diabetes: an update. Current Opinion in Psychiatry, 22(2), 211–217.

Ring, A., Dowrick, C., Humphris, G., et al. (2005). The somatising effect of clinical consultation: what patients and doctors say and do not say when patients present medically unexplained symptoms. Social Science and Medicine, 61, 1505–1515.

Robinson, R. G. (2003). Post stroke depression: prevalence, diagnosis, treatment and disease progression. Biological Psychiatry, 54(3), 376–387.

Sharpe, L., Allard, S., and Sensky, T. (2008) Five year follow-up of a cognitive-behavioural intervention for patients with rheumatoid arthritis: Effects on health care utilisation. Arthritis and Rheumatism Care and Research, 15, 311–316.

Simon, G. E., Katon, E. H. B., Lin, E., et al. (2005). Diabetes complications and depression as predictors of health service costs. General Hospital Psychiatry, 27(5), 344–351.

Trailblazers. (2010). Guidance for Health Professionals on medically unexplained symptoms (MUS): Making Sense of Symptoms; Managing Professional Uncertainty; Building on Patient's Strengths.

Turk, D. C., and Okifuji, A. (2002). Psychological factors in chronic pain. Evolution and revolution. Journal of Consulting and Clinical Psychology, 70(3), 678–690.

Van Der Ven, N. C. W., Hogenelst, M. H. E., Tromp-Wever, A. M. E., et al. (2005) Short term effects of cognitive behavioural therapy groups training (CBGT) in adult type 1 diabetes patients with poor glycaemic control. A randomised controlled trial. Diabetic Medicine, 22(1), 1619–1623.

Suggested reading for patients

http://www.rcpsych.ac.uk/mentalhealthinfoforall/problems/physicalillness/copingwithphysicalillness.aspx (this is the Royal College of Psychiatrists' website on coping with physical illness).

http://www.rcpsych.ac.uk/mentalhealthinfoforall/problems/sleepproblems/sleepingwell.aspx.

Krakow, B. (2007). Sound Sleep, Sound Mind. Hoboken, NJ: J. Wiley and Sons.

Chapter 13

Child mental health care

Aaron K. Vallance and M. Elena Garralda

Learning objectives

Appreciate that primary care has a key role in identifying, assessing and managing child mental health problems

Outline environmental (e.g. family) factors that may contribute towards child psychopathology and explain how a formulation can be used to evaluate them for a particular case and act as a means to target intervention

List features which suggest a presentation has a non-organic origin and outline the treatment principles in somatization disorder

Outline treatment options for anxiety disorders, and school and food refusal

Discuss sleep hygiene and behaviour management techniques and their underlying principles

Outline how ADHD and autistic spectrum disorder are diagnosed and the options for intervention

The World Health Organization globally, and the National Service Framework, NICE, and the National CAMHS Review in the UK, identify primary care as a key setting to address child mental health problems. There are strong arguments for this, including:

- the frequent co-occurrence of physical symptoms, psychosocial problems and psychiatric disorders in young people

- the high prevalence rates of psychiatric disorder in young people who attend primary care. Although only 2–10% of child primary care consultations are explicitly for emotional or behavioural complaints, 10–25% of younger children and 40% of adolescents who attend primary care have an underlying psychiatric disorder (Costello *et al.* 1988; Garralda and Bailey 1986; Kramer and Garralda 1998)

- the long-standing alliance families commonly have with their GPs, which could further enhance treatment effectiveness (Shirk and Karver 2003)

- primary care's critical role in preventative medicine, with large potential for averting child mental health problems. Primary care already delivers public health programmes targeting relevant risk and protective factors, such as family planning programmes, prenatal care, promotion of nutrition and child safety information.

However, challenges abound. Many young people are reluctant to discuss their emotional difficulties with their GPs and parents often do not express their concerns. Research meanwhile shows that GPs frequently avoid exploring such issues with them, despite this being a critical factor in detecting psychological problems (Martinez *et al.* 2006). GPs also vary in their construction of mental health problems: many believe that conditions such as attention deficit hyperactivity disorder (ADHD) are over-diagnosed; many report lack of confidence in diagnosis; and many are concerned about 'over-medicalizing' normal distress (Iliffe *et al.* 2004). Such concerns are understandable, but it makes it more and not less imperative for GPs to train in recognizing and managing mental health problems in young people, particularly as such disorders often go missed in primary care (Chang *et al.* 1988). While some GPs may be right in wishing to avoid talking about 'psychiatric disorders' with children and their parents, it is possible to be explicit about the nature of problems using a bio-psychosocial model and being positive about the potential benefits of treatment.

Interventions such as psycho-education, brief cognitive/behaviour therapy, medication management and parenting support are effective and can be feasibly delivered in primary care. While this book focuses on the role of the GP in primary care, the important role of health visitors and school nurses in recognizing and providing first-line management for childhood mental health problems should also be recognized. For chronic problems such as ADHD, primary care could provide long-term monitoring with intermittent involvement of specialist services for medication review or adjuvant behaviour therapy. Specialist child and adolescent mental health (CAMHS) services could support primary care in different ways: its staff could operate within primary care ('shifted outpatient' model) or provide ongoing training to primary care professionals ('consultation liaison' model). In the UK, primary mental health workers help bridge the gap between primary and specialist services, providing consultation liaison and supporting recognition of disorders and referral to specialist services.

This chapter proceeds with an exploration of aetiological factors that may contribute to child mental health problems. Various psychiatric disorders that commonly present in children attending primary care will then be discussed, including advice on assessment and management.

Family, environment and child mental health

Since genetic and environmental factors help shape normal development and psychiatric disorder, the family plays a central role in both, as the most likely provider of both genes and the formative environment. Whereas the genetic contribution is (with current technology) relatively fixed, the environmental contribution may be targeted for prevention or intervention work.

Although the family unit is an ever-changing concept in the modern Western world, the priority of parenting is the same: to protect, nurture, love and educate children. Parenting styles will differ in accordance with parental personalities and experiences, child temperament, and cultural context; however, the factors that underlie 'good-enough' parenting are the same. Parents should give affection, quality time and availability; support the basic needs of food, shelter, health and safety, as well as their child's wider emotional, cognitive, social and moral development; and provide appropriate authority through clearly communicated and appropriate house rules. Parenting needs to be tailored to the developmental age of the child. Care-givers should also try to maintain their own sense of self-esteem and personal development.

Poor parenting and other family adversities can contribute to child psychopathology. Sometimes this can occur even before the child is born, e.g. alcohol and drug consumption and smoke exposure in pregnancy may contribute to later ADHD in the child. In early childhood, attachment difficulties can impinge on later self-esteem and social behaviour; severe insecure attachment may result in psychopathology. Children often model their behaviour on their parents', which may include antisocial, risk-taking and unhelpful coping behaviours. Parental 'expressed emotion' of excessive criticism, hostility, emotional over-involvement and a lack of warmth may contribute to childhood depression, conduct disorder and the course of psychotic disorders. Other factors such as migration, bereavement, family mental illness, abuse, parental discord, divorce, sibling rivalry, family breakdown and becoming a 'looked-after' child each present a specific psychosocial challenge and conse-quent association with psychopathology.

Such factors do not operate in isolation from each other; both normal development and psychopathology involve a complex web of interacting processes, genetic and environ-mental. Furthermore, adversities may arise from outside the family. Experiences with other children are highly significant in psychosocial development. Peer rejection and bullying may reduce self-esteem and contribute to distress, school refusal and depressive or anxiety disorders. Conversely, good-quality friendships can be protective and are a good prognostic sign.

When presented with a child with a mental health problem, a formulation needs to be constructed to identify possible contributing factors:

- predisposing factors – *why this child?*
- precipitating factors – *why now?*
- perpetuating factors – *what keeps it going?*
- protective factors – *what might help?*

Child, family and wider environmental (school, peers, community) factors should all be considered. Formulations are helpful to understand the child's and family's story, to help determine the presence of any psychiatric disorder, and – perpetuating and protective factors especially – to generate targets for therapeutic intervention.

Unexplained somatic symptoms (somatization disorder)

Recurrent medically unexplained symptoms are common in children. In many cases, they are exacerbated by, or an expression of, stress, anxiety or depressive disorders (Campo *et al.* 2004). General practice is in a good position to screen for these problems, especially amongst frequently attending children, as psychological difficulties may exacerbate the presentation of or concern about physical symptoms during the consultation.

Somatization refers to when psychological distress manifests itself through bodily symp-toms, frequently compromising daily functioning. In younger children, recurrent abdominal pain and headaches are frequent; with increasing age, limb pain, fatigue and neurological symptoms become more prominent. ICD-10 disorders include *persistent somatoform pain disorder*, which involves persistent, severe and distressing pain, such as abdominal pains and headaches, and occurs in association with identifiable emotional conflict or psychosocial problems. Recurrent abdominal pain affects about 10% of children. In the majority of cases, no organic cause can be objectively demonstrated, even though the child may look in pain and appear unwell. *Dissociative or conversion disorder* may involve partial or complete loss of bodily sensations or control of movements, or pseudo-seizures; they often occur following a traumatic event. In *chronic fatigue syndrome*, the main complaint is increased fatigue after

Table 13.1. Features which suggest a non-organic origin

Lack of other significant or expected physical symptoms or signs on examination or tests. Referral to paediatrics might be warranted to exclude organic disorder. *Recurrent abdominal pain* of non-organic origin tends to be located centrally and tends not to wake the child at night

Notable psychosocial stress, e.g. family conflict. Improvement on weekends and school holidays meanwhile suggest difficulties at school

Anxious, sensitive or conscientious personality traits in the child

Family factors, such as stress, physical problems, poor family communication, and poor coping strategies. Families can, often unwittingly, reinforce illness behaviour if there is emotional over-involvement with the problem or encouragement of illness behaviour (e.g. by allowing time off school, lavishing attention or gifts, toning down disapproval of inappropriate behaviour, etc.). There can appear a fine line between what is appropriate parental care and what is unhelpful reinforcing behaviour

Concurrent psychiatric disorder. Up to 75% of children with somatization disorder in primary care may also have another psychiatric disorder, usually anxiety or depression, which may develop either before the symptoms or during its course

mental or physical effort, as well as difficulty in concentrating, bodily pains, sleeping problems and worries about deteriorating well-being.

Somatization disorders can only be diagnosed when the symptom pattern is out of keeping with the established pathophysiology, i.e. when there is no organic explanation for the presentation. That is not to say that physical abnormalities or disorders need not be present: somatization disorder is frequently preceded by actual physical problems. However, Table 13.1 depicts various features which point towards a non-organic origin.

Once a somatization disorder has been established, the most important first step is to engage the family, who may still remain anxious about the possibility of an as yet undisclosed underlying physical disorder; such concerns need to be fully discussed. Families can be sensitive to exploration of psychological issues, fearing that this implies dismissal of the symptoms as 'all in the child's mind'. Some explanation as to the overlap or link between the body and mind might help, such as how tension can give rise to pain such as headaches, or the physical effects of stress hormones. Rather than debating whether the problem is physical or psychological – a perceived division of mind and body, which is unhelpful in understanding any illness – it is more useful to direct the discussion towards how the problem can best be managed.

Intervention involves a coordinated approach with the child, family and other health or school professionals (Table 13.2).

The approach outlined in Table 13.2 is generally based on cognitive behavioural principles, which has support from NICE guidelines and an evidence base (Garralda 1999). Referral to CAMHS services may be warranted to assess and manage significant family and psychosocial factors and provide family work, to confirm the diagnosis, and where there is comorbid psychiatric disorder or significant functional impairment. Most children with somatization disorder recover in the short term, although up to a third of cases may experience ongoing symptoms albeit to a lesser degree.

Anxiety disorders

Anxiety disorders in childhood are commonly found amongst those attending primary care, particularly amongst frequent attenders, although the presentation is typically with physical symptoms (Garralda *et al.* 1999). Anxiety is an unpleasant feeling of tension or apprehension

Table 13.2. Treatment principles in somatization disorder

Targeting and reducing the contributing psychosocial stress factors
Noting daily variations in symptom severity and associated impairment in a diary
Specific techniques and coping skills to deal with individual symptoms, e.g. distraction and relaxation techniques, positive self-talk, problem-solving strategies
Modest initial goals to increase normalization of activities, with further gradual and agreed increases in daily activities
Encouraging participation in routine and enjoyable activities
Treatment of comorbid psychiatric disorder
Family work to facilitate the family's engagement in treatment, to support the child's attainment in treatment goals and strategies, to prevent symptom reinforcement, and to reduce any family stress or dysfunction that might be contributing

accompanied by physiological changes and worries or fears. It can become maladaptive if excessive or developmentally inappropriate, and can become a disorder if it causes significant functional impairment. Anxiety disorders are among the most prevalent categories of psychopathology in children, with separation anxiety and specific phobias most common before puberty.

Separation anxiety disorder is an excessive or developmentally inappropriate anxiety about separation from attachment figures or excessive worrying about the figure's welfare, causing significant distress or impairment, such as refusal to go to school. ICD-10 diagnostic criteria include an onset before the age of 6 years and duration of at least 4 weeks.

*Specific or simple phobia*s, in contrast to developmentally appropriate normal fears (e.g. of the dark, ghosts, kidnappers, animals, etc.), cause significant distress or impairment. They are characterized by excessive and unreasonable fears of clearly discernible, circumscribed objects or situations that provoke an immediate anxiety response. In children this may be manifested as crying, tantrums, freezing or clinging. Adolescents may recognize that the fear is excessive, although this may not be the case with younger children. Particularly significant for medical practice are phobias of injections and medical procedures.

Anxiety disorders in younger children are best treated by behavioural therapy, whose models generally derive from (classic and operant) conditioning theory and social learning theory. Specific techniques include systematic desensitization and exposure, relaxation training, modelling of appropriate behaviour and rewards for desirable behaviour. Some basic cognitive work may also be helpful, e.g. appraising the threat (from animals, kidnappers, etc.).

Up to 80% of children with anxiety disorders go into remission in the first year of their illness, with the highest remission rates in separation anxiety disorder (almost all children) and simple phobias. The prognosis is particularly favourable if the condition follows a recognizable precipitant, such as parental illness, and the parents can be directed to provide support.

Common behavioural disorders

School refusal

Whereas truants defiantly do something else rather than go to school, school refusal occurs with the tacit knowledge of care-givers. School refusal may relate to real or exaggerated fears or phobias about school (e.g. bullying, social phobia) or leaving home (e.g. parental illness, separation anxiety). Both child and parents may possess anxious temperaments, leading to over-protective parenting. Somatization, anxiety or depressive disorders may occur, presenting as physical complaints, particularly on weekdays.

Management involves advice and support to parents and school, and liaison with the educational welfare officer. Any underlying psychiatric disorders should be treated, and real fears and concerns need to be dealt with. Anxiety management strategies, such as using a cognitive behavioural approach, may incorporate an early graduated return to school. Protracted school refusal will require referral to CAMHS services.

Food refusal (in younger children)

Parents are commonly concerned about their child's eating habits, particularly as normal patterns of feeding vary across children or within the same child across time. Causes are often multifactorial in nature, and may include child temperament, family stress or anxiety (especially about food) and parenting behaviour. Other oppositional behaviours may also be present. Physical problems from painful teething to oral-motor delay or gastrointestinal reflux need to be excluded. Assessment includes consideration of what, when, how and how much food is presented at mealtimes:

- 'what' – *is the food age-appropriate and sufficiently varied?*
- 'when' – *are meals presented at predictable mealtimes to coincide with hunger? Are snacks given in between meals?*
- 'how' – *are meals presented in a calm unforced way, away from distractions such as television?*
- 'how much' – *are meals presented in appropriately sized portions?*

Intervention may include food diaries to establish a record of intake, growth charts to assess weight and a physical assessment to exclude any organic causes. In most cases, parents just need reassurance: as long as they are offered nutritious food, children are remarkably good at eating the right amount of food when allowed a free choice. Force-feeding is not only inefficient; it can also set up a confrontational atmosphere which perpetuates the problem. Instead, mealtimes should proceed in a relaxed atmosphere, with good feeding behaviour being rewarded with praise and attention. If families eat together, parents can model good eating behaviour and enjoyment; this particularly encourages feeding in anxious children. Reducing snacks may help, although younger children may actually prefer small frequent meals.

Sleep problems

Sleep problems are common in children, and various factors may contribute: separation anxiety, fear of darkness, displaced sleep–wake cycle, lack of bedtime routine, evening or bedroom overstimulation, and pre-sleep ruminations and worries. Assessment includes exploring the child's fears, ascertaining the family's response and screening for physical and psychiatric disorders and family stress.

Sleep relies on two conditions: the child feeling safe and calm, and the conditioning of the bedroom environment with sleep. Treating sleep problems therefore involves promoting feelings of security and establishing a regular bedtime routine (Table 13.3).

Table 13.3. Sleep hygiene techniques

Make bedroom conducive to sleep	Encourage	Avoid
Comfortable bed Correct temperature Dark quiet room; night-lights only Lack of stimulation Reassuringly familiar setting e.g. teddies, posters	30–60 minute bedtime routine to 'wind down'; e.g. bathing, stories (young children) and relaxation techniques (older children) Consistent bedtime and waking-up times An overall emotional sense of safety, positive emotions and good associations at bedtime Thinking about problems/plans earlier in day (such ruminations might otherwise occur at night when there are fewer distractions) Regular daily exercise	Overexcitement near bedtime; e.g. computer games Afternoon caffeine Excessive daytime napping Negative (e.g. punishment) or arousing (e.g. TV) associations with the bedroom Too much time awake in bed (if so, spend some quiet time in another room and then return)

Younger children frequently wake up at night; some cry because they cannot settle by themselves. Initially parents may be tempted to wait with their child until they fall asleep. However, parents should help the child learn how to settle themselves, e.g. gradually reducing the amount of time waiting with the child, whilst increasing the gaps in between. Parents can alternate nights on duty to share the burden.

Night terrors are characterized by the child sitting up in bed, eyes open, seemingly awake but disoriented, distressed and unresponsive to their parents' comfort. The child then suddenly settles back to sleep after a few minutes (usually no longer than 20 minutes) and has no recollection of the episode. Like sleepwalking, night terrors are a parasomnia resulting from deep-sleep disturbance, often 1–2 hours after sleep onset. Most night terrors need little more than parental reassurance and sleep hygiene advice, particularly as overtiredness is often a cause. Recording the timing of episodes and waking the child 30 minutes before the terror is expected ('anticipatory wakening') for about a week may help.

Defiance, tantrums and aggressive behaviour

The toddler's conceptual world is egocentric – they reside at the centre and the rest of the world is organized around them. Conceptually, they have also divorced the parental figure who provides comfort from the figure that stops them doing the things they want to do. Eventually, toddlers go through a phase where they reconcile the 'good' and 'bad' parental figures within the same parent, and realize that the world does not necessarily revolve around them. Such discoveries inevitably lead to confusion, frustration and anger, and tantrums are common in response to being told they cannot have, or do, what they want.

Assessment for aggressive or oppositional behaviour would include a screen for medical (e.g. deafness) or neurodevelopmental (e.g. language delay, autism, ADHD) conditions. Parents should record oppositional behaviour or tantrums in a diary, with attention paid to the events leading up to the episode, and those occurring subsequently, using the 'ABC' model:

- Antecedents – *what happened leading up to the tantrum?*
- Behaviour – *what did the tantrum involve?*
- Consequences – *what outcome did the tantrum 'achieve'?*

Table 13.4. Behavioural management strategies

Avoiding the antecedents	Avoiding reinforcement of the behaviour
Avoid triggering situations, if appropriate Give attention, praise or incentives (e.g. star charts) for appropriate behaviour, e.g. playing quietly, eating nicely Spend quality time as a family. Show interest in child's play Distract from undesired behaviour Give short clear specific commands, eye-to-eye, calmly but firmly, to communicate limits and consequences; e.g. 1-2-3 model: 1. I want you to … 2. When you've …, then you can get a star / watch TV 3. Now you can get a star / watch TV Or, 1. Stop that because … 2. If you don't stop …, you must go to your room / naughty step 3. Now go to your room / naughty step Children model themselves on parents; if the parents themselves aren't 'behaving', then …	Avoid rewarding undesired behaviour, such as with attention; calmly allow the tantrum to die down 'Time-out' in quiet space with low stimulation, e.g. 'for 1 minute per year of age' Follow through consistently and immediately on consequences that have already been communicated

The diary should then reveal the situations that trigger episodes and the family responses that reinforce them. Behavioural management strategies aim to reduce such episodes by targeting these two principles (Table 13.4), but it is important to remind parents that it can take time for such 'conditioning' to take affect. Such strategies are often taught on various group parenting schemes offered by primary care, social services or voluntary organizations, based on structured programmes, e.g. Webster-Stratton, 1-2-3 Magic. Such programmes have a good evidence base.

Attention deficit hyperactivity disorder (ADHD)

Diagnosis

Young children are usually lively by nature. When parents pronounce them as hyperactive, such judgement may reflect their or their cultural expectations as much as actual psychopathology. However, hyperkinetic disorder (ICD-10 classification) and the more broadly defined ADHD (DSM-IV) are recognized entities diagnosable by criterion-referenced deficits in attention, activity and impulsivity (Table 13.5).

The symptoms can also harm school performance and peer relationships, with accompanying loss of self-esteem. Affected children may drift into antisocial activities, particularly if parents, teachers and peers use coercion and punishment, which are ineffectual or breed resentment.

Aetiology

ADHD is the commonest reason for follow-up in CAMHS services. Prevalence rates are approximately 1.5% for hyperkinetic disorder and up to 5% for ADHD; males are three times

Table 13.5. ICD-based criteria for hyperkinetic disorder

Symptoms present before 7 years old, have persisted for at least 6 months, are inconsistent with developmental age, and occur pervasively across different settings, causing impairment and/or interference.

Inattention (6 out of)	Hyperactivity (3 out of)	Impulsivity (1 out of)
Not listening	Runs about excessively or inappropriately	Blurts out answers out of turn
Fails to sustain attention in tasks or activities	Difficulty remaining seated	Acting out of turn, e.g. in queues or games
Leaving tasks incomplete	Unduly noisy	Interrupts others
Avoids tasks requiring sustained mental effort	Persistent excessive motor activity	Talks excessively
Poor organization	Fidgety	(In older children, poor self control and reckless risk-taking)
Easily distracted		
Fails to focus on details		
Loses things		
Forgetfulness		

more likely to be affected. Studies have established various aetiological and risk factors, although ADHD is most likely an umbrella construct of various pathological entities. A conclusive model has yet to be proven. Studies have identified a high genetic heritability (60–90%) and various candidate genes, mostly relating to dopamine transporters or receptors. This is consistent with neurophysiological and cognitive research indicating catecholamine system, fronto-striatal and 'executive function' deficits. Significant 'gene × environment' interaction is also likely; environmental factors such as maternal prenatal smoking and alcohol, very low birth weight and extreme abuse, neglect and social deprivation have been implicated, although causality has not been conclusively confirmed. Negative parent–child relationships are more likely to be a consequence of ADHD than a cause.

Assessment and intervention

Because diagnosis depends on pervasiveness of symptoms, assessment should use multiple sources, including teachers or educational psychologists. Screening tools such as Conners' – teachers and parents' – rating scales can aid diagnosis. Direct observation is useful, although older children may control their symptoms during a clinic visit. ADHD has significant comorbidity, including oppositional defiant/conduct disorder, autistic spectrum disorder, intellectual disability, tic disorders, hearing difficulties, anxiety and depression, which need screening for.

In the UK, the management of ADHD is extensively covered by NICE guidelines (2008). Most families benefit from written information about the condition and helpful resources for support (e.g. ADDISS). As parents may have felt guilty or irritated with the child's behaviour, the alleviation of such negative emotions and consequent responses is in itself therapeutic. Depending on local services, interventions can be delivered by primary care, schools and/or voluntary organizations, as well as specialist services.

Care-givers should receive individual or group parent training, similar to those used for oppositional behaviour (e.g. Webster-Stratton or 1-2-3 Magic programmes), as well as support to reduce family stress. Schools may offer classroom behavioural interventions (e.g. offering class structure and routines; setting small achievable commands, rules and goals) and social skills training (e.g. anger management, problem-solving strategies).

NICE guidelines advise that ADHD should be diagnosed by a specialist paediatric or CAMHS services, who would also initiate the medication if necessary. GPs may, however, continue prescribing and monitoring drug treatment under 'shared care' arrangements. Various studies have confirmed that stimulant medication such as methylphenidate or dexamphetamine, and atomoxetine, are the most effective treatments for hyperkinetic disorder, although the long-term efficacy is less certain (MTA 1999). Medication should therefore be first-line treatment in school-aged children with severe symptoms, as part of a wider psychological, behavioural and educational package. It should also be used in those with moderate symptoms if behavioural interventions are refused, inaccessible or found ineffective. However, medication is not usually recommended for preschool children.

Although the precise pharmacological action of stimulant medication has not been fully elucidated, it appears to increase dopaminergic neurotransmission. Methylphenidate is rapidly absorbed, and has a therapeutic effect for 1–4 hours; sustained-release formulations offer 8–12 hours, useful for covering school hours. Doses usually start low and are then titrated upwards depending on effectiveness and side effects.

Stimulants may inhibit growth and weight, which should be measured every 6 months, although the long-term effects are not clear. Such effects may be attenuated by administering medication with or after food, taking additional snacks in the early morning or late evening, occasional drug holidays if appropriate, and consulting dietician advice. There is also an association with seizures, tics and mood and sleep disturbances. Heart rate and blood pressure should be recorded after each dose change, and every 3 months. Sustained resting tachycardia, arrhythmia or a significant persistent increase in systolic blood pressure should prompt dose reduction and paediatric referral. Note also that atomoxetine may have similar cardiovascular and growth side effects; suicidal thoughts and agitation have also been reported.

Treatment should continue for as long as it is effective and be reviewed every few months, during which the views of the child, family and teachers can be consulted. The effect of missed doses, planned dose reductions and brief periods without treatment should be ascertained.

The role of diet in the cause and management of hyperactivity is controversial. Current evidence indicates that the diets which blindly eliminate artificial additives have little effect. However, as some children may have idiosyncratic responses to particular additives, a food diary may help reveal any association and an exclusion diet and dietician referral should then be considered. There is a limited evidence base for the use of fatty acids.

Symptoms tend to decline with age, although restlessness, inattention and disorganization may persist into adolescence and adulthood. Conduct disorder is a poor prognostic indicator in ADHD. Childhood ADHD has been associated with later antisocial and criminal behaviour, drug and alcohol misuse, unemployment and relationship difficulties. This suggests that early treatment may significantly help to improve the life trajectory and prospects of a young person with ADHD.

Autistic spectrum disorders

Diagnosis

Autistic spectrum disorders (ASD) are characterized by impairments in social interaction and communication and the presence of repetitive behaviours. However, they represent a clinically heterogeneous set of conditions, with varying severity of language and cognitive impairment. Compare the highly competent IT programmer with Asperger syndrome who can mechanically detail the ins and outs of computer algorithms to anyone at length, with the severely impaired child with autism, who barely speaks but expresses himself through behavioural outbursts and head-banging. Symptoms also present differently according to developmental stage (see Case 1 versus Case 2), and a regression of skills occurs in about 25% of cases. The ICD-10 and DSM-IV classification systems describe these disorders as pervasive developmental disorders (Table 13.6).

Other difficulties are often present. Approximately one-third of people with ASD have severe learning difficulties, and one-third mild-moderate. Coordination difficulties are commonly described in Asperger syndrome. Tantrums, aggression, anxiety and self-injury are all common, particularly in response to a change in environment or routine. Hyperactivity is also a frequent feature, and may be sufficient to qualify for ADHD. Eating and sleeping problems, although typical in young children, may be particularly pronounced in children with ASD. Potential causal medical associations are found in about 5–10% of autism, e.g. Down's syndrome, fragile X and tuberous sclerosis. Epilepsy occurs in approximately 20–30% and can commence either in childhood or in adolescence. Because of the range of disorder and comorbid presentations, the functioning and needs of individual patients can vary widely.

Aetiology

Epidemiological studies have shown increasing rates of ASD, although this probably reflects increased awareness and the development of specialist services. Current research puts prevalence at 1% for ASD and 0.25% for autism, with a male:female ratio of 4:1.

Case 1

Parents are concerned about their 3-year-old son, X, who seems to be speaking less. On assessment, speech milestones (e.g. babbling and gesturing by 12 months, single words by 16 months, two-word spontaneous phrases by 24 months) were all delayed by several months, and word usage and range have notably declined in recent months. He tends not to respond to his name, follow simple directions, point or wave bye-bye; when younger he did not raise his arms in anticipation of being picked up. Although he sometimes smiles, it tends to occur out of context and his eye contact is often poor. He prefers to play by himself and can appear in a world of his own. He is very attached to his toy train and gets upset when it is taken off him; he likes to spin its wheels. He does not like being hugged and can get very upset when people touch him. He is increasingly oppositional, and frequently throws tantrums.

Case 2

Parents are concerned about their 9-year-old son, X, after a recent parents' evening at school. X had been struggling in his work, where he is increasingly falling behind, and with his peers. His reading and writing skills are below average. His speech is unusual: he often calls himself 'he', repeats the speech of others, and talks in a strange squeaky tone. He does, however, talk lots about dinosaurs, which he describes in incredible detail, even in response to an unrelated question or 'out of the blue'. He often shouts out in lessons, where he often gets into trouble. He spends break-times alone. When he tries to join group games, his peers get frustrated or make fun of him; he often lashes out at other kids in the playground. He can also get very upset when things are late, such as going to school or mealtimes, or when things have been moved around the house.

Table 13.6. ICD-based criteria for pervasive development disorder

Childhood autism requires at least six symptoms to be present across all three domains before the age of 3 years old; ASD is defined less stringently. Asperger syndrome is typified by relatively normal language development; IQ tends to be near-normal.

Qualitative impairment in social interaction	Qualitative impairment in communication	Repetitive restricted behaviours
Poor appreciation of socio-emotional cues and contexts Poor social reciprocation (e.g. in sharing interest and enjoyment with others, proto-declarative pointing …) Poor non-verbal communication (e.g. in eye contact, social smiling, facial expression …) Failure to develop quality peer relationships	Delayed development or abnormal language (e.g. ranging from odd intonation to muteness) Stereotyped and repetitive speech Difficulties in to-and-fro conversation Lack of varied and spontaneous pretend play	Preoccupations with unusual parts or sensory aspects of objects Can be oversensitive to certain sounds, touch … Stereotyped mannerisms (e.g. hand flapping) Intense adherence to routines or rituals (e.g. lining or ordering things in a certain way) An encompassing preoccupation with an interest, unusual in type or intensity

Research suggests that ASD is primarily a disorder of early brain development, starting prenatally and continuing through early life. The disorder is most likely the endpoint of several organic aetiologies. Family and genetics studies have determined a high heritability (90%) as well as a number of chromosomal regions which might harbour susceptibility genes, although significant candidate genes have yet to be conclusively identified. No single environmental factor has been determined, even though speculation gets bandied about in the media and internet, fuelling parental worries. A case in point is the MMR vaccine (Goldacre 2007): the original study has been widely criticized and subsequent extensive research has failed to support any such association (Department of Health: www.immunisation.nhs.uk/Vaccines/MMR).

Various models have been proposed to explain the underlying neuropsychological pathology. The 'theory of mind' or 'mentalizing' hypothesis proposes that people with ASD have difficulties in attributing mental states to people, with difficulty conceiving of others as having thoughts or feelings different from their own. The 'executive function' hypothesis proposes that people with ASD have difficulties in planning for future goals, with underlying deficits in organizing, working memory, cognitive flexibility and inhibiting distracting stimuli or impulses. Such models have received support from neuropsychological and neuroimaging studies, although research is currently far from conclusive.

Assessment and intervention

Assessment aims to differentiate ASD from disorders such as ADHD, global developmental delay, language disorders, hearing problems and anxiety and conduct disorders. However, no single symptom is pathognomonic and, given the wide range of symptomological expression, an extensive multidisciplinary approach is often required to make the diagnosis. Comorbid psychiatric disorders require assessment and treatment in their own right. Professionals involved in multidisciplinary teams may include a child psychiatrist, clinical psychologist, paediatrician and speech and language or occupational therapists. For preschoolers, referral is usually to child development centres; for school-aged children, local services vary but would usually involve paediatric, CAMHS or learning disability teams. The division of services can result in varying and sometimes confusing pathways of care for the child and family. It is useful to bear in mind the frequent exasperation encountered by families over the difficulty accessing services and long waiting lists (particularly if they perceive a 'postcode lottery') and the repetitive assessment meetings across different teams when they are eventually seen.

Children should be observed in both unstructured and structured settings, and ideally observed at preschool or school to assess social responsiveness. The disorder is becoming increasingly diagnosed in 4–5-year-olds, when symptoms are most typical; when assessing older children, it is useful to ask care-givers about their child's behaviour at this younger age. Various diagnostic instruments have been developed, such as the Autism Diagnostic Interview-Revised (ADI-R) for interviewing caregivers, and the Autism Diagnostic Observation Schedule (ADOS) for observing children. Physical investigations may be indicated, particularly if there are seizures, a fluctuating clinical course, or neurological symptoms and signs (Baird *et al.* 2003).

The main aims of intervention are to:

- optimize cognitive, language and social development and skills
- reduce problem behaviours relating to inflexibility, rigidity, hyperactivity, aggression or self-injury
- treat any existing comorbid psychiatric disorders
- help support families.

Early intervention may improve long-term outcomes. Intervention should be delivered as part of a comprehensive package in various settings. Schools may provide specific and structured educational and behavioural management techniques, particularly those aimed at optimizing social and communication skills. Special schools may have particular expertise, although accessibility may vary and the individual's and family's needs and wishes need to be considered.

There is some evidence for intensive behavioural intervention, such as Lovaas (applied behavioural analysis or ABA), although there is significant individual variation and accessibility can prove difficult. 'Social stories' use illustrations to help children understand social situations; social skills training may help older children. Behavioural management techniques are often effective for comorbid difficulties such as hyperactivity, aggression, anxiety and sleeping problems; psychotropic medications may help in more resistant cases, but do not tend to improve core ASD symptoms. Potential benefits need to be balanced against the increased sensitivity to side effects experienced by individuals with ASD, as well as patient and family wishes.

Like the clinical presentation, the course of ASD is diverse. An IQ of above 70 and a functional language onset before 5 years of age are good prognostic signs. A minority are able to live independently and develop a work and social life. However, autism is a life-long condition and the likelihood of complete independence remains low. Support from services and the interventions above, as well as care from family, friends and voluntary organizations, can make a difference. However, families may struggle with the knowledge that as yet there is no cure for this condition.

Summary

- General practitioners should have an active role in the assessment and management of psychiatric disorders of children and young people.
- Biological and family/environmental factors are important in the genesis or continuation of these disorders.

- General practice will have a special role in providing advice for children presenting with somatization or the common behavioural problems and in screening and providing some advice for anxiety disorders, especially amongst some frequently attending children.

- There will be a joint role with the specialist services in monitoring children with ADHD, in supporting families of children with autistic spectrum disorder and guiding them to the appropriate local diagnostic and treatment services.

References

Baird, G., Cass, H., and Slonims, V. (2003). Diagnosis of autism. *British Medical Journal*, **327**, 488–493.

Campo, J. V., Bridge J., Ehmann, M., *et al.* (2004). Recurrent abdominal pain, anxiety, and depression in primary care. *Pediatrics*, **113**(4), 817–824.

Chang, G., Warner, V., and Weissman, M. M. (1988). Physicians' recognition of psychiatric disorders in children and adolescents. *American Journal of Diseases of Children*, **142**(7), 736–739.

Costello, E. J., Costello, A. J., Edelbrock, C., *et al.* (1988). Psychiatric disorders in pediatric primary care. Prevalence and risk factors. *Archives of General Psychiatry*, **45**(12), 1107–1116.

Garralda, M. E. (1999). Practitioner review: assessment and management of somatisation in childhood and adolescence: a practical perspective. *Journal of Child Psychology and Psychiatry and Allied Disciplines*, **40**(8), 1159–1167.

Garralda, M. E., and Bailey, D. (1986). Children with psychiatric disorders in primary care. *Journal of Child Psychology and Psychiatry*, **27**(5), 611–624.

Garralda, M. E., and Chalder, T. (2005). Practitioner Review: Chronic Fatigue Syndrome in Childhood. *Journal of Child Psychology and Psychiatry*, **46**, 1143–1151.

Garralda, M. E., Bowman, F. M., and Mandalia, S. (1999). Children with psychiatric disorders who are frequent attenders to primary care. *European Child and Adolescent Psychiatry*, **8**, 34–44.

Goldacre, B. (2007). Medicine and the media: MMR: the scare stories are back. *British Medical Journal*, **335**, 126–127.

Iliffe, S., Gledhill, J., da Cunha, F., Kramer, T., and Garralda, M. E. (2004). The recognition of adolescent depression in general practice: issues in the acquisition of new skills. *Primary Care Psychiatry*, **9**(2), 51–56.

Kramer, T., and Garralda, M. E. (1998). Psychiatric disorders in adolescents in primary care. *British Journal of Psychiatry*, **173**, 508–513.

Martinez, R., Reynolds, S., and Howe, A. (2006). Factors that influence the detection of psychological problems in adolescents attending general practices. *British Journal of General Practice*, **56**, 594–599.

MTA Cooperative Group. (1999). A 14-month randomized clinical trial of treatment strategies for attention-deficit/hyperactivity disorder. Multimodal Treatment Study of Children with ADHD. *Archives of General Psychiatry*, **56**, 1073–1086.

National Institute for Health and Clinical Excellence. (2007). *Chronic Fatigue Syndrome guidelines.* www.nice.org.

National Institute for Health and Clinical Excellence. (2008). *ADHD guidelines.* www.nice.org.

Shirk, S. R., and Karver, M. (2003). Prediction of treatment outcome from relationship variables in child and adolescent therapy: a meta-analytic review. *Journal of Consulting and Clinical Psychology*, **71**(3), 452–464.

Suggested reading for patients and families

Bailey, S., and Shooter, M. (2009) *The Young Mind: An Essential Guide to Mental Health for Young Adults, Parents and Teachers.* Ealing: Bantam Press.

Baron-Cohen, S. (2008) *Autism and Asperger Syndrome.* Oxford: Oxford University Press.

Chalder, T., and Hussain, K. (2002). *Self Help for Chronic Fatigue Syndrome: A Guide for Young People.* Witney: Blue Stallion Publications.

Dunn Buron, K., and Curtis, M. (2003). *The Incredible 5-point Scale: Assisting Children with ASDs in Understanding Social Interactions and Controlling Their Emotional Responses.* Overland Park, KS: Autism Asperger Publishing Co. (a practical workbook for 7–13 year olds and their parents to help manage challenging behaviour and social skills).

Phelan, T. (2003). *1-2-3 Magic: Effective Discipline for Children 2–12.* Glen Ellyn, IL: Child Management Inc. (practical parenting techniques, also helpful in ADHD).

Webster-Stratton, C. (2006). *The Incredible Years.* Seattle, WA: The Incredible Years (practical parenting techniques, also helpful in ADHD).

Useful contacts

ADDISS (Attention Deficit Disorder Information and Support Service)
- www.addiss.co.uk
  020 8952 2800
- Royal College of Psychiatrists
- www.rcpsych.ac.uk
  020 7235 2351

The National Autistic Society (www.nas.org.uk, 0845 070 4004)

Adolescent mental health care

Raghuram Shivram and Panos Vostanis

Learning objectives

Develop an understanding of adolescent mental health problems, in particular their likely
   presentation in primary care
Enhance detection and recognition
Develop interventions for milder and less complex types of adolescent psychopathology
   within primary care
Maximize the impact of specialist mental health services through the establishment of care
   pathways and protocols, and appropriate use of other agencies

Introduction

Adolescence is a period of substantial change, and often of turmoil, between childhood
and young adult life, and this is reflected in different areas of psychosocial functioning.
Adolescents often struggle because of disparities between their cognitive, emotional, social
and physical development; experimentation, sometimes with high-risk behaviours; forming
a cultural and sexual identity; redefining their family relationships; and becoming part of a
wider peer group. Such transitions are usually resolved, as the young person moves towards
independence; however, these can also act as vulnerabilities that predispose to psychopathology.
Distinguishing between 'normal' adolescent behaviours and the onset of psychiatric symptoms can be difficult, and needs to be interpreted with caution, and in the context of their
overall functioning, life circumstances, previous history and corroborative information from
their carers or other significant adults. For example, one needs to consider the differences
between withdrawal and depression or psychosis, a pessimistic stance and suicidal ideation, a
wish to conform in their appearance and anorectic symptoms. While young people have
often been reluctant to open conversations with doctors about these 'problems of adolescence', it is all the more important that GPs and others in primary care should feel confident
to engage in conversations with young people about how they feel. Confident practitioners
can act to reassure young people that what they are experiencing is understandable or
alternatively that there may be problems which can benefit from interventions.

Case 1

The parents of a 13-year-old boy (named Y) arranged to see their GP. They described feeling
'at the end of their tether' with his behaviour, as he had been involved in fights and stealing,
and he had been arrested by the police on three occasions. They stated that he might need to
go into care if he did not improve. The GP asked to see Y, who had not been brought to the

first appointment, and suggested that the parents were honest with him about the reason for the GP's involvement. Y reluctantly came to the next appointment, and the GP screened for any underlying disorder such as depression, and checked Y's perceptions and expectations of any future help. Neither Y nor his parents thought that anybody can really help them, and they appeared to accept that he would end up in care. The GP explained why Social Services needed to be involved at this stage, to assess the family situation, liaise with other agencies (including the Youth Offending Service, who had already been involved, and Y's schools), and formulate a care plan at an inter-agency meeting. The parents agreed and the GP initiated the referral to Social Services.

Comment

Although the presentation of young people with behavioural problems is common, and can cause distress to families, this does not automatically require specialist CAMHS involvement. Understanding the reasons for the behaviours, the young person's and parents' views and the previous and current agency involvement will help determine the appropriate course of action. If there is risk of family breakdown, and consequently child protection concerns, Social Services would be the most appropriate agency. CAMHS involvement might be useful if the GP suspects a comorbid psychiatric disorder, or, if there are adequate boundaries, safety and motivation to improve communication through family therapy. This does not seem the case in this scenario, although it might be possible at a later stage.

The British Child and Adolescent Mental Health Survey (Green *et al.* 2005) detected a rate of 9.6% for all disorders among both children and adolescents, which increased with age (11.5% among 11–16-year-olds, compared with 7.7% in children aged 5–10 years). Male adolescents reported higher overall levels of disorders (12.6%) than female adolescents (10.3%). This difference was mainly accounted for by conduct disorders, whilst the reverse pattern was established for emotional disorders such as depression. These trends are consistent with findings from other countries (Costello *et al.* 2003; Fleitlich-Bilyk and Goodman 2004). Recent evidence suggests a real increase of mental health problems in Western societies, i.e. not merely explained by better recognition and likelihood of seeking help (Collishaw *et al.* 2004). This increase is mainly accounted for by adolescent depression, substance abuse, self-harm and conduct disorders. The concurrent presentation of mental health problems is not unusual in this age group; for example, depression may present together with either anxiety or conduct problems, or both. Adolescent psychiatric disorders often co-occur with learning difficulties and developmental delays.

A number of issues are important to consider in relating to adolescents within primary care. Although the majority of contacts and referrals are initiated by parents, a substantial proportion of young people may either present of their own accord or be asked to see their GP by their teacher or school nurse. This can pose ethical, clinical and legal questions, particularly when the young person does not wish their parents or carers to be involved or even informed. It is always preferable to discuss and reach an agreement in involving the family. Where this is not possible despite all attempts, the clinician needs to balance the importance of engaging the young person and respecting their wishes, if they are Gillick competent, against the risk of initiating treatment or a referral to the specialist service (child and adolescent mental health service – CAMHS) without the parents' involvement. Ethical parallels can be drawn from other health fields such as sex education (Mueller *et al.* 2008). In cases of risk such as deliberate self-harm, confidentiality may need to be breached. It is paramount not to miss child protection concerns, even if a young person appears mature or developmentally able.

In fact, such developmental discrepancies can be misleading and need to be taken into consideration in adolescents' assessment. Some young people may come across as cognitively advanced, but emotionally or socially immature, and this can make them particularly vulnerable. Engagement is also essential in the successful initiation of therapeutic interventions. Adolescents should preferably be seen on their own, even when they appear informed of the reasons for attending a primary care clinic, as their perceptions often differ from those given by their parents. When parents seek an appointment or referral without involving the young person, they should be asked to come again with the adolescent's consent, as the contrary would only compromise any future therapeutic engagement.

Adolescent psychiatric disorders have many similarities with both child and adult psychopathology that is covered in other chapters. This text focuses on those adolescent disorders and presentations that are more likely to be seen in primary care, and whose characteristics in this age group merit a different approach.

Depression

Depression occurs in 1% of young adolescents (girls = boys), which may rise up to 4% in later adolescence (higher in girls). The key features are similar to those experienced by adults, i.e. depressed mood (persistent for at least 2 weeks), irritability, poor or excessive sleep, change in appetite (usually decrease), weight changes (usually loss), self-harm thoughts, poor concentration, loss of interest in previously enjoyable activities, fatigue and negative cognitions (feeling useless, inadequate, ugly, guilty, hopeless). Young people with depression often have comorbid anxiety, conduct or eating disorders. Established causes are life events (trauma/loss), personal predisposition (genetic) and physical illness (Angold and Costello 2006). The depressive episode usually remits, but there is high risk of relapse (one-third of young people over 2–3 years). In a small proportion of young people, depressive symptoms may become chronic, and there is risk of depression persisting in adult life (Fombonne *et al.* 2001).

The recognition of depressive presentation is important for primary care practitioners, as changes can be subtle and be missed until they become severe enough to be noticed, hence more difficult to treat. Symptoms can also be masked by externalizing behaviours. Treatment includes cognitive behavioural therapy (CBT – aiming at changing maladaptive and negative ways of thinking), antidepressant medication, management of underlying family, school or social problems, brief psychotherapy, and social skills training (improving self-esteem and interpersonal relationships) (National Institute for Health and Clinical Excellence 2005; TADS 2005; Goodyer *et al.* 2007). CBT and other psychological interventions can be provided in primary care for mild to moderate depressive episodes by trained counsellors (King *et al.* 2002; Watanabe *et al.* 2006). It is important, however, to monitor the young person in case they develop more serious and entrenched symptoms or self-harm behaviours that will require involvement of specialist services (Rushton *et al.* 2000). It is also preferable that antidepressant medication is prescribed and monitored, where possible, by CAMHS. If there are waiting-list constraints and until the young person can attend an outpatient appointment, this can be initiated in primary care. Unlike adult psychopharmacological options, there is limited choice of antidepressants for adolescents. In the UK, for example, only fluoxetine from the SSRIs is currently licensed, because of recent but inconclusive indications that other SSRIs were associated with increased suicidality (Smith 2009).

Case 2

A 15-year-old girl (named Z) visited her GP because she had been feeling low in her mood. She was accompanied by a friend, who insisted that she should be seeking help. During the consultation, Z disclosed that she had been cutting her forearms for a few months, which she described as giving her a temporary relief from her feelings. Z was in agreement to be referred to the local CAMHS, but on the condition that her parents would not be informed, as she worried that they would not understand, and would be angry with her. At the first attempt, the GP failed to persuade her to give consent to involve her parents, although there was no indication of potential child protection concerns. The GP agreed to make a referral, but asked to meet with Z in the interim; she reassured Z and explained to her and her friend the importance of including her parents in future treatment. Z thought about it, and agreed when she saw her GP for the second time. When the family attended their CAMHS appointment, the parents were not surprised to hear that their daughter had been self-harming. They had suspected this for some time, but did not know how to approach her and find ways of helping; instead they felt guilty that it was their fault.

Comment

In addition to an assessment and initiation of treatment for self-harm and maybe underlying depression, the appropriate initiation of a referral by engaging the family can be crucial for a positive outcome. It is thus important to balance the young person's wishes for confidentiality, her cognitive and chronological age, ethical concerns, consideration of any safeguarding issues, and the need to involve the family in the assessment and intervention. Usually, perseverance, containment and clear communication with the young person and her carers should be sufficient at this early stage.

Deliberate self-harm

Vague suicidal thoughts can occur in up to one-third of teenagers, with an annual prevalence of deliberate self-harm (hospital-treated) of about 0.2% in the general population. The lifetime prevalence of deliberate self-harm in adolescence has been found to be between 2 and 3.5% in studies from Europe and much higher in the United States (about 9%). It increases with age, is more common in females (3:1) and low socioeconomic groups, and is often precipitated by arguments with family, friends or partner (Evans *et al.* 2004). The method is usually either by overdose of analgesics, antidepressants or other medication, or by inflicting lacerations (Hawton *et al.* 2003). There are often associated mental health problems such as depression, behavioural problems and alcohol/drug abuse (Skegg 2005); emerging personality disorder should also be considered, particularly in those with a history of abuse or abandonment and other features such as extreme emotional lability and destructive relationships. There is high risk of eventual suicide in up to 10% of the young people who self-harm (Windfuhr *et al.* 2008).

When young people present with mental health concerns in primary care, it is important to ask screening questions on self-harm history or ideation, and not to solely rely on parents' feedback. As long as the young person is engaged and the questions are asked in a sensitive manner, these are likely to bring relief, rather than increase their distress. A mental state examination can identify underlying psychiatric disorders such as depression. Reassurance and containment of anxieties and fears should be addressed at both the adolescent and their parents, before further help is sought. Clear communication with the family can alleviate secrecy, hence distortion of the young person's cognitions or acts; for example, if the young person does not wish their parents to know, or vice versa. A number of factors should be considered in order to establish the extent of risk such as the severity, perceived intent and impact, safety within the household and family relationships. In some situations, child protection procedures may need to be instigated through involvement of Social Services, i.e. if there is indication or evidence of abuse, persistent fear of returning to the family, impaired parenting capacity or other concerns about the young person's safety.

While a referral is made to emergency community or inpatient adolescent psychiatric services, depending on the degree of risk, a number of measures can be put in place to minimize this risk. All adults involved with the young person, including their teachers, should adopt a consistent, comforting and understanding approach. This may not be the best time to address underlying problems such as family conflict, as this is an emotive period, with parents and young people experiencing different and intense emotions of guilt, anger and anxiety. Safety precautions include the removal of tablets and sharp objects, and monitoring of any pharmacological treatment by the parents. Similar systems should set up if the young person lives in a children's home or hostel (Taylor *et al.* 2006), although consistency is more difficult because of the multiple carers involved.

The degree of risk will determine whether an urgent psychiatric assessment is required by the on-call service, or within the next few days at the outpatient service. There is no established intervention for self-harm, which usually depends on the underlying causes. This may involve individual cognitive behavioural or psychodynamic therapy, treatment of an underlying disorder, family therapy, or work with the school, for example if the self-harm is precipitated by bullying (AACAP 2001; Hawton *et al.* 2006). Maintaining a trusting and engaging relationship with the young person is crucial, so that they feel empowered to revisit the primary care service if in future distress, particularly if they start recognizing early signs of low mood or becoming suicidal again.

Anxiety disorders

Anxiety is a normal self-protective reaction in young life to novel and fear-evoking situations. It is the severity of distress and the consequential dysfunction that influences a clinician's decision to diagnose anxiety disorders. They are one of the commonest mental disorders seen in adolescence, with a prevalence of 4.4% and a higher representation in girls (Green *et al.* 2005). They are classified as in adults, with the main types experienced by adolescents being generalized anxiety, phobic, panic and separation anxiety disorder. They present with a combination of physical and psychological symptoms.

Phobic disorders are characterized by persistent irrational fears of specific objects or situations, which lead to avoidance behaviours that play a role in the maintenance of the anxiety. In contrast, in *generalized anxiety* disorders their worries are related to general life circumstances, be it the past, present or future, and are usually not characterized by avoidance behaviours. *Social anxiety* disorder or *social phobia* is anxiety about social situations, as adolescents fear scrutiny, embarrassment, humiliation and ridicule. This anxiety is not caused by impaired capacity in socialization, as the young people interact well with familiar people, except in severe cases. In the generalized form, all social interactions are avoided, while in the non-generalized form, anxiety is observed in specific social situations such as public speaking or eating in restaurants. *Separation anxiety* disorder is exaggerated anxiety for the young person's chronological age, in response to true or perceived separation from carers. It is a cause of *school refusal* that has to be differentiated from truancy, as they have different aetiological factors and management. *Panic disorders* present as unprovoked spontaneous attacks of severe anxiety.

Cognitive behavioural therapy is the preferred treatment for anxiety disorders, in which the cognitive element aims to convert the negative fearful beliefs to neutral realistic ones (Klein 2009). The behavioural element involves gradual exposure to a hierarchy of objects or situations that provoke anxiety and promote acclimatization, with reduction in both the anxiety response and the abnormal fearful cognitions. Behavioural therapy can be offered by most child mental health practitioners, suitably trained practice therapists and primary mental health workers (Sakolsky and Birmaher 2008). Relaxation therapy can be used as adjuvant in all types of anxiety disorders. Referral to a CBT therapist in specialist CAMHS will be needed for severe or resistant cases. Antidepressants are only reserved for severe cases of anxiety and to treat comorbid depression. These should be best commenced by a child psychiatrist and may be monitored by the young person's GP. Use of benzodiazepines should be restricted to treat severe acute anxiety for brief periods under close supervision. Mild cases of anxiety disorder have a good outcome, while chronic and severe cases are at risk of persisting or recurring in adulthood.

Case 3

The parents of a 14-year-old boy (named X) feared that the local council will take action against them for his school absence, as he had refused to go to school after staying at home for a fortnight with a viral illness. They felt frustrated and angry about their situation, and approached their GP. The GP saw X in surgery and was told that he was anxious about going to school, although he was happy when he was at home. He had not completed the course-work sent to him by his teachers, and instead played on his computer and PlayStation. X enjoyed good energy levels, appetite and sleep. His parents worried that X was being bullied at school. He was the only child, and he had similar problems when he moved from primary to secondary school. The GP made a diagnosis of separation anxiety disorder and liaised with the education welfare officer, who arranged graded entry to school. The GP also referred X for anxiety management to the local CAMHS, and asked the practice counsellor to see X's mother, who was suffering with general anxiety disorder, and was maintaining X's own worries.

Comment

It is important to work collaboratively with the family, in order to help the young person. Liaison work with the school to aid his return to school is as essential as the anxiety management with the young person. It is important to rule out underlying depression and at the same time differentiate this presentation from school truancy.

Oppositional and conduct disorders

Behavioural problems are classified as psychiatric disorders in both the ICD-10 and the DSM-IV. However, there is ongoing debate whether they constitute a mental health condition, as these young people and their families also frequently come into contact with social and education services (Vostanis *et al.* 2003). Behavioural problems are broadly divided into *oppositional* (usually of milder severity and in younger children) and the more severe *conduct disorders* (in older children and adolescents, and often associated with offending). The prevalence of behavioural problems that require assessment and treatment is about 6.5% in boys and 2.5% in girls of 5–10 years. In adolescence, the rates rise to 8.5% and 4% respectively (Maughan *et al.* 2004). There is higher frequency in urban and socially deprived areas. Well-established associated characteristics and risk factors are chronic marital conflict, family dysfunction and family breakdown, parenting (lack of affection and discipline/consistency), overcrowding, criminality of the father, exposure to violence (at home or among peers) and alcohol abuse in the family (Burke *et al.* 2002; Meltzer *et al.* 2007).

A young person may present by being argumentative, defiant, angry or spiteful/ vindictive. More severe behaviours include lying, initiating fights, cruelty to animals or people, destructiveness, fire setting, stealing, truanting, running away, robbery and violence. At least one-third of young people with behavioural problems also have learning difficulties. Other comorbid disorders are hyperactivity, depression and substance abuse (Arcelus and Vostanis 2005). It is also important to consider whether the behavioural problems are secondary to a developmental disorder such as autism or learning disability, because of impaired communication and social skills, as these children will need a different treatment approach. Although there are continuities with antisocial behaviour in late adolescence and adult life, many young people break this cycle, i.e. there are also discontinuities from further psychosocial problems, usually in the presence of protective factors such as parental warmth, school achievement, high self-esteem and friendships (Rutter 2005).

Interventions include behaviour modification, parental counselling, family therapy, social problem-solving, group therapy (for young people and/or parents) and school-based programmes (Sanders and Turner 2005; National Institute for Health and Clinical Excellence 2006; Scott 2007). Irrespective of the debate on whether behavioural problems constitute a mental health condition, young people with externalizing presentations frequently attend primary care services (Arcelus *et al.* 2001). As their acts often have substantial impact and burden on their families, schools and wider community, carers and agencies may exert additional pressure on primary care services to provide help. The adolescents themselves may not understand the reason for the request, and therefore do not wish to attend their appointment. Nevertheless, every attempt should be made to assess them before deciding on the next course of action.

If there are indications of an underlying comorbid psychiatric or developmental disorder, a referral to the local mental health service would be indicated. In the absence of psychiatric comorbidity, a good knowledge of local services, particularly if there are established protocols and care pathways, will establish which are the most appropriate for the young person and their family (Shivram *et al.* 2009). These include voluntary or youth services, family support, education services if the behaviours are school-related, youth offending, substance abuse or housing agencies. Where the needs are complex and the potential risk is high, an inter-agency meeting may be helpful in ensuring agreement and consistency among the professionals involved. Primary mental health workers operating on the interface with specialist mental health services can facilitate this process, where one single intervention is unlikely to suffice.

Eating disorders

Concerns regarding eating problems may be raised by parents, teachers or friends of adolescents. It is important to differentiate the much more benign dieting to stay slim from physical disorders that cause weight loss, and from eating disorders. Because of the effect eating disorders can have on growth and development, early identification and prompt referral to specialist service is important. Diagnostic features and sub-categories used in adolescents are the same as in adults in both the ICD-10 and the DSM-IV classification systems. Problems related to eating, weight and body image are probably on the rise, and are related to a combination of underlying difficulties with emotional and social maturity, family communication and conflict, and societal pressures on losing weight, through the peer group and the media (Sigel 2008). The aims of treatment are to encourage weight gain and healthy eating, reduce symptoms and impairment, and facilitate physical and psychological recovery (NICE 2004). The following two broad types of disorders are seen, although a mixture of the two can also occur (Birmingham *et al.* 2009).

Anorexia nervosa is the most common eating disorder in adolescence, with its peak onset being between 15 and 19 years. The average prevalence rate is 3% among girls of this age range, with a female to male ratio of 10:1. It is characterized by body weight that is less than 15% of the expected, self-induced weight loss, body image distortion and widespread endocrine dysfunction involving the hypothalamic pituitary gonadal axis, which manifests as amenorrhea in girls and loss of sexual interest and potency in boys (Herpertz-Dahlmann 2009). Usually the restricting sub-type, in which weight loss is accomplished by dieting, fasting or exercising, is seen in adolescents. The binge eating / purging sub-type, which is associated with regular binging, purging or both, is seen in later adolescence or adulthood. The main psychopathological feature is the dread of fatness, and this might continue in spite of gross emaciation. It is this that differentiates from the weight loss seen in other psychiatric disorders such as depression.

Denial of illness is common, hence there is a need for a high index of suspicion and collaborative working with family and other professionals. Detailed physical examination in addition to weight and height and laboratory investigations for metabolic effects of starvation are crucial and should be carried out by the GP prior to referral to specialist services. Early identification and prompt referral are important, before the symptoms become entrenched and there is rapid weight loss. In recent years, there has been a shift in management from inpatient to outpatient care, except for the very physically unwell adolescents. These should be admitted to units that can provide skilled re-feeding with careful monitoring, in combination with psychosocial interventions (NICE 2004). Gradual and steady weight gain with frequent meals is aimed for, alongside nutritional counselling and psychoeducation. A multi-component management package that includes physical monitoring, behavioural contracts and individual and family therapy is often preferable, depending on the severity of the illness, the cognitive ability of the adolescent and the underpinning family factors (Gowers 2008). Individual therapy involves a combination of empathetic support, education, problem-solving, cognitive analytical therapy, focal dynamic therapy, CBT to positively reframe cognitions regarding weight and body image, and interpersonal therapy. Evidence supports the effectiveness of family therapy and CBT (Le Grange and Eisler 2009; Schmidt 2009), while findings on the use of medication (antidepressants and low-dose atypical antipsychotics) remain inconclusive (Gowers and Byrant-Waugh 2004).

Bulimia nervosa usually presents in older adolescents and young adults, with recent surveys suggesting that 1% of female 11–20-year-olds meet the diagnostic criteria.

Presentation, as in adults, includes fear of being overweight, binge eating and measures to counteract the effects of eating that include self-induced vomiting, exercises and use of purgatives and laxatives. These adolescents are more likely to have impulse control, alcohol and substance misuse and mood problems. Cognitive behavioural therapy is emerging as treatment of choice (Gowers 2008).

Early-onset psychosis

The national average incidence rate of psychotic disorders is around 15 per 100 000. Schizophrenia, drug-induced psychosis, mania, severe depression and organic conditions are known causes of psychosis in adolescence. The core symptoms of psychosis in adolescents are similar to those seen in adults (Clark 2001). The symptoms and signs may, however, not be clear-cut and keep changing, stressing the need for a full diagnostic assessment, good therapeutic engagement and the need to work with diagnostic uncertainly in early psychosis.

Schizophrenia is considered a neurodevelopmental disorder with multifactorial aetiology in which genetic inheritance, developmental susceptibility and environmental factors are implicated. The incidence rises in adolescence and peaks in early adulthood. In contrast to the adult's male to female prevalence of 2:1, in adolescence an equal sex distribution is seen, possibly due to earlier onset of puberty in girls. The adolescent presentation continues into adulthood, and the same diagnostic features are used in adolescence as in adulthood in both the DSM-IV and the ICD-10. Insidious deterioration in the form of social aloofness, declining school performance and bizarre behaviour may be seen before the onset of florid psychosis. Slow onset, negative symptoms, disorganized behaviour, hallucinations and fewer delusions are seen in adolescent-onset schizophrenia. Early recognition and treatment improves outcome; in contrast, a longer duration of untreated psychosis (DUP) is associated with poorer prognosis (Marshall *et al.* 2005). DUP is the time interval between the onset of symptoms and the initiation of treatment. Indicators of poor prognosis are premorbid social and cognitive impairment, prolonged first episode and duration of untreated psychosis, and presence of negative symptoms.

There is a high risk of suicide in the early years of the psychotic illness. In bipolar affective disorder the teenager's mood can swing from severe depression to mania, and is more likely to present as rapid or mixed cycling, instead of the clear episodes of mania that are commonly experienced by adults (Giedd 2000). Early features of psychosis may be difficult to differentiate from usual adolescent behaviours, non-psychotic mental health problems or drug-induced psychosis. Young people can experience severe anxiety following trauma such as abuse or death of a family member, which may be experienced as sensory phenomena defined as 'pseudo-hallucinations', but misinterpreted as psychotic symptoms. A typical illustration is seeing the image or hearing the voice, usually at bedtime, of their loved one following their death.

Unfortunately, there is often a delay in the recognition and treatment, which can result in deterioration of symptoms and unnecessary hospitalization (Bhangoo and Carter 2009). When such admission is unavoidable, this should be in an age-appropriate adolescent psychiatric unit, and it is essential to keep compulsory admissions under the Mental Health Act to a minimum. The young person usually struggles with symptoms of psychosis, and has to come to terms with the stigma of diagnosis and the recommended treatment, and these place them at risk of disengaging from services. Following the development and evaluation of such service models in Australia, early intervention psychosis teams (PIER) for 14–35-year-olds have been set up in recent years in the UK to offer expertise with multimodal treatment packages of antipsychotic medication, psycho-education for the young person and their family, family therapy to deal with the impact of illness, social skills training and cognitive therapy to deal with resistant psychotic symptoms in suitable young persons (Joseph and Birchwood 2005; McLeod *et al.* 2007; Patton *et al.* 2007). The first 3 years following the initial onset is the critical period for interventions to reduce the impact of the illness. The majority of young people will require long-term service input that includes close monitoring, relapse prevention and effective transition to adult mental health services.

Substance abuse

The use of chemical substances by youth for their psychological effects has become a major public health issue. Many adolescents go through experimental use as part of their curiosity and high-risk peer-related activities. Some go on to use substances on a recreational basis, and this may progress to problematic use in which young people continue to take them on a regular basis in spite of negative consequences. The same definitions are used for substance dependence in adolescents as in adults in the ICD-10 and the DSM-IV. Alcohol and nicotine are most frequently used, followed by cannabis, stimulants, sleeping pills and hallucinogens, while cocaine and opiate use is less frequent and lower than in adults. Young people tend to use multiple or changing types of drugs. Availability of substances in the presence of predisposing factors such as family psychopathology, deviant peer group and family adverse circumstances results in substance misuse (Sussman *et al.* 2008). Self-treatment with substances for psychological distress is a popular hypothesis that is supported by the presence of concomitant psychiatric disorders that include mood, anxiety, conduct disorders and ADHD in these young users.

Substance misuse affects all the domains of adolescent life. Young people may become preoccupied with substances at the cost of positive growth and educational attainment. The financial stress of drug-seeking may result in indulgence in criminal activities such as stealing and prostituting to feed the habit. Health effects arising from acute intoxication include accidents, overdoses and reckless behaviours of violence, unprotected sex and blood-borne infections such as hepatitis C and HIV due to needle sharing; while chronic intoxication leads to poor nutrition and specific health hazards, according to the particular substance. Psychiatric disorders are often comorbid, with different underlying mechanisms. For example, in the last decade studies have identified adolescent cannabis use to be a risk factor for psychosis (Arseneault *et al.* 2002). There are increased rates of comorbid depression, anxiety, deliberate self-harm and risk of suicide (Hawkins 2009).

A good history with emphasis on psychosocial circumstances and a physical examination are helpful in making the diagnosis. Developing good rapport is essential, so that the young person feels comfortable in giving an accurate account. In addition, urine drug testing is a valuable tool. Although there is a need for more systematic research in adolescents, the same principles of treatment in adults are being used with young people. Multiple agencies are involved and coordinated working is vital in addressing the needs of this vulnerable group. Engagement with services can be problematic, for which reason a GP has a major role in ensuring supportive collaborative working with young people and prompt referral to specialist services. A motivational style of interviewing can help the young person to move through the stages of pre-contemplation, contemplation, determination, action and maintenance (Prochaska and Diclemente 1992). The treatment of comorbid psychiatric disorders is important, as it is to address the adverse social and financial circumstances. Individual psychotherapy, pharmacotherapy, family therapy and group education therapy programmes are part of the multimodal treatment (Galanter *et al.* 2007; Becker and Curry 2008).

Summary

- The prevalence of adolescent psychiatric disorders that require assessment and treatment is approximately 11.5%.
- These are possibly on the increase, predominantly depression, deliberate self-harm, substance abuse and conduct disorders.
- There is a high rate of comorbidity between disorders.
- Adolescents present frequently in primary care, and physical or behavioural presentations may mask psychiatric disorders.
- The distinction between 'normal' adolescent behaviours and the onset of psychiatric symptoms can be difficult, and requires careful assessment and corroborative information.
- It is important to involve the young person in their own right, as well as their family or carers.
- A psychiatric assessment should take into consideration the young person's developmental functioning (cognitive, emotional, social), which may differ from their chronological age.
- Engaging the young person from the outset is a significant predictor of successful clinical outcome.
- Ethical, confidentiality and child protection issues should be taken into consideration in the formulation of a treatment plan.
- A range of individual, family and pharmacological treatment modalities are provided by specialist mental health services.
- As multiple factors are likely to be present, other agencies may need to be involved, from the social care, education or voluntary sector.

References

American Academy of Child and Adolescent Psychiatry (AACAP). (2001). Practice parameter for the assessment and treatment of children and adolescents with suicidal behaviour. *Journal of the American Academy of Child and Adolescent Psychiatry*, **40** (suppl), 24S–51S.

Angold, A., and Costello, E. (2006). Puberty and depression. *Child and Adolescent Psychiatric Clinics of North America*, **15**, 919–937.

Arcelus, J., and Vostanis, P. (2005). Psychiatric co-morbidity in children and adolescents. *Current Opinion in Psychiatry*, **18**, 429–434.

Arcelus, J., Gale, F., and Vostanis, P. (2001). Characteristics of children and parents attending a British primary mental health service. *European Child and Adolescent Psychiatry*, **10**, 91–95.

Arseneault, L., Cannon, M., Poulton, R., et al. (2002). Cannabis use in adolescence and risk of adult psychosis: longitudinal prospective study. *British Medical Journal*, **325**, 1212–1213.

Becker, S., and Curry, J. (2008). Outpatient interventions for adolescent substance abuse: a quality of evidence review. *Journal of Consulting and Clinical Psychology*, **76**, 531–543.

Bhangoo, R., and Carter, C. (2009). Very early interventions in psychotic disorders. *Psychiatric Clinics of North America*, **32**, 81–94.

Birmingham, C., Touyz, S., and Harbottle, J. (2009). Are anorexia nervosa and bulimia nervosa separate disorders? Challenging the 'transdiagnostic' theory of eating disorders. *European Eating Disorders Review*, **17**, 2–13.

Burke, J., Loeber, R., and Birmaher, B. (2002). Oppositional defiant disorder and conduct disorder: a review of the past 10 years–part II. *Journal of the American Academy of Child and Adolescent Psychiatry*, **41**, 1275–1293.

Clark, A. (2001) Proposed treatment for adolescent psychosis: Schizophrenia and schizophrenia-like psychosis. *Advances in Psychiatric Treatment*, **7**, 16–23.

Collishaw, S., Maughan, B., Goodman, R., and Pickles, A. (2004). Time trends in adolescent mental health. *Journal of Child Psychology and Psychiatry*, **45**, 1350–1362.

Costello, E., Mustillo, S., Erkanli, A., Keeler, G., and Angold, A. (2003). Prevalence and development of psychiatric disorders in childhood and adolescence. *Archives of General Psychiatry*, **60**, 837–844.

Evans, E., Hawton, K., and Rodham, K. (2004). Factors associated with suicidal phenomena in adolescents: a systematic review of population-based studies. *Clinical Psychology Review*, **24**, 957–979.

Fleitlich-Bilyk, B., and Goodman, R. (2004). Prevalence of child and adolescent psychiatric disorders in southeast Brazil. *Journal of the American Academy of Child and Adolescent Psychiatry*, **43**, 727–734.

Fombonne, E., Wostear, G., Cooper, V., Harrington, R., and Rutter, M. (2001). The Maudsley long-term follow-up of child and adolescent depression: I. Psychiatric outcomes in adulthood. *British Journal of Psychiatry*, **179**, 210–217.

Galanter, M., Glickman, L., and Singer, D. (2007). An overview of outpatient treatment of adolescent substance abuse. *Substance Abuse*, **28**, 51–58.

Giedd, J. (2000). Bipolar disorder and attention deficit-hyperactivity disorder in children and adolescents. *Journal of Clinical Psychiatry*, **61**, 31–34.

Goodyer, I., Dubicka, B., Wilkinson, P., *et al.* (2007). Selective Serotonin Reuptake Inhibitors (SSRIs) and routine specialist care with and without cognitive behaviour therapy in adolescents with major depression: randomised controlled trial. *British Medical Journal*, **335**, 142–146.

Gowers, S. (2008). Management of eating disorders in child and adolescents. *Archives of Disease in Childhood*, **93**, 331–334.

Gowers, S., and Byrant-Waugh, R. (2004). Management of child and adolescent eating disorders: the current evidence base and future directions. *Journal of Child Psychiatry and Psychology*, **45**, 63–83.

Green, H., McGinnity, A., Meltzer, H., Ford, T., and Goodman, R. (2005). *Mental Health of Children and Young People in Great Britain*. London: Palgrave MacMillan.

Hawkins, E. (2009). A tale of two systems: co-occurring mental health and substance abuse disorders treatment for adolescents. *Annual Review of Psychology*, **60**, 197–227.

Hawton, K., Rodham, K., and Evans, E. (2006). *By their Own Young Hand: Deliberate Self-harm and Suicidal Ideas in Adolescents*. London: Jessica Kingsley.

Hawton, K., Hall, S., Simkin, S., *et al.* (2003). Deliberate self-harm in adolescents: a study of characteristics and trends in Oxford, 1999–2000. *Journal of Child Psychology and Psychiatry*, **44**, 1191–1198.

Herpertz-Dahlmann, B. (2009). Adolescent eating disorders: definitions, symptomatology, epidemiology and comorbidity. *Child and Adolescent Psychiatric Clinics of North America*, **18**, 31–47.

Joseph, R., and Birchwood, M. (2005). The national policy reforms for mental health services and the story of early intervention services in the United Kingdom. *Journal of Psychiatry and Neuroscience*, **30**, 362–365.

King, M., Davidson, O., Taylor, F., *et al.* (2002). Effectiveness of teaching general practitioners skills in brief cognitive behaviour therapy to treat patients with depression: randomised controlled trial. *British Medical Journal*, **324**, 947–950.

Klein, R. (2009). Anxiety disorders. *Journal of Child Psychology and Psychiatry*, **50**, 153–162.

Le Grange, D., and Eisler, I. (2009). Family interventions in adolescent anorexia nervosa. *Child and Adolescent Psychiatric Clinics of North America*, **18**, 159–173.

McLeod, T., Morris, M., Birchwood, M., and Dovey, A. (2007). Cognitive behavioural therapy group work with voice hearers: Part II. *British Journal of Nursing*, **16**, 292–295.

Marshall, M., Lewis, S., Lockwood, A., *et al.* (2005). Association between duration of untreated psychosis and outcome in cohorts of first episode patients: a systematic review. *Archives of General Psychiatry*, **62**, 975–983.

Maughan, B., Rowe, R., Messor, J., Goodman, R., and Meltzer, H. (2004). Conduct disorder and oppositional defiant disorder in a national sample: developmental epidemiology. *Journal of Child Psychology and Psychiatry*, **45**, 609–621.

Meltzer, H., Vostanis, P., Goodman, R., and Ford, T. (2007). Children's perceptions of neighbourhood trustworthiness and safety in their mental health. *Journal of Child Psychology and Psychiatry*, **48**, 1208–1213.

Mueller, T., Gavin, L., and Kulkarni, A. (2008). The association between sex education and youth's engagement in sexual intercourse, age at first intercourse, and birth control use at first sex. *Journal of Adolescent Health*, **42**, 89–96.

National Institute of Health and Clinical Excellence. (2004). *Eating disorders: Core Interventions in the Treatment and Management of Anorexia Nervosa, Bulimia Nervosa and Related Eating Disorders.* Quick Reference Guide. London: NICE (www.nice.org.uk).

National Institute for Health and Clinical Excellence. (2005). *Depression in Children and Young People: Identification and Management in Primary, Community and Secondary Care.* Quick Reference Guide. London: NICE (www.nice.org.uk).

National Institute for Health and Clinical Excellence. (2006). *Conduct Disorder in Children: Parent-training / Education Programmes.* Guidance. London: NICE.

Patton, G., Hetrick, S., and McGorry, P. (2007). Service responses for youth onset mental disorders. *Current Opinion in Psychiatry*, **20**, 319–324.

Prochaska, J., and Diclemente, C. (1992). Stages of change in the modification of problem behaviours. *Program of Behaviours Modifications*, **28**, 183–218.

Rushton, J., Clark, S., and Freed, G. (2000). Primary care role in the management of childhood depression: a comparison of paediatricians and family physicians. *Pediatrics*, **105**, 957–962.

Rutter, M. (2005). Environmentally mediated risks for psychopathology: research strategies and findings. *Journal of the American Academy of Child and Adolescent Psychiatry*, **44**, 3–18.

Sakolsky, D., and Birmaher, B. (2008). Pediatric anxiety disorders: management in primary care. *Current Opinion in Pediatrics*, **20**, 538–543.

Sanders, M., and Turner, K. (2005). Reflection on the challenges of effective dissemination of behavioural family intervention: our experience with the Triple P–Positive Parenting Programme. *Child and Adolescent Mental Health*, **10**, 158–169.

Schmidt, U. (2009). Cognitive behavioural approaches in adolescent anorexia and bulimia nervosa. *Child and Adolescent Psychiatric Clinics of North America*, **18**, 147–158.

Scott, S. (2007). Conduct disorders in children: parent programmes are effective but training and provision are inadequate. *British Medical Journal*, **334**, 646.

Shivram, R., Bankart, J., Meltzer, H., *et al.* (2009). Service utilization by children with conduct disorders: findings from the 2004 Great Britain child mental health survey. *European Child and Adolescent Psychiatry*, **18**(9), 555–563.

Sigel, E. (2008). Eating disorders. *Adolescent Medicine*, **19**, 547–572.

Skegg, K. (2005). Self-harm. *The Lancet*, **366**, 1471–1483.

Smith, E. (2009). Association between antidepressant half-life and the risk of suicidal ideation or behaviour among children and adolescents: confirmatory analysis and research implications. *Journal of Affective Disorders*, **114**, 143–148.

Sussman, S., Skara, S., and Ames, L. (2008). Substance abuse among adolescents. *Substance Use and Misuse*, **43**, 1802–1828.

Taylor, H., Stuttaford, M., Broad, B., and Vostanis, P. (2006). Why a 'roof' is not enough: the characteristics of young homeless people referred to a designated mental health service. *Journal of Mental Health*, **15**, 491–501.

The Treatment for Adolescents with Depression Study (TADS) Team. (2005). The Treatment for Adolescents with Depression Study (TADS): demographic and clinical characteristics. *Journal of the American Academy of Child and Adolescent Psychiatry*, **44**, 28–40.

Vostanis, P., Meltzer, H., Goodman, R., and Ford, T. (2003). Service utilisation by children with conduct disorders: findings from the GB national study. *European Child and Adolescent Psychiatry*, **12**, 231–238.

Watanabe, N., Churchill, R., Hunot, V., and Furukawa, T. (2006). Psychotherapy for depression in children and adolescents. *Cochrane Systematic Review*, **3**.

Windfuhr, K., While, D., Hunt, D., *et al.* and the National Confidential Inquiry into Suicide and Homicide by People with Mental Illness. (2008). Suicide in juveniles and adolescents in the United Kingdom. *Journal of Child Psychology and Psychiatry*, **49**, 1155–1165.

Further reading

Carr, A. (ed.). (2000). *What Works with Children and Adolescents? A Critical Review of Psychological Interventions with Children, Adolescents and their Families*. London: Routledge.

Dogra, N., Parkin, A., Gale, F., and Frake, C. (eds.). (2008). *A Multidisciplinary Handbook of Child and Adolescent Mental health for Front-line Professionals*, 2nd edn. London: Jessica Kingsley.

Fonagy, P., Target, M., Cottrell, D., Phillips, J., and Kurtz, Z. (2002). *What Works for Whom? A Critical Review of Treatments for Children and Adolescents*. New York: Guilford.

Goodman, R., and Scott, S. (2005). *Child Psychiatry*, 2nd edn. Oxford: Blackwell,.

Gowers, S. (ed.). (2005). *Seminars in Child and Adolescent Psychiatry*, 2nd edn. London: Gaskell.

Rutter, M., Bishop, D., Pine, D., *et al.* (2008). *Rutter's Child and Adolescent Psychiatry, 5th edn.* Oxford: Blackwell.

Stallard, P. (2002). *Think Good–Feel Good: A Cognitive Behaviour Therapy Workbook for Children and Young People*. Chichester: Wiley.

Vostanis, P. (ed.). (2007). *Mental Health Interventions and Services for Vulnerable Children and Young People*. London: Jessica Kingsley.

Wolpert, M., Fuggle, P., Cottrell, D., *et al.* (2006). *Drawing on the Evidence: Advice for Mental Health Professionals Working with Children and Adolescents*, 2nd edn. London: CAMHS Evidence Based Practice Unit.

Useful websites for parents

Association for Child and Adolescent Mental Health: www.acamh.org.uk.

Bullying UK: www.bullying.co.uk.

CAMHS Outcome Research Consortium, collaboration to evaluate outcomes in children's mental health services: www.corc.uk.net.

Change Our Minds: www.changeourminds.com.

Child and Adolescent Mental Health, website for professionals, young people and parents: www.camh.org.uk.

Children's Commissioner for England, promoting the views and interests of children and young people: www.11million.org.uk.

Department for Children, Schools and Families: www.dcsf.gov.uk.

FOCUS, Royal College of Psychiatrists, promotion of effective practice in child mental health: www.rcpsych.ac.uk/crtu/focus.aspx.

Health and Social Care Advisory Service, CAMHS Projects: http://www.hascas.org.uk/camhs_doh_projects.shtml/.

Mind Matters, Australia: www.mindmatters.edu.au.

Mood Gym, training programme to prevent depression, Australia: www.moodgym.anu.edu.au.

Teacher Net: www.teachernet.gov.uk/wholeschool/sen/ypmentalhealth/.

Young Minds: www.youngminds.org.uk

Mental health care for older adults

James Warner and Daniel Hacking

Learning objectives

Understand the presentation and management of depression in older people
Recognize signs and symptoms of dementia and initiate initial management of a person
  suspected of having dementia
Recognize and manage behavioural and psychological symptoms of dementia
Understand the causes and management of delirium

Older people are as vulnerable as the young to mental disorders although the epidemiology and presentation may differ compared to younger people. Many factors common in older people such as social isolation, poverty, bereavement and physical comorbidity contribute to the aetiology, and complicate the management of these conditions. This chapter focuses mainly on three mental disorders (dementia, depression, delirium) which are particularly prevalent, or have unique clinical and management characteristics, in older populations. GPs have a key role in managing mental health problems for older people who have high levels of access to primary care, and who often have trusting and long-standing relationships with practitioners. The physical comorbidity is probably the most salient mediator of quality care: while its presence increases access and therefore recognition for some, those who are housebound may lose out; physical illness can mask psychiatric problems or provide a cover for GP and patient to collude against recognition of emotional distress. The challenge is for primary care teams, including community nurses, to work together along with specialists to provide flexible care, sensitive to psychiatric diagnoses, but incorporating services related to physical and social needs.

Dementia

Epidemiology

Approximately 700 000 people currently have dementia in the UK and this is estimated to increase to nearly one million by 2021. A GP with an average list size will diagnose 1–2 new cases of dementia per year and care for between 10 and 20 people with established dementia. Approximately two-thirds of people with dementia never receive a formal diagnosis due partly to patients lacking insight or concealing their problems and partly to a reluctance of general practitioners to diagnose this condition (Knapp *et al.* 2007). Dementia increases with age; around 1in 20 people over the age of 65 will have dementia, increasing to 1 in 5 people over 80. The majority of people with dementia live at home, but it is estimated over half of care-home residents have dementia. Dementia affects all races and tends to be slightly more common in women, with an average life expectancy after diagnosis of 7–10 years. Dementia is a major source of personal distress to affected individuals and their carers in addition to being a huge burden on health and social services. In 2007, the total cost of dementia in the UK was estimated to be £17 billion (Knapp *et al.* 2007).

Symptoms and diagnosis

Dementia is not just a consequence of normal ageing. With advancing age people may find it harder to remember but this is distinct from dementia. In dementia there is usually a disturbance of more than one higher cortical function: memory, orientation (in time and/ or place), thinking, comprehension, language or judgement may be affected. In addition personality often changes. The profile of symptoms will vary according to the subtype of dementia and the individual. Dementia is distinguished from delirium (acute confusional states) because the syndrome develops over months rather than hours or days, and con-sciousness is not clouded.

In addition to these impairments of cognitive function, emotional and behavioural disturbances are very common. Collectively known as behavioural and psychological symp-toms of dementia (BPSD), these include apathy, depression, anxiety, aggression, hallucina-tions and delusions.

Diagnosis begins with suspecting something is awry and the general practitioner is often well placed to detect subtle signs, especially when people live alone. Clues may include noticing changes in a person's ability to care for themselves, confusion, disorientation or problems learning new things (for example with a change in medication). Carers (often spouses or children) may notice changes and bring the person to the GP. Insight is frequently lacking and people with dementia may demonstrate strategies to appear quite convincing. As a broad range of medical and social interventions become available, there is more of an imperative for GPs to become skilled at introducing the idea of memory loss in what can become difficult consultations.

If dementia is suspected, screening should include basic cognitive tests such as the Abbreviated Mental Test Score (AMTS) (see Table 15.1) or Mini-Mental State Examination (MMSE). A score of 8 or less on the AMTS or 24 or less on the MMSE indicates significant cognitive problems. However, there are problems with bedside tests which are culturally specific, do not account for differences in premorbid ability or sufficiently test frontal lobe function or memory. Note that higher scores (even 30/30 on the MMSE) can be achieved by people with dementia who have high premorbid intellect, and evidence of decline in cognition and function in the history is a better indication of dementia than bedside cognitive testing alone.

The differential diagnosis of dementia includes depression (depressive pseudodementia), delirium (acute confusional state), dysphasia (often due to stroke), learning disability and mild cognitive impairment. Furthermore some causes of dementia are considered reversible (for example hypothyroidism, normal-pressure hydrocephalus). Consequently any person suspected of having dementia should be referred to specialist services (old-age psychiatry, neurology or geriatric medicine depending on local services (NICE)).

Specialist assessment would normally include a history from the patient and informant, ideally in the person's home because assessing the environment can give several clues to the

Table 15.1. The Abbreviated Mental Test score

How old are you?	Exact age only
What is your date of birth?	Exact date/month
What is the year now?	Exact year only
What is the time of day?	Within one hour
Ask subject to remember an address '42, West St'	
Where are we?	Exact place name
Who is the current monarch	Current only
What was the date of the first world war?	Start or end OK
Count backwards from 20 to 1	No mistakes allowed
Can you tell me what those two people do for a living?	Recognize two roles e.g. doctor and nurse
Can you remember the address I gave you?	Point for exact recall

diagnosis. Specific investigations may include an occupational therapy assessment (to assess safety and function/activities of daily living), neuroimaging, psychometry (in-depth cognitive testing); blood tests including thyroid function, bone profile, renal function, full blood count, ESR, B12 and folate are best organized by the GP before referral.

People with dementia should have an extensive risk assessment including

- wandering/getting lost
- leaving gas or water taps running
- falls
- financial management and financial exploitation
- elder abuse.

However, these risks should be considered as part of an overall risk and benefit assessment. Where possible patients should be involved in decisions about what kind of action might be required; this will involve an assessment of mental capacity. Families and carers may also need to be involved in these decisions.

Common causes of dementia

There are many rare causes of dementia but over 95% of all cases of dementia are of four main types: Alzheimer's disease, vascular dementia, Lewy body dementia and fronto-temporal dementia. Rarer but important causes of dementia include normal-pressure hydrocephalus and alcohol-related dementia.

Alzheimer's disease

Alzheimer's disease (approximately 60% of all cases) is characterized by insidious onset and slow, generally fairly smooth decline in cognitive function. Specific gene mutations have been identified as causing AD in younger people; for the vast majority of people with AD, i.e. those over 65, the aetiology is a combination of genes (e.g. APOE) and environmental factors such as obesity, hypertension and head injury. In many people the aetiology is unclear. Alzheimer's is characterized by neurofibrillary tangles and deposition of amyloid in the cerebral cortex.

Vascular dementia

Approximately 30% of people have vascular dementia either alone or in combination with Alzheimer's disease. There are various patterns of vascular damage which may lead to dementia including a single stroke, multiple infarcts and hypoxic brain damage. Characteristic features of vascular dementia include

- abrupt onset (not invariable)
- stepwise deterioration
- fluctuating course
- vascular risk factors
  - diabetes, hypertension, obesity
- focal neurological signs
- often, greater insight than in Alzheimer's disease.

Dementia with Lewy bodies

While less than 10% of all dementia, DLB has a unique cluster of signs and symptoms including parkinsonism and vivid visual hallucinations arising around the time of cognitive impairment. The cognitive impairment often fluctuates considerably over the space of a few hours. Accurate diagnosis is necessary as antipsychotics should be particularly avoided in DLB. Diagnostic criteria include:

- primary criteria (2/3 for 'probable diagnosis')
  - fluctuating cognition or alertness
  - recurrent visual hallucinations
  - spontaneous features of parkinsonism
- supporting criteria
  - repeated falls or syncope
  - nocturnal confusion
  - transient loss of consciousness
  - antipsychotic sensitivity
  - tactile or olfactory hallucinations.

Fronto-temporal dementia

Although relatively rare (<5% of all dementia), FTD is noteworthy because of its atypical presentation. In contrast with other dementias, it often affects people under 65 and memory loss is often a late symptom. People with FTD usually present subtly with personality change, language disorders (dysphasia and loss of spontaneous conversation), disinhibition, distractibility and sometimes development of compulsive rituals.

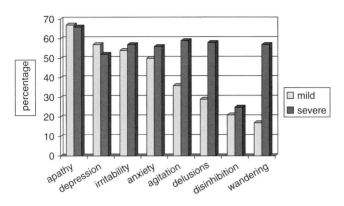

Figure 15.1 BPSD symptoms

Behavioural and psychological symptoms of dementia

Dementia is not just a disorder of cognition. Virtually everyone with dementia will experience non-cognitive symptoms. These tend to fluctuate over time and vary depending on the individual and dementia subtype. BPSD symptoms (profiled in Figure 15.1 showing BPSD prevalence for mild and severe dementia) cause great distress to the individual with dementia and their carers.

Management of BPSD should first exclude physical causes, especially if the onset is rapid or dramatic. Physical causes of BPSD include infection (commonly urinary and chest infections), pain, constipation and prescribed medication. Once physical causes have been excluded, management should include:

- environmental modification
  - sleep hygiene (avoid daytime napping)
  - social stimulation (deter care homes from sitting residents in front of the TV)
  - exercise
  - carer training
- behavioural approaches which are specifically designed to manage specific situations (see case vignette below)
- drug treatment should be a last resort and involve specialist input. Note: antipsychotics increase the risk of cerebrovascular disease and early death in people with dementia and should only be used as a last resort.

Drug treatment of dementia

Several drugs are now available for treating dementia. These include the acetylcholinesterase inhibitors (ACHIs), which increase levels of cortical acetylcholine – a neurotransmitter related to memory. Drugs in this group include donepezil, rivastigmine and galantamine. Evidence from several randomized trials suggests these drugs will have a clinically significant impact in around 1 in 4 people with dementia. Although probably effective in vascular dementia and DLB, they are only recommended by NICE for Alzheimer's disease. ACHIs are generally well tolerated but patients may experience nausea, diarrhoea and abdominal pain, which are often transient. Memantine (an NMDA partial agonist) may have some efficacy for people in later-stage dementia. NICE have issued guidance on the treatment of dementia.

NICE guidance on treatment of dementia

- Alzheimer's disease only ('standard diagnostic criteria')
- cholinesterase inhibitors only (not memantine)
- specialist diagnosis and initial prescription
- MMSE 10–20 when starting therapy (should be stopped if MMSE falls below 10)
- clinician must be sure of compliance
- follow-up every six months
- shared care protocols should be in place for ACHI use.

Management of dementia

Early assessment and treatment of dementia is important, ideally coordinated through a specialist service, but integrated with or linking to generalist primary care provision. Most people want to know their diagnosis and should be given the opportunity to hear it. People with dementia should be given the chance to learn about their diagnosis, make choices about treatment now and in the future (by setting up lasting powers of attorney and advance decisions) and sort out financial arrangements, including will writing, while they are able to. Alzheimer's societies have a huge amount of information available through their websites and helpline numbers (www.alzheimers.org.uk for England/Wales, www.alzscot.org for Scotland) and often run local support groups. Where available Admiral Nurses can provide information, advocacy and support to carers of people with dementia (www.fordementia. org.uk). All people diagnosed with dementia should be advised to inform the Driver and Vehicle Licensing Agency (DVLA) and their car insurance company; they may still be able to drive, subject to approval from the DVLA.

A range of benefits (attendance allowance, reduction in council tax) may be available and assistive technologies such as community alarms, fall monitors and GPS tracking devices may help make the home environment safer. Home care, day care, befriender services and respite care are often helpful to people with dementia and their carers. To access these resources it is helpful to arrange a needs assessment with local social services.

Case 1

Ray, a retired accounts executive, was 64 when his wife began to notice subtle changes. He stopped watching football and was no longer interested in how his favourite club (Spurs) was doing. Furthermore he began to let his appearance slip, having previously been fastidious about this. He also began to forget things such as appointments and seemed to be less able to do crosswords. At first his wife put this down to Ray retiring from work, but over the next year he began to have problems finding the right words for everyday objects and his memory got a lot worse – for the first time in 40 years of marriage he forgot their wedding anniversary. The last straw was when Ray, who had always been a gentle person, started getting up in the middle of the night and getting dressed for work. When his wife reminded him he had retired and it was 3.00 a.m. he looked bewildered and then lost his temper.

Ray would not accept there was any problem so his wife arranged for him to see his GP by suggesting he had a 'check up' now he had retired. The doctor listened to Ray (who said all was well) and his wife, who outlined the problems she had noticed. Ray was referred to local memory assessment services, who visited Ray at home and then arranged investigations including a cognitive assessment and MRI scan. The tests suggested Ray had vascular dementia. An occupational therapist suggested thicker curtains and a large clock in Ray's bedroom so he could see the time if he woke at night – this improved his early wakening. Ray was told his diagnosis, offered counselling, and encouraged to attend a support group and cognitive rehabilitation group. After attending a local Alzheimer's society support group, Ray's wife now avoids confrontation if he does get bewildered.

Specialist referral

- Anyone who shows memory loss and problems with language, planning, orientation, comprehension or thinking.

- Anyone over 50 with personality change, disinhibition, disorganized behaviour or apathy.

- Anyone with an established diagnosis of dementia who begins to exhibit behavioural or psychological symptoms not due to physical causes such as infection or pain.

Depression in the elderly

In older people depression is the most common psychiatric illness, with an estimated prevalence of 10–15% and rated as severe in 3%. Depression is under-diagnosed in older people for a multiple of reasons. For some there is a perception that depression carries a social stigma, so symptoms may not be volunteered. The diagnosis may also be masked by the presenting symptoms being of a physical rather than psychiatric nature (e.g. weight loss rather than low mood). This may be further complicated by medical comorbidity being one of the major risk factors for precipitating depression in the elderly.

There is no clear association between incidence of depression and age. It is, however, important to note that certain groups of older people are at higher risk. These include the bereaved, those with cerebrovascular disease (i.e. post stroke), Parkinson's disease, chronic physical illnesses, especially when associated with chronic pain, and people with dementia (especially dementia with Lewy bodies). As at younger ages, there is a higher prevalence in females compared to males although the sex difference narrows with increasing age.

Clinical features

The core symptoms of depression in older people are similar to depression presenting in younger people with a few important differences. The core symptoms remain a combination of low mood, lethargy and anhedonia (lack of sense of enjoyment) (Table 15.2) but all need not be present to reach a diagnosis. Sadness is commonly denied by patients and not necessary in order to make a diagnosis of depression. In the elderly, depression presents frequently at the more severe end of the spectrum with higher prevalence of psychosis (delusions and hallucinations). It is often marked by depressive thoughts such as hopelessness, helplessness, guilt, worthlessness, low self-esteem, self-blame and suicidal thoughts. Sleep disturbance is also a common presenting complaint to primary care. The elderly require less sleep so the key is whether they wake refreshed or wake anxious and fearful, keen to return to sleep but unable to do so. It is important to ensure good sleep hygiene, which includes ensuring that the patient is not sleeping during the day.

Table 15.2. Features of depression

Physical features	Psychological features
Sleep disturbance, waking early	Low mood – sustained and pervasive
Change of appetite/weight	Low mood often worse in the morning
Loss of libido	Poor memory and concentration
Being slowed up or agitated	Loss of enjoyment in life (anhedonia) Loss of motivation Feelings of guilt Hopelessness Worthlessness Suicidal ideation

Disturbance of behaviour, often with agitation or irritability (rather than psycho-motor retardation), is a common presentation of depression. Other signs may include aggression, self-neglect, malnutrition or social withdrawal. Psychomotor change may manifest as increased dependence and it is important to exclude physical causes (e.g. parkinsonism, CVAs and thyroid disturbance). If the depression is severe with much reduced mobility, (e.g. a bedbound, motionless, anorexic patient) then it is a psychiatric emergency.

It is important to exclude a physical cause for the symptoms such as dementia, hypothyroidism, occult carcinoma or any other haematological, endocrine, metabolic or space-occupying lesion.

Cognitive impairments are present in the majority of depressed older people. If this is severe it may be indistinguishable from dementia ('depressive pseudodementia'). Depressive pseudodementia differs from dementia because the onset is relatively abrupt, patients often complain about poor memory and are despairing, the assessment of cognition often results in 'don't know' responses, memories are often accessible with hints or cues from the assessor and there is often a past history of depression or an identifiable precipitant. The prognosis is variable and in some, mood and cognition respond to antidepressants. Some deficits, however, often persist after recovery and are associated with structural brain changes such as hippocampal atrophy. Perhaps related to this, depression is a risk factor for subsequent dementia (O'Brien *et al.* 2004).

Aetiology

Factors implicated in the aetiology of depression in the elderly include:

(1) disability and handicap (such as stroke and Parkinson's disease)
(2) physical illness (especially when associated with pain and sleep disturbance)
(3) sensory impairment (e.g. hearing or sight)
(4) social isolation with lack of a confiding relationship
(5) care home residents

(6) independent life events (particularly those of loss such as bereavement)

(7) existential concerns due to impending death.

There is a significant association between cerebrovascular disease and depression. Deep white-matter lesions are particularly strongly associated with depression when they occur in frontal lobes and basal ganglia, and by the fact that these lesions predict treatment resistance and poor outcome (O'Brien *et al.* 1998).

Assessment and investigations

- Psychiatric history and examination
- Collateral history from family, carers
- Physical history and examination. Targeting evidence of physical illness and contraindications to drug treatments
- Bedside cognitive assessment screen (e.g. the Abbreviated Mental Test Score, Mini-Mental State Examination, clock-drawing test)
- Depression rating scales (e.g. Geriatric Depression Scale, which is known to be valid in community and hospital settings and maintains specificity in mild to moderate dementia)
- Blood tests:
  - (i) FBC (anaemia leading to lethargy, high MCV in alcohol excess)
  - (ii) ESR (malignancy, vasculitis)
  - (iii) B12 and folate (low levels may contribute to depression or result from anorexia)
  - (iv) U & Es (uraemia, dehydration)
  - (v) Calcium (hypercalcaemia leading to depression, fatigue)
  - (vi) Thyroid function (hypo- and occasionally hyperthyroidism may present as depression)
  - (vii) Liver function (malignancy, alcohol excess)

Drug treatments

Studies have consistently shown that depression is undertreated as well as underdiagnosed in the primary care setting. Although tackling psychological and social elements of the aetiology are important facets of depression management, pharmacological treatment is often necessary.

Drug treatment is generally effective, well-tolerated and non-addictive, although patients often believe otherwise. There is significant stigma associated with taking antidepressants and this may need to be explored and addressed. Management of late-life depression is similar to that in younger adults, although older people may take longer to respond (8–10 weeks rather than 4–6 weeks). Selective serotonin-reuptake inhibitors (SSRIs), e.g. citalopram or sertraline, are effective first-line treatment in older people due to their reduced propensity for troubling side effects (e.g. urine retention and worsening confusion seen with the anticholinergic effects of tricyclics).

Provided the antidepressant dosage is optimal and the patient has been compliant, the prospects of recovery are poor if the patient has not responded in the first 4 weeks. If there has been little or no recovery, then the following steps are recommended:

- review the diagnosis (especially for organic causes of depression)
- review compliance
- optimize the antidepressant dosage
- consider psychosocial maintaining factors (e.g. family discord).

For patients who have not responded in the first 4 weeks, the choice lies between switching to an antidepressant from another class and augmenting with another substance (e.g. lithium). Switching class is the most practicable option in the primary care setting. If, however, the patient has clearly improved at 4 weeks but has not recovered then continuing the antidepressant at optimal dosage is associated with further remission in a significant proportion of patients. If there are any concerns about response, a referral to an old-age psychiatrist is warranted.

Treatment should be continued for up to a year according to the Royal College of Psychiatrists in those who respond, as in younger adults. If depression has been severe and/or recurrent then consider continuing indefinitely.

When stopping antidepressants withdrawal reactions (anxiety, mania, delirium, insomnia, GI side effects, headache, giddiness) may occur if drugs are stopped abruptly after 8 weeks or more. Therefore reduce gradually, over 4 weeks or, in those on long-term treatment, reduce over several months. When switching antidepressants 'gradual cross-tapering' is generally advised. This involves the incremental reduction of the 'old' drug and incremental increase of the 'new' drug.

Non-drug management

It is always important to address the psychological and social needs of the patient especially if there has not been a full recovery. Primary care is ideally positioned to provide optimal management of disabilities, improving pain control and achieving greater financial security for vulnerable older people. Consider stopping contributing drugs (beta-blockers, benzodiazepines, levodopa, opiates, steroids). Supportive treatment includes counselling and relief of loneliness (e.g. befriending schemes, day centres). It is important to address rational anxieties (e.g. financial, housing).

Psychotherapy has been rated as being as effective as antidepressants for mild to moderate depression and may be preferred by some. Cognitive behavioural therapy has the most evidence (Wilson *et al.* 2008). It may complement drug treatment in resistant cases but historically has often had limited availability, especially in primary care. This has led to recent initiatives such as Increasing Access to Psychological Therapies.

Electroconvulsive therapy (ECT) offers a safe, rapid and reasonably certain response in cases where rapid response is necessary. It is considered in secondary care when depression is very severe and manifests as psychosis, severe physical retardation, depressive stupor or food/fluid refusal and the patients have been intolerant to or have not responded to drug treatment. Relative contraindications to ECT include coronary, cerebrovascular and pulmonary disease.

Suicide and attempted suicide

Older people, especially men, have a higher risk of completed (rather than attempted) suicide. Men aged over 75 years have the highest rate of suicide of any age group. Following an attempted suicide, further attempts, and successful suicide, are common. In the UK, 1 in every 9 people who commit suicide is aged 65 years or over (Appleby

2001). Unlike younger people, the substantial majority of older people who attempt suicide are psychiatrically unwell at the time of the attempt, with most being depressed. Many seek contact with medical services immediately prior to the attempt although they may not express depressive or suicidal thoughts at that visit (Pfaff and Olmeida 2005).

Risk factors include being male, single (i.e. unmarried, divorced/separated or widowed), socially isolated, having financial problems, having made previous attempts and suffering recent bereavement. Suicidal behaviour is more common in institutional settings (acute and rehabilitation hospital wards, and care homes) and in people with acute or chronic pain, sleep disturbance, functional impairment, drug use and psychotropic drug prescription. At their mildest, suicidal ideas manifest as common and relatively benign doubts about whether life is worth living. At their most worrying, they are carefully considered, well formulated and strongly held beliefs that death is preferable to life, and consideration of how it could be achieved.

Suicidal behaviours may be overt or covert. Overt behaviours include intentional drug overdoses (opiates, antidepressants, paracetamol, benzodiazepines; more common in women) and self-injury (hanging, shooting, jumping, drowning; more common in men). Covert suicide is relatively more common in the elderly and includes social withdrawal, severe self-neglect and refusal of food, fluid or medication. Covert behaviour may manifest in subtle ways that encourage extensive investigation to exclude physical illness, whilst the psychiatric problem goes unrecognized and untreated.

Any person suspected of having suicidal thoughts should be referred to a specialist service as a matter of urgency.

Prognosis

It has long been recognized that elderly depressed patients have a poor outcome in terms of high mortality, with rates increased two- or three-fold above those of matched controls. Only a small proportion of the increased mortality is due to suicide; the bulk is due to current physical health problems or to the development of cardiac or cerebrovascular disease. A study from the Netherlands showed that among depressed older people attending primary care, a third remitted without relapse after 1 year, a quarter remitted but relapsed and 40% remained chronically depressed (Beekman *et al.* 1995). Many depressed patients are inadequately treated, but even in treated cohorts elderly patients take longer to respond than younger subjects and the risk of relapse may be higher.

Several prognostic factors have been described but there has been great inconsistency between studies to date and no real agreement about the consistent effects due to age or sex. Predictors of poor prognosis include long duration of illness, the presence of adverse life events following the onset of depression, medical comorbidities and the presence of cognitive impairment (more white-matter lesions on MRI and the presence of executive dysfunction) (O'Brien *et al.* 1998).

Specialist referral

Consider referral to old-age psychiatry if:

- treatment is unsuccessful after 6–8 weeks
- depression is severe (e.g. with delusions or hallucinations)
- the patient is not eating or drinking adequately

- the diagnosis is unclear (e.g. when depression and significant cognitive impairment co-exist)
- a patient is refusing treatment
- a patient is suicidal.

Case 2

Mrs X was a 67-year-old widow who had had a diagnosis of post-natal depression made following the birth of the third of her children 30 years previously that had resolved with counselling. Her much-loved husband of 45 years had died suddenly of a cardiac arrest 9 months previously and her children had noted that Mrs X had managed to arrange the funeral and had not cried. In the last few weeks her children were becoming increasingly concerned about their mother's increased forgetfulness, especially as their maternal aunt had been diagnosed with Alzheimer's in her 70s. Mrs X was forgetting appointments such as the dentist and hairdressers and would forget what she had gone to the shops to buy. On further questioning Mrs X revealed that although she denied that she felt low following her husband's unexpected death and had 'just got on with things' she had found that her energy levels were lower in recent months and she had stopped listening to the gospel music programmes she had previously loved on the radio. Her appetite had now decreased and she found herself waking 2 hours earlier than usual at 5 a.m. and was unable to get back to sleep despite feeling un-refreshed. Mrs X was aware of her recent memory problems and was concerned that she may have dementia. Physical examination and tests were unremarkable. Mrs X scored 24/30 on MMSE, losing marks on attention and concentration as well as recall. A provisional diagnosis of depression was made with associated cognitive impairment. Her symptoms improved following a trial of SSRI (citalopram 20 mg od) and referral to bereavement counselling. On follow-up appointment her MMSE had improved to 29/30 and Mrs X had returned to her previous level of functioning.

Comment

Treat depression whatever the cause, whether a true pseudodementia or a combination of dementia and depression. Avoid mislabelling a depressed patient as also demented as the management and prognoses are very different. Always screen for depression when assessing patients with cognitive disorders, including short-term memory loss alone.

Schizophrenia of late onset

Schizophrenia of late onset is uncommon and in several respects differs from early-onset type. It is more common in women than men, paranoid symptoms are often prominent and personality is well preserved. Response to antipsychotic medication is good but doses lower than in younger age groups are recommended. In some elderly people late-onset psychosis may augur dementia. See Chapter 8 for the treatment of schizophrenia.

Delirium

Delirium (acute confusional state) is characterized by changes in consciousness and impairment of cognition occurring suddenly, often over hours or days. It is nearly always caused by an underlying medical condition. Almost any medical illness can give rise to delirium if it is severe enough or if the patient is susceptible. It is a common condition in general practice particularly among elderly patients.

Presentations suggestive of delirium are:

- a sudden change in mental status with global cognitive deficit
- a fluctuating level of consciousness (typically worse at night and in the late afternoon)
- change in behaviour (may be underactive, drowsy and/or withdrawn or hyperactive and agitated)
- altered perceptions (particularly visual hallucinations)
- mood disturbance/anxiety symptoms.

Recognized risk factors for delirium include dementia, parkinsonism, stroke or other structural brain lesions, sensory impairment (vision, hearing) and polypharmacy.

Causes of delirium

The differential diagnosis of delirium includes dementia, depression and mania.

- Among the various forms of dementia, diffuse Lewy body disease (DLBD) is the most difficult to distinguish from delirium due to its frequent fluctuations in consciousness and associated behavioural disturbances. These patients can undergo multiple negative delirium investigations before their symptoms are attributed to DLBD.

- Depression may also be confused with hypoactive delirium. Farrell and Ganzini (1995) demonstrated that one-third of patients in psychiatric consultations for depression in the hospital actually had hypoactive delirium.

- Certain acute psychiatric syndromes, such as mania, can present similarly to hyperactive delirium.

The most common diagnostic issue is whether a newly presenting confused patient has dementia, delirium, or both. Information from family members, caregivers or others who know the patient is essential to clarify the patient's baseline status and the time course of symptom presentation.

Table 15.3.

General conditions	Pain, constipation, urinary retention, heart failure, hypoxia, dehydration, alcohol withdrawal
Medication	Consider new additions, sudden withdrawals, increased doses, or interactions. High-risk drugs are those with central effects, e.g. anticholinergics, H_2-blockers, benzodiazepines, L-dopa, anticonvulsants, opioids, and antipsychotics
Infection	Sepsis, pneumonia, meningitis, urinary tract infection, herpes zoster, HIV, peritonitis, neurosyphilis, endocarditis, cellulites
Metabolic abnormality	Hyponatraemia, hypernatraemia, hypoglycaemia, hyperglycaemia, hypocalcaemia, hypercalcaemia, hypomagnesaemia, hypermagnesaemia, hypercapnia, hypoxaemia, hypothermia, hyperthermia, hepatic failure, thyroid failure, renal failure
Neurological	Stroke, tumour, epidural haematoma, subdural haematoma, intracerebral haemorrhage, subarachnoid haemorrhage, non-convulsive epilepsy

Delirium is a medical emergency so treatment needs to be initiated early. In many cases the patient should be admitted to an acute general hospital. It may be considered suitable to treat at home if the dominant cause is clear, effective treatment can be given, appropriate care and supervision can be ensured and the risk of transfer to an acute environment (e.g. change of environment, less-familiar care staff) are considered to outweigh the benefits.

Identifying and treating the underlying causes of delirium is critically important. In addition, other factors, while not directly causing delirium, should also be addressed in management (e.g. correcting sensory impairments by using glasses and hearing aids, and using orienting items such as clocks and calendars). It is important to stress to patients and family members that while delirium is usually not a permanent condition, many cognitive deficits associated with the delirium syndrome can continue, abating only weeks and even months following treatment of the triggering illness.

Delirium itself is not an indication for pharmacological intervention. However, treatment with antipsychotics or sedatives may be necessary for symptoms such as delusions or hallucinations that are frightening to the patient when verbal comfort and reassurance are not successful. When medications are used, high-potency antipsychotics are preferred because of their low anticholinergic potency and minimal hypotensive effects. In elderly patients with mild-to-moderate symptoms, low doses of haloperidol (0.5–1 mg orally) should be used initially, with careful reassessment before additional dosing. Haloperidol should be avoided in older persons with parkinsonism or Lewy body dementia, and a benzodiazepine or atypical antipsychotic may be substituted. A growing body of literature demonstrates that atypical antipsychotics, such as olanzapine and quetiapine, are equally as effective as haloperidol for the management of agitation in delirium (Lonergan *et al.* 2007).

Summary

- GPs have a key role in managing mental health problems for older people who have high levels of access to primary care and lengthy relationships with practitioners.

- Dementia, depression, delirium and suicide are particularly prevalent in the elderly.

- They have specific management characteristics with regard to dosage of medication and environmental factors such as loneliness and loss.

- Dementia-like symptoms can be a feature of depression.

- Delirium requires general medical intervention.

References

Appleby, L. (2001). *Safety First: five year report of the National Confidential Inquiry into Suicide and Homicide by People with mental illness.* London: Department of Health.

Beekman, A. T. F., Deeg, D. J. H., Smit, J. H., and Vantilburg, W. (1995). Predicting the course of depression in the older population – results from a community-based study in the Netherlands. *Journal of Affective Disorders,* **34**, 41–49.

Farrell, K. R., and Ganzini, L. (1995). Misdiagnosing delirium as depression in medically ill elderly patients. *Archives of Internal Medicine,* **155**, 2459–464.

Knapp, M., Prince, M., *et al.* (2007). *Dementia UK (A report to the Alzheimer's Society on the prevalence and economic cost of dementia in the UK produced by King's College London and London School of Economics).* London: Alzheimer's Society.

Knapp, M., Comas-Herrera, A., Somani, A., and Banerjee, S. (2007). *Dementia: International Comparisons.* London: London School of Economics.

Lonergan, E., Britton, A. M., Luxenberg, J., and Wylier, T. (2007). Antipsychotics in delirium. *Cochrane Database Systemic Review*, **18**, CD005594.

O'Brien, J., Ames, D., Chiu, E., Schweitzer, I., Desmond, P., and Tress, B. (1998). Severe deep white matter lesions and outcome in elderly patients with major depressive disorder: follow up study. *British Medical Journal*, **317**, 982–984.

O'Brien, J. T., Lloyd, A., McKeith, I., Gholkar, A., and Ferrier, N. (2004). A longitudinal study of hippocampal volume, cortisol levels, and cognition in older depressed subjects. *American Journal of Psychiatry*, **161**, 2081–2090.

Pfaff, J., and Olmeida, O. (2005). Detecting suicidal ideation in older patients: identifying risk factors within the general practice setting. *British Journal of General Practice*, **55**, 261–262.

Wilson, K. C. M., Mottram, P. G., and Vassilas, C. A. (2008). Psychotherapeutic treatments for older depressed people. *Cochrane Database Systemic Review*, **1**, CD004853.

Further reading

Balwin, R. (2008). Mood disorders: depressive disorders. In Jacoby, R., Oppenheimer, C., Dening, T., and Thomas, A. J. (eds.), *Oxford Textbook of Old Age Psychiatry.* Oxford: Oxford University Press, pp. 529–556.

Illife, S. (2007). The role of the GP in managing mental illness in later life. *Psychiatry*, 7, 64–69.

Inouye, S. K. (2006). Current concepts: delirium in older persons. *New England Journal of Medicine*, **354**, 1157–1165.

Marcantonio, E. (2007). Clinical management and prevention of delirium. *Psychiatry*, 7, 42–48.

Rockwood, K. (2007). Causes of delirium. *Psychiatry*, 7, 39–41.

Thomas, A. J., and O'Brien, J. T. (2008). Mood disorders in the elderly. *Psychiatry*, **8**, 56–60.

Useful contacts and websites

Age Concern England, Astral House, 1268 London Road, London, SW16 4ER, UK. Helpline: 0800 009966. Tel: 020 8765 7200. Website: www.ageconcern.org.uk.

Alzheimer's Society, Devon House, St Katharine's Way, London, E1W 1JK, UK. Helpline: 0845 300 0336. Tel: 020 7423 3500. Website: www.alzheimers.org.uk.

Carers UK, 20–25 Glasshouse Yard, London, EC1A 4JT, UK. Helpline: 0808 808 7777. Tel: 020 7490 8818. Website: www.carersuk.org.

For Dementia, 6 Camden High Street, London, NW1 0JH, UK. Helpline: 0845 257 9406. Tel: 020 7874 7210. Website: www.fordementia.org.uk. Focuses on providing specialist dementia nurses who can offer practical advice, emotional support and skills to families and carers of people with dementia.

Public Guardianship Office, Archway Tower, 2 Junction Road, London, N19 5SZ, UK. Tel: 0845 330 2900. Website: www.guardianship.gov.uk. Responsible for providing services that promote the financial and social well-being of people with mental incapacity.

Royal College of Psychiatrists, 17 Belgrave Square, London, SW1 8PG, UK. Useful fact sheets on depression, in several languages, found at: http://www.rcpsych.ac.uk/mentalhealthinfoforall.aspx.

Useful reading for patients and carers

The Alzheimer's Society publishes a wide range of advice sheets full of practical information which are easy to understand. Many of these are available on the Society's website: www.alzheimers.org.uk.

BMA/Family Doctor books (www.familydoctor.co.uk) offer a wide range of authoritative, easy-to-understand, affordable books on health issues.

Bryden, C. (2005). *Dancing with Dementia: My Story of Living Positively with Dementia.* London: Jessica Kingsley Publishers.

Graham, N., and Warner, J. (2009). *Understanding Alzheimer's Disease and Other Dementias.* Poole: BMA/Family Doctor Publications.*

Mace, N. L. (2006). *The 36 Hour Day: A Family Guide to Caring for People with Alzheimer's Disease, Other Dementias, and Memory Loss in Later Life,* 4th edn. Baltimore, MA: Johns Hopkins University Press.

McKenzie, K. (2008). *Understanding Depression.* Poole: BMA/Family Doctor Publications.

Non-pharmacological therapies

Psychological therapies

Graeme Webster and Neill Richardson (Cognitive behavioural therapy)
Breda McLeavey and Mary Kerrisk (Problem-solving therapy)
Nigel Smith (Solution-focused therapy)
Patricia Casey (Counselling)

Learning objectives

The principles underlying cognitive behaviour therapy (CBT)
Common myths about CBT
What conditions is CBT used to treat?
What is problem-solving therapy?
Who is it used for?
Outline of a structured approach to problem-solving training
Solution-focused therapy
The underpinning theory
Focusing on the client's skills to bring about a solution
Counselling – what it is and what it is not
Basic principles of counselling
Beginning and ending therapy

This chapter aims to help generalist clinicians to gain a real understanding of the kind of therapy their patients might receive. The brief summaries explain the theory and practice of three therapies and the associated audio CD with worked examples allows one to experience the very different feel of the various therapies. This understanding will help in the discussions prior to referral, as well as contact during and after therapy.

While these are inevitably tasters, they might also motivate practitioners to participate in courses supporting the integration of some of these techniques into the 10 minute consultation. The concluding section on counselling does not include a worked example on the CD.

Cognitive behavioural therapy

The Department of Health's strategy for Improving Access to Psychological Therapy (IAPT) has incentivized local comissioners to purchase services which implement the psychological therapies within NICE guidelines for anxiety and depression. This means that CBT has come to the fore in recent months and years. It is vital for clinicians in primary care to understand CBT and how it has developed into the key modality for treating mental health problems in the community.

Cognitive behavioural therapy (CBT) is a psychotherapeutic approach combining cognitive therapy (CT) with behavioural therapy (BT). It has a relatively sound evidence base and is thus recommended for the treatment of anxiety disorders and depression commonly encountered in primary care (NICE 2004, 2009).

BT, which has emerged from the work of writers such as Skinner (1953), is concerned with behaviours and their role in maintaining problems. For example, people suffering with depression commonly withdraw from social interaction and pleasurable or rewarding activity. Not only does this result in a less rewarding life but it also provides a greater opportunity to ruminate about how bad things are, leading to further withdrawal and so on. The aim of BT in this instance would be to re-engage in previously rewarding activities and to identify new ones with a focus on building a more meaningful and rewarding lifestyle (Martell *et al.* 2001). Behavioural interventions are probably best known for their effectiveness in the treatment of anxiety disorders, developed from the early work of authors including Wolpe and Lazarus (1966) (Hawton *et al.* 1998). Fear and the resultant avoidance of feared situations are conceptualized as conditioned responses; in other words, the client has developed an automatic fear reaction when confronted with a stimulus, such as standing on a high cliff. The reward of feeling better when moving away from the edge serves to reinforce the fear. Behaviour therapists utilize *systematic desensitization* (Wolpe and Lazarus 1966) whereby the client is exposed to gradually more fearful stimuli on a hierarchy, towards their ultimate goal. Through prolonged exposure the individual becomes desensitized to the feared situation and no longer needs to engage in avoidance strategies.

CT, developed from the work of Beck *et al.* (1979), focuses on thinking styles, personal rules and assumptions and deeply held *core beliefs* about the self, others and the wider world. Beck *et al.* propose that dysfunctional core beliefs developed in childhood drive the development of rules for living and day-to-day negative automatic thoughts which play a key role in the maintenance of problems. CT uses a systematic approach of challenging distorted and biased thinking by considering all available evidence to develop more accurate and helpful perspectives. CT was initially developed as a treatment for depression, a disorder typified by self-denigratory beliefs and negatively biased ruminations. Depressed clients are encouraged to see the whole picture, paying equal attention to and accurately assessing the value of positive aspects of their lives. Attention is also given to the *internal dialogue*, which is the conversation we have within ourselves. CT has been applied to wider problems in more recent times, including anxiety disorders. Clark's (1986) work on panic disorder is one of the best examples. The misinterpretation of the physiological symptoms of anxiety is identified as the major factor in the maintenance of the problem. Therapists work with clients to develop alternative explanations for these symptoms. The new ideas are then tested in the field, allowing them to be confirmed.

Today, CBT combines both approaches in the treatment of anxiety disorders such as panic (Clark 1986) and social anxiety (Wells and Clark 1997) as well as depression (Beck *et al.* 1979). Elements of both behavioural and cognitive techniques are used to greater or lesser degrees depending on the expertise of the therapist, the specific presentation and, of course, the client's preferred approach. For example, a therapist working with a depressed client may well engage in behavioural activation as described earlier, but may also engage in cognitive work around rationalising day-to-day *negative automatic thoughts* or processing core beliefs. Although therapists regularly use established protocols to treat disorders, it is the individualized formulation which drives intervention.

The elements of CBT discussed in this chapter are illustrated in the accompanying CD.

Myths

There are some common myths relating to CBT which should be addressed.

- CBT is sometimes referred to as a 'quick fix'. This is incorrect. Therapists work with clients towards permanent fundamental changes in thinking and patterns and styles.

- Cognitive therapy is frequently mistaken for 'positive thinking'. This is incorrect. CT is more about gaining accurate, 'whole picture' perspectives. It could be said that CT is about identifying *the truth, the whole truth* and *nothing but the truth* and then changing behaviour accordingly.

- At times, CBT has been accused of not paying attention to emotions. In truth, CBT is focused on the reduction of distress in the longer term and therapists work with emotional processing as a matter of course. CBT therapists utilize the same core therapeutic principles of empathy and compassion as practitioners from other modalities (Curwen *et al.* 2000).

What is therapy like?

CBT is a collaborative approach based upon the foundation of a strong therapeutic alliance. The client is seen as the expert who possesses the knowledge of the problem and the resources to change. The therapist is therefore seen more as a guide with treatment being *done with* rather than *done to* the client. Therapists tend to adopt an inquisitive Socratic stance using *guided discovery* to collaborate with clients in developing a shared formulation (Grant *et al.* 2004). Typically, presenting problems are conceptualized using a maintenance formulation such as a five-areas approach (Williams 2001) consisting of triggers, cognitions, affect, physiology and behaviour. An example of a maintenance formulation for a depressed individual is shown in Figure 16.1.

This approach offers the client a thorough understanding of the problem in terms of the individual systems involved and, crucially, the way in which they interact with one another. Understanding how the problem works on a day-to-day level is key in identifying targets for therapy. The focus in therapy tends to be on moving forwards and for many clients a maintenance formulation will be sufficient for successful treatment. However, in more complex cases it may be necessary to develop a more comprehensive understanding of the client's development and the deeper cognitive structures which drive maintenance (Beck *et al.* 1979) and to process these within therapy. To this end, therapists may work with clients in collaboratively developing a longitudinal formulation (Beck 1995) such as the one shown in Figure 16.2.

Although formulation is undertaken at the beginning of treatment, it is an ongoing process which is constantly reviewed. For example, a change in behaviour such as re-engaging with friends may result in an improvement in mood. The mechanisms involved can be explained within the maintenance model. In short, a formulation is a model of 'how' rather than 'why' and knowing how the problem works enables clients to identify how to fix it!

CBT is a structured approach with an agenda being collaboratively set at the beginning of each session. Typically, time is taken to review the period between sessions which may then provide a topic for discussion. In general, each session is used to address a specific issue and clients are encouraged to explore their thoughts and actions, to identify problematic areas, and develop new more adaptive ideas and behaviours. Homework is then set which the client undertakes between sessions. This homework may consist of behavioural exercises such as exposure or testing out new ideas developed in the therapy session (Curwen *et al.* 2000). This is a key feature of CBT; the majority of change happens outside the therapy room.

Who is CBT for?

As has been mentioned previously, CBT can be as effective in the treatment of depression and anxiety disorders as SSRIs (Roth and Fonagy 1996). When considering CBT as a treatment

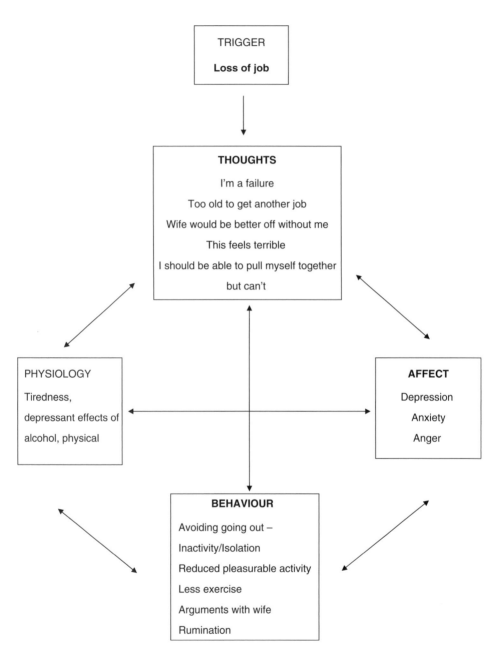

Figure 16.1. A maintenance formulation for a depressed individual

option with clients, referrers are encouraged to explain the collaborative nature of the approach and that the client must be prepared to take an active role in treatment. It may also be beneficial to discuss the general principles of graduated exposure with clients suffering with anxiety disorders.

EARLY EXPERIENCE

Critical father. Mother used alcohol.

Bullied by peers at school.

Stress made it difficult to concentrate. "Scraped through" exams.

CORE BELIEFS

"I'm stupid"

"I'm unloveable"

CONDITIONAL BELIEFS / ASSUMPTIONS

"I must do well - if I fail I'm stupid".

"if I fall out with those I love they will leave me"

COMPENSATORY STRATEGIES

Work to a high level – Perfectionism.

Avoid conflict

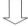

CRITICAL INCIDENT

Redundancy at work (trigger in maintenance formulation)

Figure 16.2. A longitudinal formulation

Different problems require varying numbers of sessions. There are no hard and fast rules on this although evidence has indicated the number of sessions required for following disorders:

- depression – http://www.nice.org.uk/nicemedia/live/12329/45888/45888.pdf
- obsessive compulsive disorder – minimum 10 sessions including exposure and response prevention (ERP)
- generalized anxiety disorder 16–20 (http://www.nice.org.uk/nicemedia/live/10960/29636/29636.pdf

- post-traumatic stress disorder 8–12 (http://www.nice.org.uk/nicemedia/live/10966/29769/29769.pdf

- panic disorder (with or without agoraphobia) 7–14 (http://www.nice.org.uk/nicemedia/live/10960/29636/29636.pdf.

Low-intensity interventions

The roll-out of the Improving Access to Psychological Therapies (IAPT) initiative has seen significant developments in the area of low-intensity interventions. This approach is CBT-based but focuses more on guided self-help, psycho-educational groups, computerized CBT and brief individual therapy consisting of fewer than 10 sessions. Low-intensity interventions can be extremely helpful for the vast majority of clients and are often offered as the first port of call using a stepped care approach (Clark *et al.* 2009).

Specialist applications

CBT also has far wider applications in the management of problems such as severe and enduring mental health problems (Grant *et al.* 2004), personality disorders (Young 1990), substance misuse (Beck *et al.* 1993), eating disorders and chronic obesity (Fairburn and Harrison 2003), neurological disorders, chronic fatigue syndrome and pain. Referral for CBT to treat these conditions would usually be made via the appropriate specialist service.

Problem-solving therapy

Problem-solving therapy (PST), which was originally developed by D'Zurilla and Goldfried (1971), is an evidenced-based, cognitive-affective-behavioural intervention that promotes the adoption and effective application of adaptive problem-solving attitudes and skills to solve problems in everyday living (Nezu 2004). Problem-solving was originally defined by D'Zurilla and Goldfried (1971) as: 'a behavioural process, whether overt or cognitive in nature, which a) makes available a variety of potentially effective response alternatives for dealing with the problematic situation and b) increases the probability of selecting the most effective response from among these various alternatives'. More specifically, in social problem-solving we are addressing primarily those problems in living that relate to an emotional and interpersonal context. Problems can originate from the social environment (e.g. difficulties with a partner or co-worker) or from within the person him- or herself (e.g. conflicts in goals, lack of resources, inability to manage negative emotions). Substantial research has documented the association between social problem-solving deficits and a range of psychological distress and pathology symptoms and disorders (Nezu *et al.* 2004).

Who is it used for?

PST has been shown to be suitable for the treatment of depression (Cuijpers *et al.* 2007; Bell and D'Zurilla 2009), deliberate self-harm (Hawton *et al.* 1998; Brown *et al.* 2005; Slee *et al.* 2008; Tarrier *et al.* 2008), personality disorder (McMurran *et al.* 2008), social anxiety, distressed couples, parent-child problems (D'Zurilla and Nezu 2007), obesity (Perri *et al.* 2001), distressed cancer patients (Nezu *et al.* 2003) and back pain (D'Zurilla and Nezu 2007).

PST should not be delivered merely as a skills-teaching programme, but conducted in a therapeutic context where the complexities of interpersonal problems and emotional experiences are addressed (Nezu *et al.* 2009).

Problem-solving skills training

The problem-solving skills training programme consists of a minimum of six sessions held at intervals of 1 week, plus one booster session held 2 to 3 weeks later. A structured approach to problem-solving, which breaks it down into steps that form a complete process, is central to the success of problem-solving training.

The training model used is based on the five general stages of problem-solving; i.e. general orientation; problem definition and clarification; generation of options; decision-making; implementation and evaluation. Each skill involved is presented as part of an overall problem-solving process. The model is presented in the CD accompanying this book.

Session 1: general orientation

This addresses how people generally approach their problems. A positive orientation to problems is enhanced by training in the following:

> *Feelings of upset and distress are cues for identifying a problem, rather than signs of personal inadequacy or failure.* This helps to discriminate between external features of the problem (e.g. an argument) and internal emotional features of the problem (e.g. the anger felt towards the other person), so that the person does not become overwhelmed and feel hopeless.
>
> *Recognizing that a gap exists between how a situation is and how one would like it to be* points to the existence of a problem.
>
> *Acknowledging feelings of emotional upset while at the same time inhibiting the tendency to react impulsively to problems or to avoid problems* allows one to engage in problem-solving instead.
>
> *Accepting that having problems is fundamentally normal, despite their novelty or severity,* helps to reject the belief that problems are a sign of one's own inadequacy. It also helps to reduce the likelihood of impulsive or avoidant reactions when confronted with a problem.

Session 2: defining and clarifying problems

This deals with clearly defining the nature of the problem and identifying a realistic goal.
In carrying out this problem-solving stage, six main strategies are used:

(1) *Gathering all the facts and information about the problem (including how others feel).* Here the client is introduced to the 'investigative reporter' approach. They are told that they will deal with this aspect of problem-solving just as a reporter investigates a story, asking the questions who, what, where, when and how, and using only facts, not assumptions, hearsay or unsubstantiated opinions. A good reporter looks for evidence to support his/her facts.

(2) *Setting out these facts in clear specific language.* This is particularly important when an individual is experiencing high levels of emotions such as sadness, anger or hopelessness. Often the feeling is seen as the problem, for example, *'I feel awful'. There is often a sense of relief when a person is told that of itself this is not the problem, but is a cue for recognizing that a problem exists. Setting out the facts helps the individual to create some distance from overwhelming feelings.*

(3) *Separating the facts from the opinions.* Here the client learns that by making sure that they are solving a real problem, and not one that they just think is real, they ensure that they will be working on relevant solutions, not solutions that are irrelevant and inappropriate. It is important to focus on positive as well as negative aspects of the

problem, and the long-term as well as short-term issues. This prevents seeing the problem as a crisis. After gathering all the information, only what is relevant, factual, and useful becomes the focus of attention.

(4) *Identifying those factors that are actually causing the problem: comparing existing and desired states of affairs.* By answering questions like an investigative reporter (who? what? when? where? how?) the facts become clearer. Then it is easier to identify the gap between the existing situation and the desired outcome.

(5) *Setting out one or more realistic goals to solve the problem.* Often a goal can be stated beginning with the phrase *'If this problem were solved it would mean that ...'* It is also important that goals set are attainable, otherwise the likelihood of failure is increased and the person's sense of hopelessness or helplessness is worsened.

(6) *Stating the obstacles.* In setting realistic goals, the individual must state the obstacles that are currently preventing them from reaching the desired goal(s). These obstacles might involve a skill deficit, a lack of resources, uncertainty, fears, or interpersonal conflicts. This is very important, as later work on generating options will be focused on directly overcoming these obstacles in order to meet the desired goal(s).

Session 3: generating options

This involves learning to develop a wide range of options for dealing with each problem, thus increasing the likelihood that the most effective option will be among them. Identifying a number of effective options also means that the problem can be worked on from a number of different angles, further increasing the likelihood of successfully solving the problem. The theoretical underpinnings are related to the brainstorming method, with its four rules of quantity of ideas, ruling out criticism, combining ideas, and creativity. Session topics include training in the difference between 'what' you can do to solve a problem (strategies) and 'how' to do it (tactics).

The therapist needs to particularly emphasize the necessity of generating as many different options as possible. Training in this skill will help to protect clients against hopelessness, as they are now able to think of several alternatives that can be drawn upon to cope with a problem.

Session 4: making decisions

This deals with using skills that will enable them to critically evaluate their options for dealing with a problem, so that they have a better chance of selecting the most effective option(s). In evaluating the usefulness of each option, the client has to decide its value as a solution in terms of reaching the desired goal. They have already set out details of the facts, obstacles, sub-problems and missing information, from the problem definition and clarification stage. They can now use this information to guide them in evaluating their options. The main skill taught at the decision-making stage is to predict consequences for each option or combination of options, based on their advantages and disadvantages. In order to do this, the criteria focused on for each option are:

(1) their view on the likelihood of this option attaining their goal, as set out during the problem definition and clarification stage

(2) to what extent they believe that this option will successfully overcome the identified obstacles.

A second skill taught at this stage is assessing the likelihood of being able to carry out their particular choice of option. In many cases, they will have selected an option that they believe will enable them to reach their goal and to overcome obstacles, but they may be unable to carry it out. This points up further obstacles or sub-problems (e.g. inability to cope with criticism or anxiety) that may need additional therapy to develop further skills such as assertiveness or anxiety management.

Session 5: evaluating outcome

It is crucial that the client's implementation of their chosen solutions is then evaluated in terms of:

(a) the effects of the solution they have carried out

(b) how the actual outcome compares with their original goal.

Where a problem is effectively solved, it reinforces a more positive orientation to problems and a sense of confidence in their ability to cope with future problems. If time is not given to concentrating on the actual outcome of the implemented solution, this learning is reduced. When a problem is not resolved to a reasonably satisfactory degree it is important that he/she is set to return to the problem-solving process at whatever stage is appropriate (e.g. redefining the problem, generating more options, etc.) until a satisfactory outcome is reached. Three tasks are involved in evaluating solution outcome and these are addressed separately during the session:

(1) evaluation of the effectiveness of the solution

(2) positive reinforcement for having gone through the problem-solving process

(3) if not reasonably satisfied with the outcome, getting set to resume problem-solving until a satisfactory outcome is reached.

Session 6: concluding the programme

This is used to encourage clients to:

(1) resume the problem-solving process if a satisfactory outcome has not been reached

(2) end the process with self-reinforcement if they are reasonably satisfied with the outcome

(3) anticipate and prepare for future problems. This is important in preventing relapse (using old methods of responding to problems that are ineffective).

A booster session, where the ongoing use of problem-solving skills and any difficulties encountered are discussed, will help to ensure that problem-solving skills developed in the therapy programme continue to generalize and strengthen over time.

Solution-focused therapy

Solution-focused therapy (SFT) is a relatively new talking model that comes from a tradition which believes that questions and conversation are powerful in themselves: 'How we tell our story matters' (Hedtke and Winslade 2004). It differs considerably from problem-solving. Rather than breaking down a problem into components, 'solutions' are derived by thinking and talking about the detail of what it is like when things are or could be better. This section should be read in conjunction with the CD accompanying this book.

SFT was developed in the USA in the early 1980s initially by De Shazer (1985), and then, in the UK, at the Marlborough Family Centre, and later at BRIEF in London by George, Iveson and Ratner (2001).

The model was developed via practice rather than from theory and is a pragmatic and forward-thinking approach, rather than one which is interested in the past. The past is not avoided and neither is conversation about the problem, but they are not the main emphasis. The past, for example, might be used to explore a time when the patient felt that life was more like they would want it to be. Alternatively they may want to focus on a problem which might be listened to with an ear to identifying and verbalizing how the patient coped, or what they think they have learnt that will be helpful to them when they no longer have this dilemma.

Underlying SFT are a number of assumptions, some of which can feel counter-cultural to much medical training; in particular, the ideas of noticing when things are better rather than when they are at their worst, believing that patients are the agents of their own change and that all patients have what it takes to resolve their problems.

The clinician is no longer an expert or the agent of change in sessions. Instead the patient is seen as the expert on their situation and their lives and decides what to work on and when the work is finished.

Questions focus mainly on what is working already and how the patient would like life to be different. Clinicians are also asked to do the impossible, which is to avoid offering advice or suggestions! By resisting this, any solutions and changes that are identified are owned by the patient. It removes pressure from clinicians to identify solutions and avoids putting patients in the position of feeling that they have let down the 'expert' by not following advice. Indeed when failure does occur it is often because the ideas come from the clinician's background and have no fit or resonance with the patient.

Some key principles

The model has a number of underlying principles that I believe make it helpful in a primary care setting.

- Attempting to understand the cause of a problem is not a necessary or particularly useful step towards resolution. Indeed, discussing the problem may be actively unhelpful to some patients.

This is particularly true with patients who return repeatedly to surgery with the same general complaints. To continue to regularly allow the same conversation to happen can maintain the problem. The beginnings of a solution lie in doing something different! Even something as small as sitting in a different position in the room or using a different office can change dynamics. The notion of 'problem-free talk' fits with this. Explore other areas of a patient's life in which they feel more competent to uncover potential resources and strengths.

- Where a client wants to get to is more important than where they have come from.

From this perspective, the worst thing a clinician can do is ask someone what brought them there or especially 'how are you'. These questions both invite long conversations about problems.

Henden (2008) describes the 'five o'clock rule' for sessions. If you imagine a clock face, with the hands at five o'clock, then the amount of session content that is problem-focused should represent no more than the proportion of the clock face shown between the two hands. The rest of the session, the majority, should focus on what the client wants, and what is working already. Once we allow early sessions to become problem-dominated this will become a habit and can add to the maintenance of the problem.

Instead start sessions with future-focused questions based on the session you are about to have, e.g. 'What are your best hopes from meeting with me today?' 'How will you know if this session is helpful to you?' 'If meeting with me today was helpful, what would be different that would tell you'. These questions come under a general heading of 'getting down to business.'

The model is a goal-setting approach which has a number of tools to do this, most notably the miracle question, which invites the patient to imagine waking up in a morning when the problems have gone, but they don't know. An exploration then takes place of what life would look like in this preferred future. Another key goal-setting technique is the use of scales to explore what a patient is doing that is helpful to them to keep them up at, say, a 4 (on a scale where 10 is the best things can be and 1 is the worst), which shows that things are not the worst they could be, and what would needs to happen to move them up just one point on the scale.

- However fixed a problem pattern appears to be, there are always times when the client is doing some of the solution.

Following on from this, try to spend time exploring how life is when the problem is less prominent. SFT would believe that all patients have what is necessary to deal with their problems. Our role as professionals is to help them to uncover this and it is reasonable to assume that when things are better, some of the solution is happening. The work of the session then becomes focusing on that time and what is different then.

By looking for detail and lingering within these exceptions we can make them bigger and more significant, as they can become invisible alongside the much stronger narratives that are reinforcing the problem. If you feel a need to set tasks, then better to set noticing tasks around these times and what is different. What does the patient want to keep from these times?

- Sometimes only the smallest of changes is necessary to set in motion a solution to a problem.

This is a systemic idea (see Chapter 17), but in essence it suggests that we are all interconnected with each other and whilst we are not always working with the most powerful part of a system and some patients look for change in others, small change that could lead to greater things is still possible.

We can all notice problem spirals; how one problem can sometimes seem to create another and another. It seems logical that, if this happens one way round, then it can happen the other way too.

So SFT is not just about looking for dramatic 'positive' changes. Instead we can become interested in the ordinary, the mundane, the tiny details, a change in the time of getting up, what cereal you might eat, what you might notice, what you might say to one person in your family. And these small changes can become attainable readily and may ultimately cue the patient to identify further goals which they want to achieve. Always try to identify the possible benefits of change about the person in therapy, or at least explore the effects that change may have on that individual, e.g:

'So what would you like to be different?'
'I would like my mum to stop shouting at me.'
'And if that happened, what would you be able to do differently?'

'Well I might pay a bit more attention to her.'

Subsequent questions can proceed in two directions ...

(1) 'And if you did that what difference would that make?'

Or ...

(2) 'Tell me about a time when you paid more attention to your mum. What was different then?'

- Whatever the client is doing, it is their best attempt to deal with their situation at that point in time.

This perspective means that if a patient has learnt that anxiety is prevented by avoiding difficult situations, then avoiding your session may become an attempted solution. Similarly talking to a clinician for an hour may seem like a solution if afterwards they feel better because of the attention they received. Alcohol and drug addiction can also be seen as attempted solutions. So, if the clinician is able to see behaviour in this 'half full' way, it can lead to a view of the patient as a constructive ally rather than a person who is resistant, avoidant or self-destructive. By accepting the person as they are and the problem as it is, the patient may be enabled to arrive at their own solution.

Counselling

Counselling is a term that can loosely be used to describe those therapies which do not utilize drugs. For some, counselling encompasses CBT as well as other non-pharmacological interventions such as Gestalt therapy, interpersonal therapy and so on. The present chapter focuses specifically on the client-centred, *non-directive* approach of Carl Rogers, since this is one of the more accessible techniques and is also the most commonly used. Confusion exists between supportive 'therapy' and counselling. The former has limited aims, these being generally to provide a listening ear and to help at times of crisis. There is no specific focus for therapy, whereas in counselling a particular area of difficulty is being remedied and in the process the individual grows.

There are also differences between counselling and psychotherapy in that the various forms of psychotherapy (psychoanalytic, humanistic and so on) are concerned with gaining insight into the causes of problematic behaviours and symptoms. The focus is on the past, on relationships and traumas and particular use is made of interpretations. In addition, defence mechanisms such as denial, sublimation, etc., are explored. Unlike counselling, which can be relatively brief and problem-focused, psychotherapy is lengthy and insight-focused. In recent years the shift has been towards brief interventions.

Who is counselling for?

Non-directive counselling can be used for any area of life in which an individual wishes to bring about change. Not everybody is suited to this type of therapy and the attributes required for success are as follows.

(1) The capacity to express himself emotionally and have a basic acceptance of the role of psychological and emotional issues in his life – commonly referred to as psychological mindedness.

(2) The absence of any gross instability such as schizophrenia or major personality difficulties is essential since relapse or decompensation may occur in these patients during therapy.

(3) A desire for help at the outset is an advantage but not essential since this may crystallize during the sessions.

(4) Those who have a tendency to dependence on others may transfer this to the counsellor and frustrate attempts at establishing mature behaviour.

(5) The person must be flexible enough to have some capacity for change. Those who are intransigent are unlikely to benefit.

The evidence base for benefit is limited, however. An economic analysis found antidepressants to be superior to generic counselling in a randomized trial of antidepressant therapy in those with mild-moderate depression (Miller *et al.* 2003). In a study comparing general practitioner 'treatment as usual' against counselling for those with chronic depression there was some evidence of limited superiority in those referred for counselling but there was an attendant increase in treatment costs also (Simpson *et al.* 2003). However, a meta-analysis of seven studies confirmed the superior clinical effectiveness of counselling compared with treatment as usual in the short term but not the long term (Bower *et al.* 2003). Clearly more studies are required, in order to resolve these conflicting findings.

Beginning counselling

Counselling is not a non-specific treatment, but a method of dealing with problems by utilizing expression of feelings and reflection. It is essential to clarify the problems from the outset. In many patients the source of difficulty may be vague and uncertain or the problems may continually shift. This pattern will make counselling difficult.

A further prerequisite is to set achievable and realistic goals. If this is neglected, therapy may become interminable, with all the problems of dependence that this entails. Allied to this is the time limit that is set.

Active therapy

The components of counselling may be divided into two parts – listening and intervening.

Listening

This is the largest part of counselling and often the most difficult to sustain since speech is central to our interactions with others. While it may appear to be passive this is incorrect and it is best described as 'active inactivity'. The therapist is attentive to his client and is not distracted by peripheral stimuli. Attention is paid to the actual content of what the client says but also to the hidden agenda. Aspects of *language* to which attention must be paid include speed, volume and hesitations. This may throw light upon embarrassments, sources of tension and conflicts. The words, phrases and metaphors used must also be noted, for their idiosyncratic use or non-use may reveal areas of difficulty. For example the terminally ill patient who never uses the word cancer but refers to the illness as 'it' may be having problems accepting the diagnosis. *Non-verbal cues* are also important and the body language of the client often discloses much about their personality and problems. For example, the person who fidgets when certain topics are raised may have difficulties in that area. Observing this may be the only clue to the cause of the distress, especially if problems are strongly denied by the client.

Intervening

This refers to the more obvious aspect of the client–counsellor interchange and can be divided into the verbal interchanges that facilitate the client in talking about issues and those that are therapeutic in themselves.

Facilitating communication – the patient's flow of speech may be hesitant in the early stages of counselling. *Open questions* like 'Tell me about your problem' are more likely to provoke spontaneous disclosures than are closed, interrogative questions. The habit of asking many questions and of being verbally active during sessions, known as floorholding, serves only to stifle spontaneity. The other extreme from the interrogative interview is the totally free-floating interchange. This is best avoided also since the diffuseness it generates may suggest to the client that the therapist is aloof or unfocused.

Echoing either parts or the whole of the client's last sentence, *offering empathetic comments* and *summarizing* are all useful in facilitating communicating with the counsellor.

Closed questions are necessary to clarify uncertainties while *confrontational questions* such as 'Do you still love your husband?' are useful at times but should not be used early in therapy as they may appear insensitive and alienate the client.

Therapeutic interventions – a large component of counselling is concerned with exploring and allowing the *expression of feelings* and thereby effecting change. The most common of these are anger, guilt and grief. Most commonly they have been suppressed and the therapist's role is to encourage their expression. The effect of these on the personal, emotional and spiritual life of the sufferer is considerable. The therapist at times has to give permission to the client to be angry, sad or guilty. This *permission-giving* component is important for those who are ashamed of how they feel. Equally important is the terminating of the anger or guilt or sadness; e.g. a widow may feel guilty because she is beginning to enjoy life again without her husband. One of the dangers of counselling, or indeed any form of psychological treatment, is that emotions are churned up and vented but there is often no facility for healing these. Thus, discussing death with a seriously ill patient may be unhelpful if the therapist is not available to facilitate resolution of the emotion that has been generated. There are times when the therapist may have to decide that further discussion of the problem is unhelpful and that continuing to do so may provoke rather than resolve unwanted emotions.

Exploring feelings may be relatively easy where the patient is in touch with their emotions. On the other hand the well-defended patient may deny any emotions at all even where they would ordinarily be expected, e.g. losing a spouse. A few simple techniques can be used to provoke emotion, including the description of emotional scenes, e.g. the wedding day or the funeral. The 'empty chair' technique is also useful in these circumstances. The client is asked to imagine the person to whom the emotion refers sitting on the empty chair (it is important to actually place an empty chair beside the client as this brings the setting to life) and to direct their conversation to this. For example, the client who feels angry with her son for leaving home will be advised to imagine him sitting on the chair and to articulate her resentment. This is a form of abreaction and, as with any emotional expression, may be associated with a dramatic catharsis. The therapist who feels unable to deal with this should avoid further counselling until he has become more skilled, since emotional outpourings are commonplace, especially in the bereaved or in those who have been sexually abused.

During therapy clients must be encouraged to use the *correct terms* for the situations or events they are describing. Thus, the bereaved person who describes her loved one as having 'passed on' may be fearful of the word 'dead'. Similarly, the girl who has been sexually abused may speak of 'it' or 'you know' when she means penis or penetration. Euphemisms have a particular purpose, i.e. to modify the emotional content of the words to which they refer.

Explaining the reasons for an abnormal piece of behaviour may be helpful at times. For example, the housewife who constantly shouts at her children may in fact be angry with her spouse and 'taking it out' on her family. The client who understands this may then be able to deal with her feelings more appropriately. This is known as interpretation and should be used with caution and even with reluctance. It may give the therapist a spurious sense of knowledge, but used inexpertly can make also make him seem just silly.

Ending therapy

Terminating treatment should not come as a surprise to the client since a time limit will have been contracted at the outset. Inevitably, however, therapist and client get close and due warning has to be given of the plans to terminate treatment. This should be mentioned in passing at some time during the last three or four sessions to allow disengagement to occur. The client may often produce new problems at this point in the hope of prolonging therapy. Assurance must be given that further therapy will be forthcoming at a later date should the need arise. In general those who have difficulties with separation are also likely to find separation from the therapist difficult. The skilled and sensitive counsellor is keenly aware of this and facilitates separation, which should occur without misgivings or anxieties. In the author's experience the patient frequently fails to attend for the final appointment.

Summary

- Cognitive behavioural therapy has grown in importance with recent strategies aimed at improving access to psychological treatments.
- The evidence base in a number of conditions is good and as such it is recommended most frequently by NICE.
- Elements of cognitive and of behavioural strategies are used alone or in combination depending on the condition being treated and the requirements of the individual.
- The CBT movement continues to investigate treatment methods and use randomized control trials to test the effectiveness of interventions.
- Formulation-driven CBT can require up to 20 sessions to achieve recovery in complex conditions such as OCD, PTSD, GAD and depression.
- Low-intensity variations are also used and these take the form of computerized CBT, psycho-education, guided self-help and brief therapies.
- Problem-solving therapy aims to promote adaptive problem-solving skills to solve problems of everyday life.
- It can be used to deal with a range of problems in a variety of settings from obesity and social anxiety through to distress in cancer patients.
- It is highly structured and takes the person through various stages of problem-solving in a stepped manner.
- These include identifying the problem, identifying possible solutions, examining obstacles, testing the solutions and evaluating the outcomes.
- Solution-focused therapy is a short-term psychological approach.

- In a primary care setting it benefits from having very little jargon, works with the person as they are and does not try to identify external or internal processes.

- It can be utilized as a brief intervention or as a focus and a theoretical basis for clinical work.

- It can enable new thinking, especially around the patient's ability to resolve their own problems.

- Counselling is based upon the principle that exploration of conflicts and expression of emotion bring about resolution of the symptoms.

- The beginning of therapy should be confined to defining the problem and organizing details of the sessions. The middle stage is when most emotional work is done and the end of therapy should not come as a surprise to the patient.

References

Beck, A. T., Rush, A., Shaw, B., and Emery, G. (1979). *Cognitive Therapy of Depression*. New York: Guilford Press.

Beck, A. T., Wright, F. D., Newman, C. F., and Liese, B. S. (1993). *Cognitive Therapy of Substance Abuse*. New York: Guilford Press.

Beck, J. (1995). *Cognitive Therapy: Basics and Beyond*. New York: Guilford Press.

Bell, A. C., and D'Zurilla, T. J. (2009). Problem-solving therapy for depression: a meta-analysis. *Clinical Psychology Review*, **29**, 348–353.

Bower, P., Rowland, N., and Hardy, R. (2003). The clinical effectiveness of counselling in primary care: a systematic review and meta-analysis. *Psychological Medicine*, **33**(2), 203–215.

Brown, G. K., Ten Have, T., Henriques, G. R., et al. (2005). Cognitive therapy for the prevention of suicide attempts: a randomized controlled trial. *JAMA*, **294**, 563–570.

Clark, D. M. (1986). A cognitive approach to panic. *Behaviour Research and Therapy*, **24**, 461–470.

Clark, D. M., Layard, R., Smithies, R., et al. (2009). Improving access to psychological therapy: initial evaluation of two UK demonstration sites. *Behaviour Research and Therapy*, **47**(11), 910–920.

Cuijpers, P., van Stratan, A., and Warmerdam, L. (2007). Problem-solving therapies for depression: a meta-analysis. *European Psychiatry*, **22**, 9–15.

Curwen, B., Palmer, S., and Ruddell, P. (2000). *Brief Cognitive Behaviour Therapy*. London: Sage.

De Shazer, S. (1985). *Keys to Solution in Brief Therapy*. New York: Norton.

D'Zurilla, T. J., and Goldfried, M. R. (1971). Problem solving and behavior modification. *Journal of Abnormal Psychology*, **78**, 107–126.

D'Zurilla, T. J., and Nezu, A. M. (2007). *Problem-Solving Therapy: A Positive Approach to Clinical Interventions*, 3rd edn. New York: Springer.

Fairburn, C. G., and Harrison, P. J. (2003). Eating disorders. *The Lancet*, **361**, 407–16.

George, E., Iveson, C., and Ratner, H. (2001) *Problem to Solution*. London: BT Press.

Grant, A., Mills, J., Mulhern, R., and Short, N. (2004) *Cognitive Behavioural Therapy in Mental Health Care*. London: Sage.

Hawton, K., Arensman, E., Townsend, E., et al. (1998). Deliberate self harm: systematic review of efficacy of psychosocial and pharmacological treatments in preventing repetition. *British Medical Journal*, **317**, 441–447

Hedtke, L., and Winslade, J. (2004). *Remembering Lives: Conversations with the Dying and the Bereaved*. New York: Baywood.

Henden, J. (2008) *Preventing Suicide: The Solution Focused Approach*. Chichester: Wiley.

Martell, C. R., Addis, M. E., and Jacobson, N. S. (2001). *Depression in Context: Strategies for Guided Action*. New York: Norton.

McMurran, M., Nezu, A. M., and Nezu, C. M. (2008). Problem solving therapy for people with personality disorders: an overview. *Mental Health Review Journal*, **13**(2), 35–39.

Miller, P., Chilvers, C., Dewey, M., *et al.* (2003). Counselling versus antidepressant therapy for the treatment of mild to moderate depression in primary care: economic analysis. *International Journal of Technology Assessment in Health Care*, **19** (1), 80–90.

Nezu, A. M. (2004). Problem solving and behavior therapy revisited. *Behavior Therapy*, **35**, 1–33.

Nezu. A. M., Wilkins, V. M., and Nezu, C. M. (2004). Social problem-solving, stress and negative affective conditions. In Chang, E. C., D'Zurilla, T. J., and Sanna, L. J. (eds.), *Social Problem Solving: Theory, Research and Training*. Washington DC: American Psychological Association, pp. 49–65.

Nezu, A. M., Nezu, C. M., and McMurran, M. (2009). Problem solving therapy. In O'Donohue, W. T., and Fisher, J. E. (eds.), *General Principles and Empirically Supported Techniques of Cognitive Behavior Therapy*. Hoboken, NJ: Wiley, pp. 500–505.

NICE. (2004). *Anxiety: Management of Anxiety (Panic Disorder, with or without Agoraphobia, and Generalised Anxiety Disorder) in Adults in Primary, Secondary and Community Care*. London: National Institute for Health and Clinical Excellence.

NICE. (2009). *Depression in Adults: Full Guidance*. London: National Institute for Health and Clinical Excellence.

Padesky, C. A., and Greenberger, D. (1995). *Mind over Mood: A Clinician's Guide*. London: Guilford Press.

Perri, M. G, Nezu, A. M, McKelvey, W. F., *et al.* (2001). Relapse prevention training and problem-solving therapy in the long-term management of obesity. *Journal of Consulting and Clinical Psychology*, **69**(4), 722–726.

Roth, A., and Fonagy, P. (1996). *What Works for Whom?: A Critical Review of Psychotherapy Research*. New York: Guilford.

Simpson, S., Corney, R., Fitzgerald, P., and Beecham, J. (2003). *Psychological Medicine*, **33**(2), 229–239.

Skinner, B. F. (1953). *Science and Human Behavior*. New York: Macmillan

Slee, N., Garnefski, N., van der Leeden, R., Arensman, E., and Spinhoven, P. (2008). Cognitive-behavioural intervention for self-harm: randomised controlled trial. *British Journal Psychiatry*, **192**, 202–211.

Tarrier, N., Taylor, K., and Gooding, P. (2008). Cognitive-behavioral interventions to reduce suicide behavior: a systematic review and meta-analysis. *Behavior Modification*, **32**, 77–108.

Wells, A., and Clark, D. M. (1997). Social phobia: A cognitive approach. In Davey, G. C. L. (ed.), *Phobias: A Handbook of Description, Treatment and Theory*. Chichester: Wiley, pp. 3–26.

Williams, C. (2001). *Overcoming Depression; A Five Areas Approach*. London: Arnold.

Wolpe, J., and Lazarus, A. (1966). *Behavior Therapy Techniques*. Oxford: Pergamon.

Young, J. E., (1990). *Cognitive Therapy for Personality Disorders: A Schema Focused Approach*. Sarasota, FL: Professional Resource Press.

Useful websites

www.brief.org

www.ebta.nu

Useful material for patients

Nezu, A. M., Nezu, C. M., and D'Zurilla, T. (2007). *Solving Life's Problems: A 5-Step Guide to Enhanced Well-Being*. New York: Springer.

Useful contact information

British Psychological Society, St. Andrews House, 48 Princess Rd. East, Leicester, LE1 7DR, UK. Tel: 0116 2549568. Email: enquiries@bps.org.uk.

The Psychological Society of Ireland: info@psihq.ie (this website also provides information on other related bodies in the UK and Europe).

Systemic family therapy

Nigel Smith

Learning objectives

A basic understanding of the background and influences that led
  to the development of family therapy
Knowledge about five main schools of family therapy
An introduction to some basic concepts and tools from family therapy
  that maybe helpful in considering patients in a primary care setting

Why consider families, partners and relatives?

In Western society we traditionally tend to see people's health as lying within the individual. This way of considering health problems has passed through into mental health issues. The tradition follows through the medical model and into psychodynamic ideas of the self, and can ignore social and familial context, a vital element of most mental health issues. However, while general practitioners' medical training ensures a bio-medical lens for most problems, an emphasis in postgraduate education on the bio-psychosocial model and getting to know families over years in practice can invite family doctors to be alert to the dynamics and influence of family systems. Many are keen for a framework to understand the issues and a few have gone on to train in family therapy.

The individualist approach to mental health care has a number of social and economic side effects. In terms of cost, this can be seen both by the repeated 'breakdown' of patients with mental health issues and in the knock-on effect of health issues for relatives over time.

'Revolving-door patients', as they are sometimes referred to, often have the context of their problems ignored, and whenever they become unwell are taken out of their home environment to some sort of hospital venue, 'treated', mainly with medication, where they improve, only to be sent back to the same situation and where, with time, they break down again. The cost and time implications of this are obvious.

Likewise, the second cost implication sits around the health of close family members who, through dealing with these issues over time, can suffer much more frequently with stress-related problems, depression and physical health issues. And of course, in their turn, relational issues can present themselves often in small unsolvable health issues.

Research in the United States (Crane 2008) showed the considerable cost of mental health issues within the family and support networks, and how these costs could be considerably reduced by family interventions, which, on the surface, can look expensive. It is unfortunate that, in the way that funding within primary and secondary mental health in this country is so separate, this cost implication is not noticed or valued.

The social cost of these problems on families and social networks is obvious also. These issues can apply to families where there is a member experiencing a major mental health issue, but are also relevant to couple issues, marital problems and difficulties with teenagers. They also apply to the emotional effects of long-term physical illness on the wider family.

This chapter gives a brief outline of the main models of systemic family therapy and considers a number of elements of them which might be considered helpful tools within the primary care setting. It does not attempt to teach a whole approach to working with families, which, as a psychotherapy, is complex and time-consuming. However, this should not put practitioners off trying to be helpful in small but significant ways, and for many couples and families this is all they need.

Family therapy developed from interests as diverse as studies in the 1950s of psychosis and its development (see Bateson *et al.* 1956 and Leff *et al.* 2003), the development of theories of cybernetics in engineering (see Goldenburg and Goldenburg 1996) and work on understanding attachment styles in young children (see Bowlby 1969).

Schools of systemic family therapy

In very simple terms, there can be said to be five schools of systemic family therapy, and these will be related briefly here, in order of their historical development, though they do not really represent a linear time line, other than in terms of their conception. Today, many are still practised, in a variety of ways, and most family therapists would describe themselves as in some way eclectic in their practice. Alongside this time line, there has also been a gradual shift from an 'expert' to a 'non-expert' position, in which therapists have moved from seeing themselves as the agents of change, to seeing instead the patient or family as able and responsible for progress and change. Below is a brief description of each. At the end of the chapter there are some suggested texts for each model. It is also worth noting that there are other models of family work, not described here, that do not fit so much under the systemic umbrella, such as psychoanalytical family work and family management models which work from a more behavioural perspective.

Structural therapy (main proponent – Salvador Minuchin)

Structural family therapy, the earliest recognizable model, developed in the 1960s. As its name suggested, it had a belief that there were certain structures and boundaries that ought to exist in a family and around a family. In this sense it was very normative, but in simple terms it believed that parents should be the dominant subsystem in a family and that a family had a boundary around it that acted in a kind of homeostatic way, keeping the family in shape and structure and protecting it from radical change.

Problems occurred in families at times of trauma, e.g. serious illness, life stages, such as births, deaths, marriage or retirement, when a family might struggle to readjust to the changes, or when some of the structures and boundaries in the family were seen as wrong or dysfunctional, such as a household where it was obvious that one of the children was 'in charge'. Important systemic ideas such as *coalitions*, when two family members united in a negative way against another member, and *triangulation*, when a third party was brought into a difficulty that existed between two family members, were developed in this model (Dallos and Draper 2010).

Therapists in this model were very expert and directive, and would work to strengthen a more healthy structure within the family.

Strategic therapy (main proponents – Milton Erickson, Jay Haley, Jonathan Weakland)

Strategic family therapy was interested in the patterns of attempted solutions that revolved around a specific problem within a family. Aetiology and the symptoms of the problem were not of concern, but instead therapists explored symptoms and problems in order to 'identify the specific recurring sequences of interaction in which a symptom is embedded' (Hayes 1991). Thus the content was less interesting to them than the process and there was a belief that, in attempting to resolve a problem, families tended to make them worse. The seed of the problem and therefore the potential 'cure' lay within the interactional patterns of the family. Therapy involved taking a close look at how the family interacted and then devising 'strategies' to interrupt or change these patterns.

Where it was possible to intervene directly, this was always preferred, through setting tasks for the family to interrupt normal patterns of behaviour, but, where the family could not see the dynamics or felt powerless to effect change, then the therapists would develop more indirect methods, such as reframing (see later) or *paradoxical interventions*, in which, for example, prescribing more of the behaviour that was no longer wished for could allow a family to begin to feel that they could take some control over it and make choices.

Milan therapy (main proponents – Mario Selvini Palazzoli, Luigi Boscolo and Paolo Bertrando)

The Milan group of therapists working in the 1980s developed a model that saw real therapeutic power simply in the asking of questions. They saw the family as the agents of change, an idea that can be useful to hold onto in a primary care setting as it can relieve the clinician from the idea that they have to find some sort of 'expert intervention' to a difficult situation. Instead, it suggested that by being more thoughtful about the questions we ask, we can be helpful to a relational situation.

They developed a rigorous system of developing *hypotheses* of what they thought might be happening within the family and then using *circular questioning*, a process of asking questions that linked either generations or people in the family, or questions that try to grade situations in a 'most' or 'least' way, rather than a more 'all' or 'nothing' way.

They tried for the first time to take a 'neutral position', believing that as soon as the therapist sat down with the family they immediately became part of the family's system, rather than being able to sit outside it and make objective suggestions. They would finish sessions by feeding back symptoms as having positive roles or functions within the family.

The idea of circular questioning was a significant development in systemic therapy. Questions were asked in a way that fed back from information gained in conversation with the family (Dallos and Draper 2010). So, for example, if John says that he has been upset by the way Jane has spoken to him, rather than asking him why, a therapist might ask Jane why she thinks what she said makes John feel upset. This gives different layers of information about Jane's perceptions of John and her insights into her own behaviour and gives an opportunity to explore whether she understands John's perception of her. Other types of circular questions may seek to consider less/more positions within the family (e.g. 'who most understands you, who least understands you?'), or to make generational connections (e.g. 'How do you think that your own mother would have dealt with this?').

Solution-focused therapy (main proponents – Steve de Shazer, Insoo Kim Berg, Bill O'Hanlon)

Solution-focused therapy developed as a radical departure from problem-focused models of therapy. It asserted, as an underlying principle, that all clients and patients had what it took to resolve their problems (George *et al.* 1999). This was not the role of the therapist, who instead acted as a facilitator who encouraged the family to focus on the things they did well, and what worked rather than what did not.

Within this model, therapy focuses mostly on where a client wants to get to, rather than where they have been, and, through some detailed goal-setting, again led by the patient, it explores in a pragmatic and detailed way what this future would look like, and how the family would know when they got there.

It is again a model that believes in the power of questions in their own right to elicit change and seeks to avoid an expert position. In this respect the construction of questions can become important as they offer opportunity to families to consider situations in new or different ways. Solution-focused therapists would start by trying to get a very clear and detailed sense of what the family's 'best hopes' from meeting would be. Questions would then tend to focus on what the family do well already, what is going on when things feel better (rather than at their worst), what would be different if the problems that they brought in were no longer around and how they would know when they no longer needed any help.

The therapist also tries to avoid giving advice or making any suggestions of what a patient or family should do, relying instead on their making sense of the conversation for themselves and initiating change, often outside sessions.

Narrative therapy (main proponents – Michael White, David Epston)

Narrative therapy is a more complex model to describe, but worth a little time here as it is very much part of popular current practice, and its underlying ideas and beliefs influence a lot of systemic practitioners at this time.

It is called a 'post-modern' model of working. From this perspective, its proponents would reject the idea that there is such thing as objective, scientific truth; one of the fundamental beliefs of our modernist, reductionist society.

Instead, narrative therapy works on the belief that truth is socially constructed (Burr 2003) based on the conversations and stories that we tell and how, within our culture, we make sense of these. These ideas, stories, narratives and influences, filtered through language, then translate to the culture of each family in how people understand and make sense of their lives and the problems they encounter.

If a Western European person saw a man talking to himself and appearing to hear voices, then the observer may well conclude that he has a mental health problem. This is what he or she has seen and heard through the *objectification* of certain behaviours and actions. These observed behaviours have meaning for her, filtered through the language that she has to use and her upbringing, through media and cultural beliefs, and lead her to conclude that this person would need medical intervention. Someone from a different culture and language might well have a different socially constructed belief that this person is spiritually blessed, or possessed by demons, for example. From these different perspectives, a medical practitioner would not be an appropriate person to call. Within each culture their view would be seen as the 'truth', and a different 'expert' would be sought.

In the development of this approach, Michael White was influenced not only by the ongoing developments and movements in therapy, but also by art, literature and philosophy (particularly the ideas of power and control of Michel Foucault). Post-modern therapy saw our modernist society, in which the truth was seen as a measurable underlying fact, as misleading and blaming towards individuals who lived within it. There are societal pressures, norms and beliefs that people are forced to live up to. These have profound and often unnoticed influence on us. In particular sufferers of mental health problems are often perceived as 'weak' despite living day to day with problems that would destroy most of us.

The pressure of advertising and the media is a good example of this, which presents all women as needing to look slim and attractive, so that so many women cannot live up to this (anorexia), or perpetuates the societal belief in the need for us to 'stand on our own two feet', be independent, which, if we are unable to do this, can give us a message that we are inadequate and in some way a social failure. This can be a strong message for people who suffer from mental health difficulties and reinforces the idea that this problem sits in the individual rather than society having some responsibility for these difficulties.

Narrative therapists are interested in the *re-storying* of people's lives through a consideration of the stories and beliefs that might sit within the family. They believe that people often tell a story of themselves that cherry-picks events in their history, reinforcing the current story they tell of themselves. This is described as a thin description of themselves, missing out other stories and experiences that might contradict their current view of themselves. Thus, a person who feels depressed may notice stories and events that happened in their life that re-enforce their belief that they have always been depressed. The problem with this is that there is also an inevitable future for this, which is to always be depressed. By looking for 'unique outcomes' in a person's life, that is, stories and events that contradict this dominant narrative, therapy can help to begin to find richer descriptions of individual or family life that may begin to supplant this thinner narrative and suggest a different outcome. These stories are there already, but subjugated, hidden by the dominant narrative.

Again, narrative therapists are not the experts here, but facilitate conversation, use the 'telling' and 're-telling' of stories to uncover new meaning with families. Some of this 're-telling' happens via 'reflecting teams' of colleagues sharing a more personal understanding of what they have heard in the session, or 'outsider witnesses', people who have been through similar experiences. Therapeutic letters might also be used to reinforce ideas or narratives discovered in sessions, and therapists might try to move problems into a third-person place, so that the person is separated from the problem. In doing this, the belief is that the person can be more liberated from the oppressive label of the problem (schizophrenic, personality disorder) and can instead stand up to and make sense of a problem that they have. This process is called 'externalization'.

Useful tools and ideas for application in primary care

In this last section I will introduce some core systemic ideas that I feel might be either relevant or useful in primary care when faced with either a family or a couple in difficulty, or indeed an individual where it becomes apparent that there are familial dynamics within their presentation.

In doing this I am, again, not wishing to suggest that it is possible to do family therapy.

I do believe, however, that there are aspects and elements of the field that can either be helpful, or useful, in considering problems presented to a clinician, or be helpful in small ways to families or patients within the field. I will present each of these as individual ideas for consideration. Some I will consider in some detail, some as a specific tool to use in a short session. My hope from this is that staff in primary care settings might feel empowered to try something in a small way that makes a difference to both their thinking of a situation and that of their patient, or have an increased awareness of situations that might benefit from a referral to a family therapy service.

Genograms

A genogram is the name given to a form of family tree or map used by family therapists, both to gather information, usually relating to at least three generations of a family, and as a therapeutic tool to map family structure and patterns, meaning and events that may be significant within families. They can be good 'icebreakers' in early sessions, or powerful pictorial representations of families, which elicit emotional reaction. They are a helpful way of 'doing' rather than 'talking' that can be helpful to family members who find it hard to sit comfortably within a talking space, stereotypically, for example, teenage boys.

At a basic level these would show the names and ages of all family members, marriage/relationships, divorce and death. They can bring up issues that might not have been obvious through conversation. Patterns can sometimes emerge that might bring about new information and insight. For example, a woman may not have made the connection between the difficulties in dealing with her teenage daughter and her own mother leaving home when she was 12.

An example of a genogram is shown in Figure 17.1. This initially shows this basic information for the family of Bill, who came into services with a long-term problem of chronic pain in his chest that, eventually, became understood as a psychological problem.

Other information was then added that might be helpful in identifying or exploring patterns. For example, in mapping 'illness patterns' within the family of a woman who came in to clinic with her daughter, concerned that her daughter was 'depressed', it became clear that there was a generational pattern of women in the family suffering from depression. Her mother, an aunt and one of her grandmothers had all been diagnosed with some form of depression.

When we explored the reasons why she felt that her daughter might be depressed, she began to match events to things that had happened in her own childhood, such as her daughter getting upset at starting at a new school, and her own very traumatic experience of being left at a boarding school at a very young age. There seemed a pattern, almost a tradition, that at least one woman in each generation had to hold 'depression' for the family. Since the young girl's older sister had not shown any signs of having this problem, mum had been watching out for this even more with her second daughter.

We externalized 'depression' and its influence on different women in the family over the generations and identified differences that allowed us to consider an alternative narrative in which her worries were based more on her past and less on the current reality of her daughter. We came across an alternative idea that depression might not be a 'family heirloom', but each episode might, instead, be unique and unrelated. The young girl's mother was then able to allow her 'depression' to become the last in the family. The genogram was very helpful in mapping and discussing these thoughts and ideas. So, if we go back to Bill's family, we can map on health issues to the genogram which might help us to consider patterns, in a generational or gendered way.

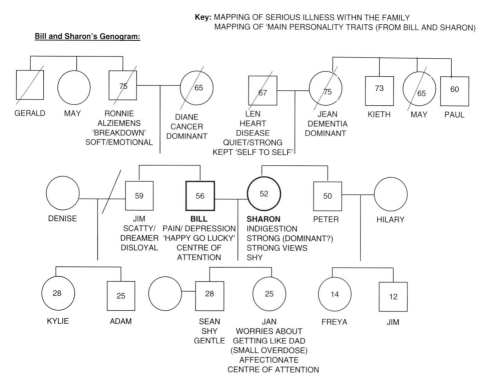

Figure 17.1. A genogram

With Bill's family, we were also able to map some 'qualities' that sat in a gendered way within the generations. This began to help us think about other meanings and ideas to what might be sitting in Bill's chest.

Hopefully, through these examples it is clear that many things can be usefully mapped within a family; illness, qualities, geography or culture for example.

Drawing out circularities (structural/strategic family therapy)

When we have problems in relationships we tend to see them in terms of cause and effect. For example, if we take a somewhat stereotypical example within a married couple, lets call them Emily and Bob: Bob might say of his wife, 'She nags me so much that I end up just ignoring her'. From this we can see that there is a relationship between what Bob believes (that Emily is nagging him) and what he does (ignoring her), between his beliefs and his actions. As he believes that Emily is nagging him he takes action to avoid this, maybe going out a lot or withdrawing in front of the television.

This statement is called a 'linear causality' and is very common in the way we speak about problems with our relationships. With it there is a clear implication of blame. Emily is seen by Bob as to blame for any problems or for his behaviour as she 'nags' him. Thus, in trying to deal with this situation in such a black and white way, we can be drawn into seeing it either in the same way and therefore look at ways of stopping Emily nagging or take a sympathetic

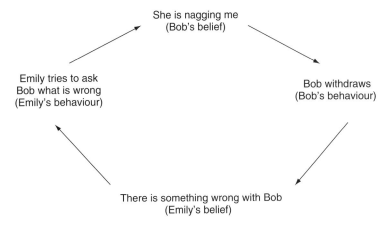

Figure 17.2. Circular causality

view of Emily and therefore suggest Bob is to blame instead. In drawing either conclusion we tend to put ourselves in a place of only having one line of resolution.

A 'circular causality' describes how patterns can become maintained through a loop of beliefs and behaviour. By adding beliefs and patterns of behaviour to form a self-maintaining circle of thoughts and actions we are able to add insight and what I would see as useful 'therapeutic doubt' into a black and white rigid belief, and also to remove blame from a system. Circularity emphasizes interdependence (Dallos and Draper 2010).

So to do this we need to add what Emily believes that she is doing and what Bob is thinking.

We can then draw this circularity, as in Figure 17.2.

Adding these other thoughts and actions immediately adds layers of meaning and understanding to the situation. It suddenly becomes more of a situation of misunderstanding than one of a victim and a perpetrator. It gives us many more areas to work on, so that rather than feeling that we can only work on Bob's actions or his beliefs of Emily's behaviour, we can also consider with him, or better still with the couple, which element of the circle or which action and belief connection is most accessible or straightforward to work on. And it is reasonable to assume that, if Bob understands Emily's approaches in a different way, he will behave differently, which will bring about new meaning. The circle is also much less blaming as it becomes difficult to work out where the circle starts or ends.

In some examples that are more problematic we can see how valuable this idea is and that it is something that we can map out with patients or couples. It can then be used to encourage them to think about where they might best be able to effect change, or what might happen if they did or believed something different.

Case 1

Ella, who was 18, was self-harming and feeling powerless and misunderstood. She was told by everyone that she had to stop cutting or nothing would change. She was told this often in a very blaming way. For example, her GP told her that she was a 'very silly and naughty girl', and that she was a big worry to her father (blame-laden linear causality). As she could not find a way to stop cutting, indeed felt ambivalent to stopping it as she got some release from it, and as it served a function in keeping her safe, she couldn't stop it as she had nothing to replace it. Her sense of failure was immense. She felt very stuck.

Early in our work together we drew out this simple circularity on a white board relating to the thoughts and action between Ella and her family (Figure 17.3):

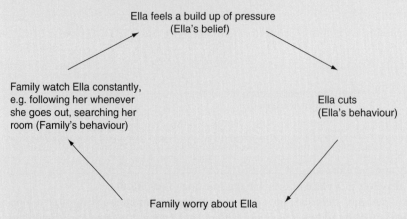

Figure 17.3. Case 1: circular causality

From this circularity we were able to consider other parts of the circle we might more easily work on, rather than Ella's 'ingrained' belief, reinforced by others, that she had to stop cutting. Instead she chose to work more on the feeling of pressure, initially choosing to work on other ways of relieving this, for example, by vomiting (something she already did when she felt unable to cut; not so helpful, but different) or by running very fast when she felt it, up and down stairs or round the block. In doing this we chose not to make a big issue about her cutting, but instead sought to understand why she did it and worked on that instead.

This emphasis led to a disclosure to me of past sexual abuse and to some very deep and difficult work for her, which eventually, led to the end of her cutting, but as almost the last thing to change for her. Throughout this I was careful never to give her my ideas of what she might do or to tell her what to do, but instead to hold a belief that she had what it took to resolve the difficulties for herself, which, over time, she did.

Rating scales (solution-focused therapy)

A small but significant commonality between circularities and scaling questions is that they can both be powerful in changing black and white 'yes or no'/'good or bad' views of situations into greyer both/and, more or less considerations which allow more possibility to see change and difference.

Many of us use rating scales, but from a more systemic perspective we can use them as a therapeutic tool in their own right, both in considering why things aren't currently worse than they are, and in goal-setting, by considering what a person needs to do to move themselves up one point on a scale, to consider where they need to be to stop seeing us, or to consider a notion of a preferred future along the scale where life is no longer so problem-saturated.

With couples we can use them to explore where they each feel things are on a scale of 1 to 10, where 1 is really problem-saturated and 10 is where things are the best they could imagine them being. Most people tend to answer somewhere around 4 or 5. This allows us to explore with them what it is that is keeping them *up* at that number rather than down at that number. This invites our patients to consider this position from the perspective of why they are not lower on the scale and what useful things are contributing to keeping them up there. It is important to look for detail in answers given, to offer as much insight for the couple as possible about the small, ordinary or even mundane things that they are doing that might be helpful and things they might wish to keep as they work to rid themselves of their problems.

This element can also be helpful in seeing an individual patient. One of the main reasons why a session can run over time is that we get too caught up on asking people how they have been or asking them how they are. This is particularly the case with a patient who is maybe coming in regularly with no real sense of a specific problem, but instead presents with unspecified difficulties.

So, instead of beginning with asking how a person is, or waiting for them to begin to tell you what is 'wrong', ask them, 'On a scale of 1 to 10, where 10 is life without the issues/problems that they are bringing and 1 is the worst things could be or have ever been, where are you today?' If a person gives you a 4 then this immediately gives you the information that they are not at the worst they can be.

The 10 minute session is then taken up with an exploration of what is keeping the patient *up* at the number they said. This needs to be explored in as much detail as possible. If they begin to explain why they are down at the number, listen to this and acknowledge it, as it is important to show that this has been heard, then gently restate the question about what is keeping them up there; what is stopping them being at the number below?

For the last part of the consultation, explore with them what they would be doing if they found themselves just one point up on the scale. Always stay with any answers that are given, looking for concrete detail: how would that feel? What would you be doing? What would others notice that would tell them that change had occurred? What things would you still want to be doing that you are doing now? Detail allows for the developing of richer goals with small elements that can then be more noticeable for the client. Finish by asking them to come back and to notice when life is most like how they have described it.

Externalizing problems (narrative therapy)

Sometimes, problems can become so oppressive to the sufferer that they begin to identify more and more with the problem. In the end they see themselves as the problem. Both in families and in society in general we can reinforce these ideas. People working within our services can also play their part in reinforcing this belief. In education, children who find it hard to concentrate or settle might be seen as 'trouble'. This is then how they are described, even to their faces, 'you're trouble'. In mental health I would like to say that calling someone a 'schizophrenic' or an 'anorexic' was a thing of the past, but I am not so sure. What this sort of language does is place someone's identity into the problem, so that the 'person then becomes the problem'. From this perspective, the more I believe that 'I am' the problem, the harder it is for me to do anything about it. If I am the problem then there is nothing I can do to affect it and this label is blame-laden.

Externalizing attempts to place the problem in the third person, and by talking about it in this way can place it back where it belongs, as a problem that the person needs to deal with.

So, to formularize this, we invite the patient to find a name for the problem that has meaning for them, map the influence of the problem on the patient and then begin to look for what they do that stands up to the problem.

For example:

- Naming the problem

  What name would you give to this problem that you live with?
- Mapping the influence of the problem

  When did sadness first come to visit your family?

  What does worry tell you will happen to you if you go outside?

  How does it get between you and your son?

  Who most helps worry to get stronger?

From this we would try to consider the strategies, deceits and tricks that the problem might use to get on top of the patient.

When anger has your ear, what does it say to you?

What other lies does depression tell you?

When is it most able to trick you into thinking that?

What hopes would this problem have for your life?

This language can feel quite strange to us as a way to discuss a problem. However, it can have a strong impact on empowering a person who may feel powerless to change something that they see as themselves.

Mapping the success of the patient

Here we would look to begin to ask questions that show a sense of the failure of the problem to always succeed in dominating the person. So, some examples of these might be:

Tell me about a time when you could have listened to worry but you didn't. What was different when you did that?

Who most stands with you against anger?

What are you doing when sadness feels at its weakest?

Within this process we are aiming to help the patient, and their family, to feel some agency over their lives again, and to develop a sense of collaborative practice.

Positive connotation and reframes (strategic/Milan/ solution-focused therapies)

A positive connotation or a reframe can work in a number of different ways.

Earlier in the evolution of family therapy, a reframe might just have been a therapist finding a different way of seeing a problem as an intervention. For example, a woman who was expressing a lot of anger might be reframed as being feisty. In talking to an arguing couple a reframe about their being good communicators of how they are feeling might be used.

Reframing black and white descriptions of an escalation within a situation combined with presuppositional language might be considered here from a solution-focused perspective. For example, a patient might come in for consultation saying that everything is awful now, the worst they have ever been, and there is no longer hope anymore. A response to this which gives a slight reframe might be: 'It sounds like things are pretty tough at the moment.' (The words 'pretty tough' show empathy whilst at the same time reducing the situation from awful and the worst. Most clients will agree with you, allowing for this subtle shift whilst feeling you have understood them. 'At the moment' is presuppositional language in that it makes an assumption that you know that things will get better, that this is just for now, which can be a powerful tool in itself.)

On from this, we could ask a question that elicits a resource held by the patient: 'So given that things up to now have been pretty tough for you, how have you been getting by?' or 'what made you able to get in to see me today?' ('Up to now' is also presuppositional language in that it suggests that something is going to change from this meeting.)

We can then make an exception-finding request such as: 'Given things are so bad, tell me about a time recently that has not been quite so difficult.' (This is again presuppositional in that it suggests that there are times when the patient experiences some difference rather than asking whether there is. If we ask, 'has there been a time recently when things have not been quite so difficult?' we ask a closed question which, if someone is in a difficult place, invites a 'no', and shows our own doubt that there will be an exception to be found.)

At a simple level it can work to begin to remove some black and white thinking that can very often stop change and lead to negative escalation; to begin to try to co-construct a different understanding of a problem or way of looking at it.

From this we might ask a presuppositional future-focused question such as 'when things get back to a more normal place for you, what do you imagine you will be doing that will tell you?'

From this solution-focused therapy perspective, noticing strengths, resources and things that a patient does well can be fed back in any small or informal conversation (try to do this in a thoughtful, questioning way: 'have you always been such a thoughtful person?' or 'sounds like you're a good person to have as a friend'; in saying these in a slightly questioning sort of way we can avoid taking on too expert a position in which we tell a person what is 'good').

Within the Milan school of therapy this was taken to a further level where therapy teams would try to positively connote all behaviour and actions in the family as having a purpose and a reason, and in this way are contributing to the maintenance and cohesion of the family (Palazzoli *et al.* 1980).

In conclusion, at a time when it is perhaps hard to access secondary mental health services, except for those patients who are severely unwell, it feels appropriate to begin to consider ways in which primary care staff can be helpful to patients in need of relief and support.

Summary

- Systemic family therapy is a complex psychotherapy.
- Systemic theory can give us insight into the context of how problems develop and are maintained by using genograms and examining circular causality.
- Basic tools and techniques can be learnt.
- Reframing the problem and altering the 'black and white' perspective can facilitate ways for moving forward.

References

Bateson, G., Jackson, D., Haley, J., and Weakland, J. (1956). Toward a theory of schizophrenia. *Behavioral Science*, **1**, 251–264.

Bowlby, J. (1969). *Attachment and Loss*, Vol. 1. London: Hogarth Press.

Burr, V. (2003). *Social Constructionism*. Hove: Routledge.

Crane, R. (2008). The cost effectiveness of family therapy: a summary and progress report. *Journal of Family Therapy*, **30**, 399–410.

Dallos, R., and Draper, R. (2010). *An Introduction to Family Therapy. Systemic Theory and Practice*. Buckingham: Open University Press.

George, E., Iveson, C., and Ratner, H. (1999). *Problem to Solution*. London: BT Press.

Goldenburg, I., and Goldenburg, H. (1996). *Family Therapy: An Overview*. Pacific Grove, CA: Brooks/Cole.

Hayes, H. (1991). A re-introduction to family therapy – clarification of three schools. *Australian and New Zealand Journal of Family Therapy*, **12**, 27–43.

Leff, J., Alexanda, B., Asen, E., *et al.* (2003). Modes of action of family interventions in depression and schizophrenia: the same or different? *Journal of Family Therapy*, **25**, 357–370.

Palazzoli, M., Boscolo, L., Cecchin, G., and Prata, G. (1980). Hypothesizing – circularity – neutrality: three guidelines for the conductor of the session'. *Family Process*, **19**(1), 3–12.

Further reading
Structural family therapy

Minuchin, S. (1974). *Families and Family Therapy*. Cambridge, MA: Harvard University Press.

Strategic family therapy

Haley, J. (1976). *Problem Solving Therapy*. San Francisco, CA: Jossey-Bass.

Milan family therapy

Palazzoli, M., Cecchin, G., Prata, G., and Sorrentino, A. M. (1978). *Paradox and Counter Paradox: A New Model in the Therapy of the Family in Schizophrenic Transaction*. New York: Jason Aronson.

Solution focused therapy

Macdonald, A. (2007). *Solution-Focused Therapy: Theory, Research and Practice*. London: Sage.

Narrative therapy

Morgan, A. (2000). *What is Narrative Therapy? An Easy to Read Introduction*. Adelaide: Dulwich Centre Publications.

Useful websites

The British Association of Family Therapy: www.aft.org.uk/.

Genograms: www.genopro.com/genogram/examples/.

Expressed emotions: www.personalityresearch.org/papers/mcdonagh.

Narrative therapy: www.dulwichcentre.com.au/.

Solution-focused therapy: www.brief.org.uk/.

Family matters, a systemic family therapy service that is based in primary care: www.familymatters-plymouth.co.uk.

Chapter 18

Sexual disorders

Gerard J. Butcher

Learning objectives

Increase understanding of sexual functioning and by contrast the nature of
  sexual dysfunction
Recognize the causes of sexual dysfunction
Have a clear understanding of how to assess an individual or couple presenting with a sexual
  dysfunction
Be knowledgeable about the treatment of various types of sexual dysfunctions and know how
  such treatment may be implemented in the primary care setting
Identify appropriate educational resources around sexual functioning that will be of potential
  benefit to the general practitioner and individuals and couples
Demonstrate an understanding of related problems of a sexual nature, to include persistent
  genital arousal disorder, sexual addiction, Internet pornography addictions, paraphilia, gender
  identity disorder and sexual dysfunction in non-heterosexual relationships

Introduction

Sex is good for your health! A report in the BMJ (Lindau and Gavrilova 2010) into the
benefits of an active sex life has suggested that higher levels of sexual activity between couples,
especially as they get older, are associated with good health and vice versa. In general, it was
also concluded that interest and participation in sexual activity was higher for men than
women and this gender gap widened with age.

It has been estimated that the number of individuals who actually seek help for sexual
problems is at variance with the numbers suffering silently, with consequent emotional pain,
and who may never seek access to potentially beneficial therapies (de Jong *et al.* 2010).
Therefore the practitioner working in primary care is in a unique position to ask the appropriate
questions that can start their patients along the road to hope for their problems in this arena
to be resolved. However, when working in primary care, it is important to know that patients
presenting with concerns about their sexual functioning may require more time than the
normal consultation due to feelings of guilt or shame or simple confusion or misunderstanding.

The human sexual response is a complex area involving a combination of cognitive,
emotional and physiological processes. In recent times much debate has been generated in
the area of categorization and classification of the sexual dysfunctions. Previously the focus
has been on disorders of desire, arousal, orgasm and pain. However, there is increasing
dissatisfaction with this model and there is also an argument that the previously accepted

model of classification of the sexual response cycle (desire followed by excitement leading to a plateau phase followed by orgasm) needs some refining and there is now an acceptance that this understanding of the sexual response cycle is very limiting and even inaccurate. The focus is now shifting toward an understanding of underlying mechanisms and transdiagnostic processes (de Jong *et al.* 2010) as studies emerge that raise implications for our understanding of sexual functioning leading to changes in therapy approaches (Brotto *et al.* 2010).

In addition, in recent years a major development in the effective treatment of sexual dysfunction has been the introduction of oral medications that enhance erectile response in men. There is ongoing research on the potential of oral medications for women but results to date on effectiveness have proved inconclusive.

Prevalence

The prevalence of sexual dysfunction is uncertain. Results from studies vary widely, with some community samples suggesting rates as low as 10% among men and 25% among women or as high as 52% of men and 63% of women, depending on which study you read. Overall though, it is accepted that rates of sexual dysfunction are relatively high in the general population and that these increase with age and chronic ill-health (Wincze *et al.* 2008).

Causality

The reasons for a sexual dysfunction are varied. The most important criterion that may need consideration from the perspective of primary care is the degree of what is called 'manifest personal distress' in DSM-IV (APA 2000). The degree of personal distress is most likely to be the reason associated with a patient making the journey to the general practitioner and requesting help in this area. In any exploration of sexual dysfunction, biological risk factors that can have a direct or indirect impact on sexual functioning must be taken into account. The factors cited most commonly include alcohol, medications (antihypertensives, antidepressants and antipsychotic drugs), diabetes and vascular disease (Wincze *et al.* 2008).

For many people, when it comes to sexual functioning throughout their lifetime, it is not unusual for temporary difficulties to arise due to life circumstances (life stressors, childbirth, menopause, etc.) and where this is the case, simple reassurance may be all that is required along with a note to follow this up over time. For some couples though, as difficulties persist and distress begins to manifest continually in a sexual context, patients may present for help having fallen into negative cognitive and behavioural patterns with each other, resulting often in a restricted sexual repertoire, with performance demands and fear of failure being reported frequently. Also, unrealistic expectations of sex (e.g. 'sex is all about intercourse') and/or a high sex drive on the part of one partner can cause considerable distress for the other. Both lack of physical attraction towards one's partner and feeling unattractive in oneself cannot be underestimated as a causative factor in sexual difficulties and specifically addressing such issues will be necessary if these problems are present (Wincze *et al.* 2008).

For many others, difficulties concerning sex may have been present since the onset of sexual activity and there are many and varied reasons for this. Shame and embarrassment may manifest as background features of sexual dysfunction. Equally, a lack of understanding of sexual functioning due to poor initial sex education can lead to myths and misunderstandings on various aspects of sexuality. Negative rigid religious and dysfunctional beliefs about sex (de Jong *et al.* 2010) or maintaining stereotypical views on male and female roles regarding sexual behaviour can not only cause sexual problems but will interfere with an ability to change when it comes to addressing these issues.

General mental health status needs to be high on the agenda during initial assessment. Issues such as low self-image, mood instability and a tendency toward worry and anxiety are all negatively correlated with a satisfactory outcome in a sexual encounter. For women in particular, general well-being and the emotional relationship with her partner are found to be the two most important factors associated with the absence of sexual distress (Basson 2005). Distress between couples, not related to sexual activity per se, can play a significant role in their sex life along with a past or present history of infidelity. In these instances it will be more appropriate for such couples to engage in relationship counselling aimed at resolving their distress. Up to 40% of those complaining of sexual difficulties also have concurrent depression (Johannes *et al.* 2009). In addition, the use of antidepressant medications among this population is associated with sexual problems being manifest. Comorbid depression in the context of chronic ill health has also been reported as a factor in sexual dysfunction (Basson *et al.* 2010a). However, although women suffering with depression can experience lower initial desire for sex, their ability to experience arousal and enjoyment of sex has been highlighted and both desire and arousal can be enhanced by learning how to cognitively adopt positive sexual schemas (de Jong 2009).

The role of disgust associated with sexual activity as a causative factor in sexual problems leading to undermining sexual arousal and desire is also worth mentioning. In an exploration of the role of disgust, it is suggested that as bodily products and odours are among the strongest disgust elicitors among humans and given the central role of the sexual organs in sexual behaviour, then feelings of disgust and disgust-related appraisals may arise during sex. For some, sexual behaviour too may remind them of animalistic behaviour that may have associations with disgust. A third category of disgust is termed 'socio-moral disgust'. This may be linked to perceptions about what may or may not be considered to be morally correct behaviour when it comes to various types of sexual activity (de Jong *et al.* 2010). All or any of these disgust experiences may lead to avoidance or interference with arousal and enjoyment of sex.

Of course the impact of childhood sexual abuse on patients can play a considerable role in sexual functioning, with one review concluding: 'There is evidence that survivors of childhood sexual abuse are significantly at risk of a wide range of medical, psychological, behavioural, and sexual disorders' (Maniglio 2009, p. 647).

Assessment

A comprehensive assessment of medical, sexual and psychosocial history is recommended for the treatment of sexual dysfunction (Basson *et al.* 2010b). Self-report questionnaires can be very helpful in gathering information quickly and there are several standardized ones that will provide useful information to the clinician. Among others, The Sexual Satisfaction Scale for Women (SSS-W; Meston and Trapnell 2005) and The International Index of Erectile Function (IIEF; Rosen *et al.* 1997) are both widely used self-administered questionnaires. When it comes to the clinical interview, Basson (2005) and Rösing *et al.* (2009) have a number of good suggestions on how assessment can be approached. The following suggestions are a combination of these.

(1) Taking time to gather enough information for an adequate assessment is essential. Sex and discussion about sexual matters may be a taboo subject for the couple, so overcoming these barriers is an important starting point. When talking with the couple,

asking them first to explain the problem in their own words is usually best as this can be a useful strategy to assess relative degrees of knowledge about sexual matters. Ideally, the couple need to be assessed individually as well as a couple, partly to determine, in a sensitive manner, whether or not there is any information that an individual does not wish to be shared with the partner. One way of exploring this is to ask directly, 'Is there anything else we may not have covered today that might be helpful for me to know?' This type of question may bring to the fore issues of childhood sexual abuse, unwanted sexual experiences, extramarital affairs or problems with gender orientation. Then clarify details with direct questions, giving options rather than leading questions. Assess motivation to change – are the couple willing/ able to take the time and effort to change certain aspects of their life that may be interfering with a good sex life?

(2) Specific questions covering the context within which sexual problems can arise along the following lines are required: how is their emotional intimacy? How useful are the sexual stimuli? How erotic is the context? Are attempts restricted to bedtime, when one or both partners need to sleep? What frequency of sex is expected or attempted? Are there concerns about birth control, safety from STIs or privacy? Are the sexual skills of the partners adequate? Is their mutual communication about their sexual needs problematic?

(3) Asking the couple why they are seeking help *now* can be relevant to gaining information about the level of distress for either or both partners. Also, asking about attempts they may have made toward resolving their problems so far can provide useful information. On an individual level, ask 'couple-centred' questions such as: 'how does your partner experience the situation?' 'How is the sexual dysfunction affecting your relationship?'

(4) Explore any history of illnesses, treatments and medication, including mental health issues.

(5) Gathering information about significant factors affecting the sexual relationship is necessary, for example, around reproduction (are the couple actively trying to conceive?; what impact does this have on the sexual relationship?); desire for sex – how equal or otherwise is this between the couple? Explore the health of the relationship in general. This will help determine whether the problem is primarily a sexual one or whether it is masking other problems that have not been addressed. In addition, are there any other non-sexual factors that may be impacting the relationship, e.g. work problems? Explore sensitively potential cultural or religious opposition to treatment methods. Guided masturbation exercises, for example, are often recommended as part of treatment toward helping individuals become more comfortable with their bodies, in the treatment of pain or aversion problems in women and premature ejaculation in men. In such instances it may be helpful to point out to the couple that masturbation need only be used as a short-term therapy technique designed to help the individual or couple achieve a treatment goal.

(6) Take a detailed history of sexual behaviour and experience, including genital and non-genital sexual activity, masturbation, sexual preferences (gender, age, practices), fantasies, behaviours and self-image. Issues pertaining to self-image can have a significant impact on sexual dysfunction.

(7) Take a general life history.

(8) A medical examination is usually necessary to rule out likely physical causes for a sexual dysfunction. These physical investigations will be detailed further on in relation to each type of sexual dysfunction.

General treatment approach

Education

In the primary care setting, the role of educating the patient is critical when it comes to dealing with sexual problems and education is considered to be a cornerstone of sex therapy to help deal with a variety of misunderstandings that are regularly seen in this area. Being able to point the patient/couple in the right direction may be very helpful before considering potentially expensive drug therapies. Dealing with myths around male and female sexuality can be a good starting point. Typical myths include ideas such as: a man is always interested in and ready for sex; real men do not have sexual problems; the bigger the penis, the better sex you will have; normal women have an orgasm every time they have sex; nice women are not really that interested in sex; a woman's sex life ends with menopause; masturbation is bad and someone with a sexual partner should not masturbate, etc. (Wincze *et al.* 2008, p. 639). Many couples may benefit from being given some direction regarding appropriate reading material. Bearing in mind too that some may have literacy problems, or may indeed just not be 'readers', advice on a suitable DVD or website material may be helpful. A list of relevant books, information on DVD and websites is given at the end of this chapter.

The right environment

A scene in the film adaptation of Roddy Doyle's book *The Snapper* (published by Vintage Press, 1991) shows one of the main characters asking his wife in a rather crude fashion if she is interested in having sex. She responds (much to his surprise) in the positive. He replies 'I'll brush my teeth!' and she says 'Mmm – that would be nice!' When it comes to sex it can be surprising how often couples expect to enjoy good sex without paying much, if any, attention to getting the environment right. Discussion between the couple of positive and negative factors affecting their level of arousal and interest is an essential exercise as part of therapy with, at times, surprising results as they may learn for the first time what is important to their partner sexually. Such factors might start with personal hygiene and may be as simple as a preference for a partner to brush their teeth before sex or whether or not to have a shower beforehand (some individuals like to feel 'clean' before sex, others may be turned on by the smell of their partner and can prefer their partner not to wash before sex). Other common discussion points include smoking, alcohol, drugs, tiredness, setting for sex, music, timing, lingerie, etc. In fact, the potential list is probably endless but the main point is for couples to communicate and thus maximize the number of positive environmental factors in their sexual encounters. Many couples believe sexual functioning is an automatic process without realizing the need to attend to the more basic issues that ensure their relationship is on a good footing (Wincze *et al.* 2008). Good communication between partners plays a significant and positive role in maintaining sexual satisfaction in relationships. In addition, mutual self-disclosure about sexual preferences contributes to relationship satisfaction, in turn leading to greater sexual satisfaction (MacNeil and Byers 2009).

Sensate focus exercises

The role of sensate focus exercises has long been established as a standard part of treatment for couples with sexual difficulties by Masters and Johnson (1966). At the heart of sensate focus is an objective that aims to remove the pressure on a couple to 'perform' by asking the couple to agree not to engage in sexual intercourse until a later stage and in its very early stages not to engage in any sexual touching for an agreed time. Instead, the couple are given instruction on learning to focus on pleasurable sensations with an emphasis on *pleasure* and not on the sexual aspect, although arousal may understandably occur. It is essential that the couple understand the rationale behind sensate focus exercises, otherwise there is a risk of early termination of treatment by the couple. Clear instructions are important and agreement should be quickly reached on the following:

(1) What the exact nature of each exercise is.
(2) Time to engage in the exercises should be set aside up to three times a week, allowing a minimum of 15–30 minutes each time.
(3) The goals of the exercises are to focus on and be aware of physical sensations and communicate the effect to the partner, positive or negative.
(4) At first, all genital stimulation is banned, as the couple will gradually move toward this as a goal.

Sensate focus plan

Stage 1: the couple may wish to start with their clothes on engaging in some gentle non-sexual touch through clothes before proceeding to being naked together. The couple take turns touching each other in a non-sexual manner. The person doing the initial touching is to explore the partner's body without touching breasts or genitals. The person being touched feeds back to the partner what is or is not enjoyable and comfortable, giving clear instructions on what they want more or less of. The couple then switch roles. This exercise is repeated two or three times over the first week.

Stage 2: this starts with doing the same exercises as in stage 1 but gradually moving to touching breasts and genitals. Again the focus is on feeding back to the partner what is enjoyable and comfortable but the couple must not yet proceed to sexual intercourse. The goal is to enjoy the time together and focus on the sensations being experienced. Efforts are not focused on reaching orgasm. This exercise is repeated two or three times in the week, with the partners moving gradually to mutual touching.

Stage 3: the couple start with stages 1 and 2 before gradually moving toward sexual intercourse. However, the couple are instructed to start with the 'woman on top' position and aim at first for containment of the penis in the vagina without movement or thrusting. This can be especially important for men with premature ejaculation problems as, often, previous attempts at intercourse involving the 'man on top' may have resulted in 'failure'. Equally, for most women who are anxious about possible pain or who have any phobic avoidance problems, this position allows them to retain control of the degree of entry of the penis into the vagina. The goal at this point is to enjoy the experience of the sensations during containment and continually feeding back to the partner what is being experienced. Gradually the couple can move slowly toward thrusting and rotating movements, with the focus still on the personal sensations being experienced. At any point where either partner experiences discomfort or anxiety, it is helpful to have agreed on a pre-arranged 'signal' indicating that one or the other wants to stop at that point. This may involve moving back to stage 2 exercises for a time before continuing on to stage 3.

Specific disorders and their treatment

Male sexual dysfunctions

In all cases, before moving to treatment, men and their partners need to be reminded that occasional difficulties in ejaculating and gaining and maintaining an erection are normal and can pass without any treatment. Being tired, drunk, hung-over or anxious for any reason can cause such difficulties. Additionally, those working in general practice need to be aware that there is increasing evidence of some men seeking and using oral medications that enhance erectile response simply as a recreational drug, thus allowing them to engage in high-risk sexual behaviour without clear evidence of erectile dysfunction (Fisher *et al.* 2010). This has been noted especially among users of marijuana/cannabis (Eloi-Stiven *et al.* 2007) and among men who have sex with men it appears that sildenafil use has become a stable fixture of their sexual culture (Paul *et al.* 2005). In the majority of cases, though, it must be noted that many of these men appear to source these drugs outside contact with their health care provider.

Physical examination and laboratory testing must be tailored to the patient's complaints and risk factors. It is now recommended that all men presenting with erectile dysfunction, hypoactive sexual desire and retarded ejaculation be screened for testosterone deficiency (Buvat *et al.* 2010). According to the British Society for Sexual Medicine (BSSM) a full clinical assessment may help to: uncover diabetes (as ED may be the first symptom in up to 20%); detect dyslipidaemia, which might not otherwise dictate treatment according to primary coronary prevention guidelines but may be the major reversible component in the patient's ED; reveal the presence of hypogonadism, a reversible cause of ED, which can be sometimes managed without the need for specific ED therapy and which has other long-term health implications; identify occult cardiac disease – ED in an otherwise asymptomatic man may be a marker for underlying coronary artery disease as symptoms of ED present on average 3 years earlier than symptoms of coronary artery disease (Heidelbaugh 2010). A free download of the BSSM guidelines in this regard is available at www.bssm.org.uk/downloads/default.asp.

1 Erectile dysfunction

According to the European Association of Urology (EAU) guidelines on erectile dysfunction (ED) and premature ejaculation (PE), ED is highly prevalent, and 5–20% of men have moderate to severe ED (all EAU guidelines can be downloaded free from the EAU website: http://www.uroweb.org/guidelines/online-guidelines/). ED shares common risk factors with cardiovascular disease. Diagnosis is based on medical and sexual history, including validated questionnaires. Specifically, a fasting serum glucose level and lipid panel, thyroid-stimulating hormone test and morning total testosterone level are recommended as part of a diagnostic workup. Obesity, a sedentary lifestyle and smoking greatly increase the risk of ED (Heidelbaugh 2010)

Medical treatment of ED is based on phosphodiesterase type 5 inhibitors (PDE5-Is), including sildenafil, tadalafil and vardenafil. PDE5-Is have high efficacy and safety rates, even in difficult-to-treat populations such as patients with diabetes mellitus. Treatment options for patients who do not respond to PDE5-Is or for whom PDE5-Is are contraindicated include intracavernous injections, intraurethral alprostadil, vacuum constriction devices or implantation of a penile prosthesis (Hatzimouratidis *et al.* 2010). From a psychological perspective though, consideration may be given to other factors, including a change in lifestyle. Of interest, for example, is the possible connection between frequency of sexual intercourse and ED. One study among males aged 55–75 years concluded that regular intercourse (i.e. more than once a week) can have a significant impact on reducing the risk of erectile dysfunction (Koskimäki *et al.* 2008). Among men with ED, it has been reported that attentional focus and erotic thoughts during sexual activity play a significant role in maintaining desire and arousal and this has implications for our understanding of problems that arise for men in maintaining an erection (Carvalho and Nobre 2011). If medication is prescribed it can be usefully psychologically for the man to first use the medication when masturbating as expectations of the medication may be very high and, if used directly in a male who has had long-term problems, anxiety about performance may be quite strong. Doing this several times will help to reduce performance anxiety but the use of sensate focus exercises needs to be incorporated into the treatment process as previously described before the couple attempt to have intercourse. For some men, it may also be that they will now experience strong erections without medication and they should be encouraged to occasionally begin sexual activity without taking the medication and allow for the likelihood of sexual intercourse without medication (Wincze *et al.* 2008). Although this may not be possible for all, a good number of men, depending on health, etc., may then experience full erections on a regular basis without use of medication.

2 Ejaculatory incompetence/delayed ejaculation/anejaculation

For some men their experience of sex may be impacted by not being able to ejaculate during sexual intercourse or possibly only after prolonged intercourse (30 minutes plus). On the surface, this may be thought of as not always being a source of dissatisfaction for a partner, though many women in such relationships realize there is something wrong and this can have a deleterious effect on their own enjoyment of sexual activity as they may believe they are somehow 'failing' to satisfy their partner. In addition, in couples who wish to have a family, levels of anxiety and distress between the couple can be considerable. The frequency is accepted as being relatively rare compared to other male sexual disorders, being reported in less than 3% of males, and men with this condition are often considerably distressed and lacking in sexual confidence (Perelman and Rowland 2006).

Causes

Delayed ejaculation may have a biogenic and/or psychogenic aetiology (Rowland *et al.* 2010) but it can very occasionally be due to certain neurological conditions or a side effect of some drugs, notably antidepressants (Segraves 2010). From a psychological perspective the causes can include the man not being attracted to his partner, unresolved or unacknowledged anger toward a partner, a prior event experienced by the individual as traumatic (a partner having an affair or being discovered in the act of masturbation or sexual activity, e.g. by a parent) or a strict religious background that results in the individual believing sex is sinful. A neurological examination is important as part of assessment. If ejaculation has never occurred in the man's lifetime (e.g. through masturbation, wet dreams or sexual intercourse) it is possible that some underlying urological disorder may be present and in such instances referral to an appropriate specialist is necessary.

Treatment

Taking a couple through the basics of a sex therapy approach as described earlier usually helps to reduce the element of performance anxiety, especially with the 'ban' on intercourse being in place. Under such circumstances the couple are encouraged to increase their communication to the point where the female partner understands the type of stimulation that is ideal for her partner. This may involve the man demonstrating clearly for his partner the type of stimulation he requires. He would be expected to show her how he successfully masturbates and then clearly feeding back to her in a positive manner his experience of allowing her to stimulate him. Under such circumstances, the couple engage in external stimulation close to the point of orgasm with sexual intercourse only taking place at that time. At an earlier stage though, ejaculation through masturbation may be better achieved near to the entrance to the vagina before intercourse is attempted. A positive outcome is dependent upon a number of factors including short history of the problem, some previous history of sexual satisfaction during intercourse, positive feelings of sexual desire and love for one's partner and an absence of other serious psychological problems (Lue and Broderick 2007).

3 Premature ejaculation

Premature ejaculation is the problem most commonly complained of by men with a sexual dysfunction. It is defined as the persistent or repeated occurrence of ejaculation before, during or shortly after penetration, over which the individual has little or no control and not accompanied by a feeling of orgasmic satisfaction (APA 2000). In surveys, up to 25% of men report having this condition with associated distress (Rösing et al. 2009).

Causes

Although this is a common problem, there is surprisingly little research into the causes. However, a combination of biological and psychological factors is considered in causation. From a biological perspective, penile hypersensitivity, hyperexcitable ejaculatory reflex, increased sexual arousability, possible endocrinopathy; genetic predisposition and 5-hydroxy-tryptamine (5-HT) receptor dysfunction have all been suggested. Psychologically, anxiety, social phobia, relationship problems, infrequent sexual intercourse and lack of sexual experience are all cited as contributing factors (Linton and Wylie 2010).

Treatment

Very often, expectations of patients (and their partners) with premature ejaculation need to be dealt with first as part of an overall psycho-educational approach. In particular, it would appear important that patients are aware of what the normative latency to ejaculation is. Most men ejaculate within two to eight minutes of commencing sexual intercourse. Factors that influence latency to ejaculation include age and the length of time since last ejaculation. For some patients, masturbation some time prior to partner sexual activity can be of benefit. During sexual activity, the benefits of taking it slowly during intercourse and the use of the 'female-superior' or 'woman on top' position can help to delay ejaculation, as this can have the effect of taking some of the pressure off the male to 'perform' in the male superior (the so-called 'missionary') position. In addition, specific behavioural techniques that have been reported to be helpful in delaying ejaculation are the 'stop-start' and 'squeeze technique'. It is important to bear in mind that successful use of these techniques requires a certain level of commitment between the male and his partner. The 'stop-start' technique involves the male being stimulated either before or during sexual intercourse to the point just prior to ejaculation, and then stopping. Once the sensations have subsided, stimulation starts again to the same point before ejaculation. With practice, the length of time taken before having to stop gradually increases. The squeeze technique involves the male or his partner using the fingers and thumb to squeeze the head (glans) of the penis to cause the ejaculatory response to subside (Linton and Wylie 2010). These techniques may also be practised by the man alone during masturbation and may thus help to build confidence in ejaculatory control, especially if the normal practice is to masturbate to ejaculation very quickly. Both partners need to be reminded that it takes time and effort for these techniques to be successful and the couple have to be prepared to be fairly light-hearted in their approach and allowance for trial and error is important.

Some medications have been reported to be of benefit for those with premature ejaculation. Delayed ejaculation has been reported as a side effect of many antidepressant medications and they have been commonly prescribed to be taken some 6 hours before anticipated sexual activity, but it may take some experimentation to discover the optimal dose (Wincze et al. 2008). This has led to recent studies on identifying a possible pill for premature ejaculation and dapoxetine (Priligy), an SSRI, has recently been reported to be effective in satisfactorily increasing the latency to ejaculation (Hatzimouratidis et al. 2010).

Female sexual dysfunction

Sexual problems among women increase with age and are closely associated with illness and drug use and are associated with decreased sexual satisfaction (Lindau and Gavrilova 2010). Previous understandings of female sexual dysfunctions and their classification have been heavily criticized and recent research findings have brought changes to our understanding of both origins and treatment (Brotto et al. 2010; de Jong et al. 2010). Female sexual dysfunctions are classified according to pain, arousal, desire and orgasm, though there may be considerable overlap. For example, a patient presenting with avoidance of sex due to fear of pain or penetration may also have problems with arousal and low desire.

Due to the relative success of oral medications in the treatment of erectile dysfunction in males, much attention has been paid to a search for a similar drug in women with a sexual dysfunction. Reviewing the research findings to date however, Chivers et al. (2010, p. 46) concluded: 'we predict that peripherally-acting drugs that only increase genital response will not be effective treatments for female sexual arousal disorder, except in those cases where women experience subjective sexual arousal without concomitant vaginal vasocongestion and lubrication'. This has generated much debate and there is an argument that seeking to understand and treat female sexual dysfunctions in the same manner as male sexual dysfunctions (i.e. that a pill will cure all ills) is a failure to recognize the complexity of female sexual arousal.

1 Pain-related disorders

The reality for some women is that simple reasons for pain can exist but are often unreported. One not uncommon example cited is post-partum pain, but health care professionals may neglect to ask any questions about this during routine checkups after delivery (Abdool et al. 2009). Boardman and Stockdale (2009) have described sexual pain as generally under-recognized and poorly treated. Sexual pain disorders include dyspareunia (superficial and deep), vaginismus, vulvodynia, vestibulitis and noncoital sexual pain disorder. Pelvic floor muscle dysfunction has been found in women with provoked vestibulodynia (PVD) and successful treatment using physical therapy exercises has been reported (Gentilcore-Saulnier *et al.* 2010).

The diagnosis of vaginismus is defined in DSM-IV (APA 2000) as recurrent or persistent involuntary spasm of the musculature of the outer third of the vagina that interferes with intercourse. However, doubt has been expressed on whether such spasm occurs in all cases and it has recently been proposed that the diagnoses of vaginismus and dyspareunia be collapsed into a single diagnostic entity called 'genito-pelvic pain/penetration disorder'. Diagnosis is further refined according to the following five dimensions: percentage success of vaginal penetration; pain with vaginal penetration; fear of vaginal penetration or of genito-pelvic pain during vaginal penetration; pelvic floor muscle dysfunction; medical comorbidity (Binik 2010). The benefit of altering these criteria means that therapy can be directed more clearly at the source of the disorder. For example, if fear or avoidance of phobic proportions is the more obvious problem (rather than pain), then difficulties related specifically to penetration can be targeted in treatment (de Jong *et al.* 2010).

Psychological reasons for experiences of genital pain can play a significant role in maintaining the problem. For example, low or disrupted arousal leading to attempts at penetration without sufficient lubrication could be the reason why pain is occurring. Fearful preoccupations associated with penetration will also play a role (e.g. 'it will not fit'). Under such circumstances sexual arousal will be inhibited and this may 'elicit defensive contractions of the pelvic floor muscles, which in turn may interfere with attempts of having sexual intercourse' (de Jong *et al.* 2010, p. 25). Such fearful preoccupations about sex will probably result in a vicious cycle of low arousal and pain.

Treatment of pain-related disorders

In the first instance it is important to determine what conditions cause the pain. As previously stated, if the problem is due to a lack of adequate lubrication due to insufficient arousal, then attention to this aspect of sex is important and where education can play a significant role with a couple. Many women with vaginismus also report problems in use of tampons and most likely will report a history of avoidance of gynaecological examination. It is helpful if the patient draws up a hierarchy of difficult situations graded according to difficulty or anxiety experienced. The patient at first will be encouraged to work alone, without her partner, and starting with the least difficult item on the list will be given a series of 'exposure-based' instructions. As many aspects of sexual activity can provoke a fear response in these patients, this may mean starting with items such as looking at a photograph of male and/or female genitalia. The patient is asked to record her thoughts and anxiety level associated with each stage. In session the therapist can work to help the patient challenge any negative thoughts experienced when engaging in the exercise and with repeated exposure anxiety levels would be expected to decrease. It is important that the patient gives an adequate amount of time to allow anxiety to decrease. Once anxiety levels associated with a particular activity are lowered, the patient is encouraged to move on to the next step in the hierarchy. At the stage at which the partner is included in the therapy process, it is essential that the partner fully agrees with the condition that the woman decides the level of exposure she can tolerate and at any time she can decide to discontinue the exercise (e.g. due to discomfort or a very high level of anxiety). It is essential for a sufficient level of trust to be established early on so that later stages when attempts at intromission are made can be more likely to succeed. For some patients the use of a dildo (these can be purchased in graded sizes) or vibrator can be of benefit, especially when they are working alone at first, as they can engage with the experience of insertion without the possible 'pressure' of their partner.

2 Disorders of arousal

According to DSM-IV-TR (APA 2000), the essential feature of sexual arousal disorders is persistent or recurrent inability to attain or to maintain arousal until completion of sexual activity – that is, an adequate lubrication–swelling response (vasocongestion of pelvis, vaginal lubrication and expansion, and swelling of the external genitalia). The disturbance must cause distress or interpersonal difficulty and must not be due to another axis I disorder or to the effects of a substance or a general medical condition. As previously discussed, this along with other definitions of female sexual dysfunction is being challenged, as in medically healthy women it is suggested that impaired genital responsiveness is not a valid diagnostic criterion as sexual problems these women report are clearly not related to their potential to become genitally aroused (Laan *et al.* 2008).

Causes

The following features figure significantly in causation: feelings of lack of safety during a sexual encounter, fears of pregnancy or STI, an insufficiently erotic situation or even more mundane factors such as the time of day or not enough time being given to the sexual act. Specific sexual worries concerning fears of not being sufficiently aroused or worries about reaching orgasm or a partner's performance also interfere with arousal and interest being sustained during sexual encounters (Basson 2005). In those presenting with low or disrupted sexual arousal, a lack of knowledge about how to become aroused can be a contributing factor along with a lack of requisite communication skills or insufficient knowledge about their own and/or their partner's anatomy – all leading to a lack of appropriate sexual stimulation (de Jong *et al.* 2010). To complicate matters further, in a meta-analysis of studies in the area of sexual arousal, a statistically significant gender difference in agreement between self-reported and objective genital measures emerged, with men being more able to clearly identify subjectively their levels of sexual arousal than women. Among women it would appear that they can have physiological-genital sexual arousal but subjectively report feeling unaroused (Chivers *et al.* 2010), although it has also been suggested that women may be more aware of their level of physiological arousal than previously assumed (Waxman and Pukall 2009). The possible reasons for a lack of awareness of arousal states are varied. Some suggestions are that learning and attention to genital arousal are culturally different between men and women. Other cognitive factors may also play their part in arousal. Negative body image among women, for example, has been associated with problems in sexual arousal and sexual functioning (Nobre and Pinto-Gouveia 2006).

Treatment of arousal disorders

The possible sources of the arousal difficulties must first be established. If the difficulty is related to dysfunctional or rigid beliefs, then these can be dealt with using an educational and cognitive approach to challenge these beliefs. Ensuring that the right conditions for a positive sexual experience are met, as already discussed, will play an important role here. For example, adequate time given to being stimulated before attempts at intercourse are made will obviously be helpful. If the woman has a high level of self-consciousness or embarrassment about her body, then use of a graded exposure-related exercise along with an exploration and modification of negative thoughts about her body will be helpful. A very useful exercise on this topic can be downloaded by or for patients at www.wholeliving.com/article/body-consciousness-raising-plan.

Mindfulness-based approaches have also shown promise in the treatment of low arousal disorders as these techniques may result in longer-term changes in attentional focus; these changes, in turn, may improve sexual response (Brotto *et al.* 2008; de Jong 2009).

3 Hypoactive sexual desire disorders

Sexual desire disorders have been reported as 'probably the most difficult to manage, and yet they are seen more frequently than any other sexual disorders in patients presenting for sexual therapy' (Riley and May 2001, p. 1849). Hypoactive sexual desire disorder is characterized by 'persistently or recurrently deficient (or absent) sexual fantasies and desire for sexual activity' (APA 2000, p. 541). Dissatisfaction has been reported with this definition as it is considered that desire for sex and sexual fantasy are not universal experiences (Carvalheira *et al.* 2010). It is considered that sexual desire in a woman may often be 'neutral' or absent at the initiation of a sexual encounter, but can be triggered by a variety of (non-sexual) factors, such as emotional intimacy (current status of relationship with partner, desire to express love and give and receive pleasure) and general well-being. Thus, being sexually stimulated in an appropriate context leads to psychological and biological processing and then leads to subjective arousal and responsive sexual desire (Basson 2005). It has also been reported that women's motivation to engage in sex is influenced by a variety of factors associated with their past sexual experiences, the type of relationship they are in and lifestyle factors related to their career and family demands (Meston *et al.* 2009).

The relevance of a cognitive dimension has been shown to be an important factor where disorders of sexual desire are concerned. Carvalho and Nobre (2010) reported on cognitive factors (mainly automatic thoughts during sexual activity) being the best predictors of sexual desire in women. Certain dysfunctional beliefs (e.g. 'it is wrong to enjoy sex') will also undermine sexual desire (de Jong *et al.* 2010).

Physically, urinary incontinence can significantly impact women's interest in and enjoyment of sex and a combined pelvic floor rehabilitation programme has been shown to improve sexual functioning and quality of life (Rivalta *et al.* 2010). Surgical interventions for breast cancer impair a woman's quality of life across several dimensions, including sexual health, and targeted interventions are required in such cases (Biglia *et al.* 2010). Radical hysterectomy also impacts women's sexual functioning negatively (Serati *et al.* 2009).

Treatment

The use of transdermal testosterone patches in the management of low sexual desire among post-menopausal women has been shown to be very beneficial in various large-scale studies, though long-term safety data are still being gathered (Krapf and Simon 2009). As is the case for treating arousal disorders, many couples will need to be prepared to engage in a variety of change strategies to increase desire. This can include exploring with the couple the degree to which boredom with their sexual routine may be both a causative and maintaining factor, challenging negative or faulty attitudes to sex and increased open communication about what each finds attractive (or not) during sexual activity. The use of erotic literature can play an important role for the couple, though couples with very conservative attitudes may be offended by such suggestions and the therapist needs to be very aware of this possibility (Wincze *et al.* 2008).

Case 1

Tina (aged 47) and Martin (aged 54) presented to the clinic with a variety of sexual concerns mainly focused on Tina's apparent loss of interest in and desire for sex. Both agreed that the impact of raising three children in the past 20 years of marriage had taken its toll on their relationship and that with each birth, Tina's level of interest declined. At initial assessment, sexual activity was limited to once every 3–4 weeks with Tina admitting that this was usually in response to a feeling of inherent guilt she experienced at 'not being a good-enough wife'. Her desire was usually to try and 'get it over with' as quickly as possible. Martin was very aware of Tina's feelings but admitted to feeling very frustrated. He was upset too that he had developed premature ejaculation, in part he believed because he was very aware of Tina's feelings and 'not wanting to bother her too much'. He was also bothered by the fact that most of his sexual experience these days was 'solo' sex, i.e. masturbation. Although he had no inherent problem with masturbation on an occasional basis, his preference was for a better sex life with his wife.

During further questioning it emerged that Tina had often experienced in the past that sex could have been better. She stated that she would prefer Martin to look after his health better – he was overweight and often smoked just before they went to bed. She admitted both these issues affected her interest in him sexually. Martin expressed surprise at this as he was not aware she felt this way. Furthermore she complained that sex was over far too quickly and this often left her feeling dissatisfied and less interested. She stated that she had not discussed these issues with Martin before this as she was afraid of hurting his feelings. Full medical investigations revealed that both were in reasonable health and Tina was not yet menopausal. This raised further discussion about Tina's interest in sex as she was concerned about the possibility of becoming pregnant and Martin was not in favour of using condoms.

All the above gave much cause for discussion in the initial sessions. They both found it helpful to be able to talk about their problems in an open manner. Martin agreed to take better care of his health and they started to walk together daily. He said that entering therapy for their sexual difficulties also gave him an incentive to quit smoking and he commenced a smoking cessation programme. Both agreed to, and enjoyed, the sensate focus exercises. Taking the pace more slowly was very helpful to them both and they were able to use the 'stop-start' technique to improve Martin's ability to delay ejaculation. They found some of the recommended reading materials very beneficial too. Having satisfactorily sorted out the concerns about contraception and as the relationship and communication issues improved, Tina found her interest in sex was much better. They realized too that given the inherent problems of having three teenagers around the house, they needed to be more creative about ensuring they had time together. Six months follow-up showed that they had been able to maintain a much better relationship overall and the sexual worries were no longer an issue.

4 Orgasmic dysfunction

Orgasm is defined as 'a sensation of intense pleasure creating an altered consciousness state accompanied by pelvic striated circumvaginal musculature and uterine/anal contractions and myotonia that resolves sexually-induced vasocongestion and induces well-being/contentment.' (Meston *et al.* 2004, p. 66). Female orgasmic disorder is considered to be the persistent or recurrent delay in, or absence of, orgasm following a normal sexual excitement phase that causes marked distress or interpersonal difficulty (APA 2000). In couples where the woman has anorgasmia, it is not unusual to find a high level of anxiety around discussion of sexual matters. In many cases the woman may not be receiving adequate stimulation due to either her own or her partner's lack of knowledge. Along with the aforementioned sensate focus exercises, cognitive behavioural approaches that promote positive attitude change, education and specific behavioural exercises such as mirror exercises and guided self-stimulation/masturbation, possibly using a vibrator, are utilized in treatment. As is the case in the treatment of disorders of arousal, it is essential that the couple are prepared to work together in improving communication skills. It is essential too that the therapist ensures the couple are both fully knowledgeable about their sexual functioning and it should not be assumed, for example, that a patient will fully understand what is meant by the term 'masturbation'. Equally, the couple may need to be educated on aspects of orgasm and reassurance that clitoral orgasm is not in any way 'inferior' to a vaginal orgasm (Wincze et al. 2008).

Case 2

Laura, a 31–year-old woman, attended stating that she had difficulties in achieving orgasm. She had been involved in two previous stable sexual relationships and had been with her present partner (Pete) for the past 10 months. Although interested in sex, she stated she had never experienced orgasm during sexual stimulation or intercourse. Over time, she noticed her interest could be difficult to maintain and she admitted to some degree of frustration. She was, however, 'shy' about discussion of sexual matters and tended to lie to her partner about achieving orgasm during sex. Assessment revealed that sexual matters had never been discussed in her formative years. Laura was an only child. At menarche, at age 13, her mother had what Laura described as an 'awkward' discussion with her about menstruation and told her to be careful of men. In general, she said, the message from her mother regarding sex was that it was 'disgusting' and recalled both her parents quickly switching channels if anything of a sexual nature was on TV along with negative comments about sex. It wasn't until she left home and went to college that she became aware of sex in a more positive manner from discussion with her peers. With a 'patient' boyfriend she found that she was interested in sex, but said she could never really relax enough to allow orgasm. Often she could experience a heightening of arousal during sexual activity but tended to become quite anxious and was aware of 'shutting down inside', partly because she was fearful of what might happen if she 'lost control', though she was unable to be any more specific about what such a loss of control would look like.

Laura agreed to discuss the situation with her current partner, Pete, and they both started to attend the clinic. Assessment revealed that, although describing himself as sexually experienced, her partner's level of knowledge about sexual matters was quite limited and he was uncertain too about how arousal occurred in a woman. Therapy sessions focused initially on education of the couple, working toward increasing their knowledge of the anatomy of the sexual organs and information on arousal. Discussion of relevant reading material was helpful to both in this regard although at first Laura expressed excruciating embarrassment at such open and frank discussion. Both were encouraged to look at their own genitals using a mirror and then to talk with each other about the experience. Laura expressed some amazement that this would be normal for any woman but eventually agreed and reported back positively about the experience once she had repeated the exercises three or four times. Although both initially agreed to participate in sensate focus exercises, they quickly broke the 'agreement' on the ban on intercourse due to Pete's expression of frustration. Time was taken to explain the importance of taking it slowly if the goals of therapy were to be achieved. Laura and Pete were both given instruction on self-stimulation and information they gained during this time was very useful to them when they were carrying out the sensate focus exercises, as they communicated sensations to each other during mutual masturbation. Despite this, Laura still had difficulty achieving orgasm, although she admitted her arousal levels were much better than anything she had previously experienced. After discussion, they agreed to purchase a vibrator at an 'Ann Summers' shop in their locality, with Laura insisting on Pete accompanying her for this purchase. He was agreeable, though a little surprised at the anxiety it raised for him. Following discussion on the use of the vibrator, orgasm was experienced by Laura, 'almost by surprise', she said, the next time they were doing the sensate focus exercises. Laura thought that the intensity of the stimulation that the vibrator delivered was helpful in this regard. They also used the vibrator when they had moved on to intercourse using the 'female-superior' position. After this, Laura was much more relaxed during sex and regularly experienced orgasm during physical stimulation by Pete. At follow-up 4 months later, both expressed ongoing satisfaction with the sexual relationship and Laura continued to experience orgasm frequently.

5 Persistent genital arousal disorder (PGAD)

Persistent genital arousal disorder (PGAD) has been reported in the literature for more than a decade now and it is a condition that generates much debate, stirring a great deal of interest in the tabloid press. In reality, there is a very mixed picture as some women with this condition do not report any distress but many do (Laan *et al.* 2008). Some researchers have suggested that PGAD with and without distress be considered two different disorders (Weiss and Brody 2009). In some cases it would appear that PGAD can be caused by a variety of medical conditions such as pelvic congestion (Thorne and Stuckey 2008) but in general it is considered to be idiopathic in origin. The main feature is the report of persistent feelings of vaginal congestion and other physical signs of sexual arousal in the absence of any awareness of sexual desire provoking or accompanying this arousal. Orgasm usually results in short-term relief only and the feelings of persistent arousal will lead the woman to engage in some form of sexual activity or masturbation to relieve the sensation of vaginal congestion. Feelings of arousal may persist for hours, days or even months (Leiblum and Nathan 2001). Women with PGAD can be young or old, premenopausal or using postmenopausal hormone replacement therapy, married or single. These women require a great deal of sympathy when presenting for help as they are often embarrassed and distressed by their symptoms.

Sexual addiction

The term 'sexual addiction', also proposed as being 'hypersexual disorder' by Kafka (2010), is used to describe the behaviour of a person who has an unusually intense sex drive or an obsession with sex. It is generally thought of as a problem related to impulse control. Sex and the thought of sex tend to dominate their thinking, making it difficult to work or engage in healthy personal relationships. Distorted thinking, often rationalizing and justifying their behaviour and blaming others for problems, is not unusual in sex addicts. In general, denial is a key issue and excuses for their actions are a common feature. Risk-taking behaviours (e.g. unsafe sex, or sex in places where they may be publicly caught) are frequently found. It is also not unusual for them to engage in compulsive masturbation, extramarital affairs and engagement in consistent use of computer sex (Levine 2010). The problem of sex addiction is in general seen as male-oriented and many experience severe psychological problems as the problem persists.

Generally, a person with a sex addiction gains little satisfaction from the sexual activity and forms no emotional bond with his or her sex partners. In addition, the problem of sex addiction often leads to feelings of guilt and shame. A sex addict also feels a lack of control over the behaviour, despite negative consequences (financial, health, social and emotional). These behaviours have a significant impact on their personal and intimate relationships.

Treatment is focused on controlling the addictive nature of the behaviour and helping the person develop a healthy sexuality. Treatment includes education about healthy sexuality, individual counselling and marital and/or family therapy. Support groups and 12-step recovery programmes for people with sexual addictions can be of benefit.

Cybersex or Internet pornography addiction

Many families and couples are increasingly experiencing a loved one engaging in cybersex or Internet pornography addiction, often causing marked personality changes in the individual (Landau *et al.* 2008). The prevalence of such problematic use of the Internet is unknown due to the generally private and often secretive nature of Internet usage. Given the increasing acceptance of pornography in Western cultures as something approaching a 'norm', it may also be difficult to determine the point at which engagement with Internet pornography can be defined as problematic. It has been identified that teenagers who view sexually explicit websites display higher sexual permissiveness scores compared to those who do not engage in such viewings and they also appear more likely to engage in multiple sexual relationships (Braun-Courville and Rojas 2009). In the United States of America, adolescents of both sexes with access to the Internet are reported, in one study, to engage in sexual relationships earlier than their peers who do not have Internet access (Kraus and Russell 2008).

Given that standard protocols for evaluation and treatment of problematic Internet use have yet to be defined, this raises further problems for assessment. In spite of the recognition of problematic Internet pornography viewing, and a variety of suggested interventions being proposed, there are no systematic studies available to date on an optimum treatment approach (Twohig and Crosby 2010). However, general principles of treatment would suggest the best course to take involves recognition that such use of the Internet is most likely reflective of an underlying psychopathology (Recupero 2008). Any treatment approach therefore should be geared toward identifying underlying psychopathology and, on entering therapy, an emphasis on principles of treatment used in dealing with problems of an addictive nature. An experimental trial by Twohig and Crosby (2010) on six adult males utilizing acceptance and commitment therapy (ACT) has shown some promising results, with a reduction of 85% in viewing being reported and maintained at 3 month follow-up, along with improvements in various measures of quality of life. More systematic and randomized trials are required.

Paraphilias

Definitions of normality vary across cultures and this can cause problems when attempting to define and collect adequate data regarding the paraphilias (Bhugra *et al.* 2010). The use of the Internet has fostered a large amount of growth in sexually deviant behaviour (Holt *et al.* 2010). The course is in general chronic in nature. In general, those with a paraphilia have associated fantasies, urges and behaviours. Common paraphilias include exhibitionism, fetishism, voyeurism and sado-masochism. Paedophilia, a sexual interest in prepubescent children, is a condition that has a high rate of recidivism. Drug therapies have been shown to be useful in some cases. In all cases, specialist treatment is required that is usually outside the remit of the general practitioner.

Gender identity disorder (transsexualism)

Gender identity is the individual's basic experience of being a man or a woman. Gender identity disorder is understood to be experienced by the individual as a conflict between the individual's actual physical gender and the gender that person identifies him or herself as. Significant discomfort with their biological gender is a hallmark of the disorder. Many with gender identity disorder, despite having normal genitalia and sexual characteristics, identify themselves as being of the opposite gender. In other cases, the genitalia may be quite ambiguous and this raises questions regarding their gender.

What contributes to our sense of gender remains uncertain, though one recent MRI study supports the assumption that brain anatomy plays a role in gender identity (Luders *et al.* 2009). People with gender identity disorder may act and present themselves as members of the opposite sex.

Symptomatically, those with gender identity disorder can experience varying levels of disgust with their own genitalia, state that they want to be the opposite sex, may dress like the opposite sex, are usually quite severely distressed by their gender and experience quite high levels of social isolation. Among children, more than half may have a comorbid psychiatric disorder (Wallien *et al.* 2007). Early diagnosis leads to a better outcome and the general practitioner may be the first 'port of call' by anxious parents. Treatment for children usually involves referral to an appropriate psychiatric service and both individual and family therapy is recommended for children. Sex reassignment by both surgical and hormone means is an option that many want to consider, and patients need to be clearly advised of potential complications following surgery (Sohn and Bosinski 2007). Problems with gender identity may also persist post-surgery and ongoing psychological support may be required as a consequence (Shafer 2008).

Sexual dysfunction in non-heterosexual relationships

There is a dearth of research into sexual dysfunction among non-heterosexuals. Among homosexual men, although the prevalence of premature ejaculation has been reported to be similar to that found among heterosexual males, erectile dysfunction appears to be more common (Breyer *et al.* 2010). In the same study, Breyer *et al.* (2010) report that the incidence of sexual dysfunction in lesbians was less prevalent than among heterosexual and bisexual women. The diagnosis and management of sexual dysfunction in bisexuals, gay men, lesbians and transgendered individuals should not be any different from those in heterosexual relationships although issues such as possible ambivalence about sexual identity and difficulties negotiating transition points in life are factors that need consideration during assessment and treatment (Bhugra and Wright 2007). It has been suggested that many primary health care providers may find dealing with sexual issues in same-sex relationships difficult due mainly to ignorance of lesbian and gay lifestyles and sexual practices (Hinchliff *et al.* 2005).

Summary

- Recent research has increased our understanding of the underlying mechanisms and processes involved in positive sexual functioning. Sexual difficulties are common within the general population and these problems tend to increase with age and poor health.

Although psychological issues are common reasons for the presence of sexual dysfunction, a number of biological risk factors are causative and the presence of erectile dysfunction in men may hide an underlying, serious medical problem such as diabetes or heart disease.

- A comprehensive assessment of an individual's medical, sexual and psychosocial history is recommended for treatment of sexual dysfunction. A clinical interview and various physical investigations are usually necessary. Assessment of the general relationship between the couple is vital to rule out what may be primarily a relationship, rather than a sexual, problem.

- Education of couples and ensuring the environment is right for positive sexual experiences are both an essential part of the process of treatment. The couple in each case need to be aware of the time commitment required from them for a successful outcome. Although there are general treatment principles that must be followed (e.g. sensate focus exercises; exploration of dysfunctional beliefs, etc.), each case will usually require a tailored intervention depending on the nature of the problem. Oral medications are playing an increasing role in the treatment of male sexual dysfunction. The relevance of treating pain-related sexual dysfunction in women has gained increased attention.

- Further research into understanding persistent genital arousal disorder among women is necessary and such a presentation needs to be dealt with sympathetically.

- Among males, sexual addiction is gaining increased attention and can have enormous negative effects on an individual across many areas of their life. The focus of treatment is on helping the individual develop a healthy sexuality and addressing underlying psychopathology.

- Internet pornography addiction is proving problematic for many individuals, affecting relationships among families and couples. A variety of treatments have been proposed but no full clinical trials have been carried out.

- The use of the Internet has fostered much growth in sexually deviant behaviours and the course of paraphilia is usually chronic and unremitting. Such cases require specialist treatment.

- Gender identity disorder has a better outcome if diagnosed early and it is not uncommon for initial presentation to occur in childhood. Referral of both the individual and the family to an appropriate psychiatric service is necessary.

- The diagnosis and treatment of sexual dysfunction in non-heterosexuals should not differ from that among the heterosexual population, although possible ambivalence about sexuality needs consideration. There is still very little available research into the prevalence of sexual dysfunction among non-heterosexuals.

References

Abdool, Z., Thakar, R., and Sultan, A. H. (2009). Postpartum female sexual function. *European Journal of Obstetrics, Gynecology and Reproductive Biology*, **145**(2),133–137.

American Psychiatric Association. (2000). *Diagnostic and Statistical Manual of Mental Disorders*, 4th edn. Washington DC: APA.

Basson, R. (2005). Women's sexual dysfunctions: revised and expanded definitions. *Canadian Medical Association Journal*, **172**(10), 1327–1333.

Basson, R., Rees, P., Wang, R., Montejo, A. L., and Incrocci, L. (2010a). Sexual function in chronic illness. *The Journal of Sexual Medicine*, 7(1 Pt 2), 374–388.

Basson, R., Wierman, M. E., van Lankveld, J., and Brotto, L. (2010b). Summary of the recommendations on sexual dysfunctions in women. *The Journal of Sexual Medicine*, **7** (1 Pt 2), 314–326.

Bhugra, D., and Wright, B. (2007). Sexual dysfunction in gay men and lesbians. *Psychiatry*, **6**(3), 125–129.

Bhugra, D., Popelyuk, D., and McMullen, I. (2010). Paraphilias across cultures: contexts and controversies. *The Journal of Sex Research*, **47**(2), 242–256.

Biglia, N., Moggio, G., Peano, E., *et al.* (2010). Effects of surgical and adjuvant therapies for breast cancer on sexuality, cognitive functions, and body weight. *The Journal of Sexual Medicine*, **7**(5), 1891–1900.

Binik, Y. M. (2010). The DSM diagnostic criteria for dyspareunia. *Archives of Sexual Behavior*, **39**(2), 292–303.

Boardman, L. A., and Stockdale, C. K. (2009). Sexual pain. *Clinical Obstetrics and Gynecology*, **52**(4), 682–690.

Braun-Courville, D. K., and Rojas, M. (2009). Exposure to sexually explicit websites and adolescent sexual attitudes and behaviors. *The Journal of Adolescent Health*, **45**(2), 156–162.

Breyer, B. N., Smith, J. F., Eisenberg, M. L., *et al.* (2010). The impact of sexual orientation on sexuality and sexual practices in North American medical students. *The Journal of Sexual Medicine*, **717**, 2391–2400.

Brotto, L. A., Basson, R., and Luria, M. (2008). A mindfulness-based group psychoeducational intervention targeting sexual arousal disorder in women. *The Journal of Sexual Medicine*, **5**, 1646–1659.

Brotto, L. A., Bitzer, J., Laan, E., Leiblum, S., and Luria, M. (2010) Women's sexual desire and arousal disorders. *The Journal of Sexual Medicine*, **7**(1 Pt 2), 586–614.

Buvat, J., Maggi, M., Gooren, L., *et al.* (2010). Endocrine aspects of male sexual dysfunctions. *The Journal of Sexual Medicine*, **7**(4 Pt 2), 1627–1656.

Carvalheira, A. A., Brotto, L. A., and Leal, I. (2010). Women's motivations for sex:

exploring the diagnostic and statistical manual, fourth edition, text revision criteria for hypoactive sexual desire and female sexual arousal disorders. *The Journal of Sexual Medicine*, **7**(4 Pt 1), 1454–1463.

Carvalho, J., and Nobre, P. (2011). Predictors of men's sexual desire: the role of psychological, cognitive-emotional, relational, and medical factors. *Journal of Sex Research*, Feb 25, 1–9. **8**(3), 754–763.

Carvalho, J., and Nobre, P. (2010b). Sexual desire in women: an integrative approach regarding psychological, medical, and relationship dimensions. *Journal of Sexual Medicine*, **7**(5), 1807–1815.

Chivers, M. L., Seto, M. C., Lalumière, M. L., Laan, E., and Grimbos, T. (2010). Agreement of self-reported and genital measures of sexual arousal in men and women: a meta-analysis. *Archives of Sexual Behavior*, **39**(1), 5–56.

de Jong, D. C. (2009). The role of attention in sexual arousal: implications for treatment of sexual dysfunction. *Journal of Sex Research*, **46**(2–3), 237–248

de Jong, P. J., van Lankveld, J., Elgersma, H. J., and Borg, C. (2010). Disgust and sexual problems – theoretical conceptualization and case illustrations. *International Journal of Cognitive Therapy*, **3**(1), 23–39.

Eloi-Stiven, M. L., Channaveeraiah, N., Christos, P. J., Finkel, M., and Reddy, R. (2007). Does marijuana use play a role in the recreational use of sildenafil? *The Journal of Family Practice*, **56**(11), E1–4.

Fisher, D. G., Reynolds, G. L., and Napper, L. E. (2010). Use of crystal methamphetamine, Viagra, and sexual behavior. *Current Opinion in Infectious Diseases*, **23**(1), 53–56.

Gentilcore-Saulnier, E., McLean, L., Goldfinger, C., Pukall, C. F., and Chamberlain, S. (2010). Pelvic floor muscle assessment outcomes in women with and without provoked vestibulodynia and the impact of a physical therapy program. *The Journal of Sexual Medicine*, **7**, 1003–1022.

Hatzimouratidis, K., Amar, E., Eardley, I., *et al.* (2010). Guidelines on male sexual dysfunction: erectile dysfunction and premature ejaculation. *European Urology*, **57**(5), 804–814.

Heidelbaugh, J. J. (2010). Management of erectile dysfunction. *American Family Physician*, **81**(3), 305–312.

Hinchliff, S., Gott, M., and Galena, E. (2005). 'I daresay I might find it embarrassing': general practitioners' perspectives on discussing sexual health issues with lesbian and gay patients. *Health and Social Care in the Community*, (**4**), 345–353.

Holt, T. J., Blevins, K. R., and Burkert, N. (2010). Considering the pedophile subculture online. *Sex Abuse*, **22**(1), 3–24.

Johannes, C. B., Clayton, A. H., Odom, D. M., *et al.* (2009). Distressing sexual problems in United States women revisited: prevalence after accounting for depression. *Journal of Clinical Psychiatry*, **70**(12), 1698–1706.

Kafka, M. P. (2010). Hypersexual disorder: a proposed diagnosis for DSM-V. *Archives of Sexual Behavior*, **39**(2), 377–400.

Koskimäki, J., Shiri, R., Tammela, T., *et al.* (2008). Regular intercourse protects against erectile dysfunction: Tampere Aging Male Urologic Study. *American Journal of Medicine*, **121**(7), 592–596.

Krapf, J. M., and Simon, J. A. (2009). The role of testosterone in the management of hypoactive sexual desire disorder in postmenopausal women. *Maturitas*, **63**(3), 213–219.

Kraus, S. W., and Russell, B. (2008). Early sexual experiences: the role of Internet access and sexually explicit material. *Cyberpsychology Behavior*, **11**(2),162–168.

Laan, E., van Driel, E. M., and van Lunsen, R. H. W. (2008). Genital responsiveness in healthy women with and without sexual arousal disorder. *The Journal of Sexual Medicine*, 5, 1424–1435.

Landau, J., Garrett, J., and Webb, R. (2008). Assisting a concerned person to motivate someone experiencing cybersex into treatment: application of invitational intervention: the arise model to cybersex. *The Journal of Marital and Family Therapy*, **34** (4), 498–511.

Leiblum, S. R., and Nathan, S. (2001). Persistent sexual arousal syndrome: a newly discovered pattern of female sexuality. *The Journal of Sex and Marital Therapy*, **27**(4), 365–380.

Levine, S. B. (2010). What is sexual addiction? *The Journal of Sex and Marital Therapy*, **36** (3), 261–275.

Lindau, S. T., and Gavrilova, N. (2010). Sex, health, and years of sexually active life gained due to good health: evidence from two US population based cross sectional surveys of ageing. *BMJ*, **340**, c810.

Linton, K. D., and Wylie, K. R. (2010). Recent advances in the treatment of premature ejaculation. *Drug Design Development and Therapy*, **18**(4), 1–6.

Luders, E., Sánchez, F. J., Gaser, C., *et al.* (2009). Regional gray matter variation in male-to-female transsexualism. *NeuroImage*, **46**(4), 904–907.

Lue, T. F., and Broderick, G. A. (2007). Evaluation and management of erectile dysfunction and premature ejaculation. Chapter 22 in Wein, A. J. (ed.), *Campbell-Walsh Urology*, 9th edn. Philadelphia, PA: Saunders Elsevier.

MacNeil, S. and Byers, E. S. (2009). Role of sexual self-disclosure in the sexual satisfaction of long-term heterosexual couples. *Journal of Sex Research*, **46**(1), 3–14.

Maniglio, R. (2009). The impact of child sexual abuse on health: a systematic review of reviews. *Clinical Psychology Review*, **29**(7), 647–657.

Masters, W. H., and Johnson, V. E. (1966). *Human Sexual Response.* Boston: Little Brown.

Meston, C. M., Hull, E., Levin, R. J., and Sipski M. (2004). Disorders of orgasm in women. *The Journal of Sexual Medicine*, **1**(1), 66–68.

Meston, C., and Trapnell, P. (2005). Development and validation of a five-factor sexual satisfaction and distress scale for women: the Sexual Satisfaction Scale for Women (SSS-W) *The Journal of Sexual Medicine*, **2**(1), 66–81.

Meston, C. M., Hamilton, L. D., and Harte, C. B. (2009). Sexual motivation in women as a function of age. *The Journal of Sexual Medicine*, **6**(12), 3305–3319.

Nobre, P. J., and Pinto-Gouveia, J. (2006). Dysfunctional sexual beliefs as vulnerability factors to sexual dysfunction. *Journal of Sex Research*, **43**(1), 68–75.

Paul, J. P., Pollack, L., Osmond, D., and Catania, J. A. (2005). Viagra (sildenafil) use in a population-based sample of U.S. men who have sex with men. *Sexually Transmitted Diseases*, **32**(9), 531–533.

Perelman, M. A., and Rowland, D. L. (2006). Retarded ejaculation. *World Journal of Urology*, **24**(6), 645–652.

Recupero, P. R. (2008). Forensic evaluation of problematic Internet use. *The Journal of the American Academy of Psychiatry and the Law*, **36**(4), 505–514.

Riley, A., and May, K. (2001). Sexual desire disorders. Ch. 63 in Gabbard, G. O. (Ed.), *Gabbard's Treatments of Psychiatric Disorders*, 3rd edn. Washington DC: American Psychiatric Publishing.

Rivalta, M., Sighinolfi, M. C., Micali, S., De Stefani, S., and Bianchi, G. (2010). Sexual function and quality of life in women with urinary incontinence treated by a complete pelvic floor rehabilitation program (biofeedback, functional electrical stimulation, pelvic floor muscles exercises, and vaginal cones). *The Journal of Sexual Medicine*, **7**(3), 1200–1208.

Rosen, R., Riley, A., Wagner, G., *et al.* (1997). The International Index of Erectile Function (IIEF): a multidimensional scale for assessment of erectile dysfunction. *Urology*, **49**, 822–830.

Rösing, D., Klebingat, K. J., Berberich, H. J., *et al.* (2009). Male sexual dysfunction: diagnosis and treatment from a sexological and interdisciplinary perspective. *Deutsches Ärzteblatt International*, **106**(50), 821–828.

Rowland, D., McMahon, C. G., Abdo, C., *et al.* (2010). Disorders of orgasm and ejaculation in men. *The Journal of Sexual Medicine*, **7** (4 Pt 2), 1668–1686.

Segraves, R. T. (2010). Considerations for a better definition of male orgasmic disorder in DSM V. *The Journal of Sexual Medicine*, **7** (2 Pt 1), 690–695.

Serati, M., Salvatore, S., Uccella, S., *et al.* (2009). Sexual function after radical hysterectomy for early-stage cervical cancer: is there a difference between laparoscopy and laparotomy? *The Journal of Sexual Medicine*, **6**, 2516–2522.

Shafer, L. C. (2008). Sexual disorders and sexual dysfunction. Chapter 36 in Stern, T. A., Rosenbaum, J. F., Fava, M., Biederman, J., and Rauch, S. L. (eds.), *Massachusetts General Hospital Comprehensive Clinical Psychiatry*, 1st edn. Philadelphia, PA: Mosby Elsevier.

Sohn, M., and Bosinski, H. A. (2007). Gender identity disorders: diagnostic and surgical aspects. *The Journal of Sexual Medicine*, **4**(5), 1193–1207.

Thorne, C., and Stuckey, B. (2008). Pelvic congestion syndrome presenting as persistent genital arousal: a case report. *The Journal of Sexual Medicine*, **5**, 504–508.

Twohig, M. P., and Crosby, J. M. (2010). Acceptance and commitment therapy as a treatment for problematic internet pornography viewing. *Behavior Therapy*, **41** (3), 285–295.

Wallien, M. S., Swaab, H., and Cohen-Kettenis, P. T. (2007). Psychiatric comorbidity among children with gender identity disorder. *Journal of the American Academy of Child and Adolescent Psychiatry*, **46**(10), 1307–1314.

Waxman, S. E., and Pukall, C. F. (2009). Laser Doppler imaging of genital blood flow: a direct measure of female sexual arousal. *The Journal of Sexual Medicine*, **6**, 2278–2285.

Weiss, P., and Brody, S. (2009). Female sexual arousal disorder with and without a distress criterion: prevalence and correlates in a representative Czech sample. *The Journal of Sexual Medicine*, **6**, 3385–3394.

Wincze, J. P., Bach, A. K., and Barlow, D. H. (2008). Sexual dysfunction. Chapter 11 in Barlow, D. H. (ed), *Clinical Handbook of Psychological Disorders*, 4th edn. New York: Guilford Press.

Recommended websites

The following are websites that couples can be guided to.

The online medical library at www.merck.com is an excellent reference source on issues of sexual dysfunctions. There are separate sections covering men's and women's health issues that have detailed explanations on sexual health problems.

www.men.webmd.com/guide/sex-fact-fiction–a good website for men to explore aspects of sexual difficulties.

www.sexuality.about.com–a general website that is useful to both sexes.

A very good 'sex and relationships' website address that has guided instructions on sensate focus exercises is available at: www.sex-and-relationships.com/pages/LH/sensate-f.html.

Recommended DVDs for individuals and couples

Produced in association with 'Relate', some individuals and couples may benefit from **'The Lovers' Guide'** series of DVDs, especially if they are unlikely to spend time looking through a self-help book because of time restrictions or literacy problems. Most of the DVDs have a specific focus on relationship building and can serve as a very informative educational resource on sexual matters. The DVDs are reasonably priced and are available from many DVD shops or can be purchased online at www.amazon.co.uk.

It is important to bear in mind these DVDs are very explicit and it is best to ascertain in advance of any recommendation the individual's or couple's personal, cultural or religious sensitivities to watching nudity and sexual behaviour in this format.

Recommended books for couples

The Good Vibrations Guide to Sex by Cathy Winks, Anne Semans and Phoebe Gloeckner; published by Cleis Press; 3rd revised edition (2002). This is considered to be a fairly substantial book that can be recommended to any couple containing useful reading on basics regarding sexual anatomy, communication, masturbation, sexual fantasies.

Relate Guide to Sex in Loving Relationships (Relate series) by Sarah Litvinoff; published by Vermilion (2001). The benefits of this book are that it contains quizzes and specific talking points for couples who may have difficulties communicating about sex and gives pointers to very practical tasks that will help to revive a couple's sex life.

The Sex-starved Marriage: A Couple's Guide to Boosting Their Marriage Libido by Michele Weiner Davis; published by Simon & Schuster Ltd (2004). A useful book for couples who may have been avoiding dealing with the painful issue of sexual problems in their lives, addressing especially factors such as communication problems, poor body image and depression. Gives worthwhile discussion points and practical advice to the couple.

Sexy Mamas: Keeping Your Sex Life Alive While Raising Kids by Cathy Winks and Anne Semans; Inner Ocean Publishing Inc; 2nd revised edition (2004) is a book that many couples with children may find encouraging and practical.

Chapter 19

Care for people with enduring and complex common mental health problems

Learning objectives

Defining the problem using the three Ds model
Epidemiology of complex mental health problems
Developing individualized care
Developing collaborative care, assertive follow-up and mental health promotion

The literature on primary care mental health has tended to focus on those with common mental health problems and to a lesser extent on those with psychosis, including bipolar disorder. This leads to the impression that most common mental health problems are new-onset, whereas as many as 60% are recurrent (Vuorilehto *et al.* 2005) and many are enduring. Depression and other problems are beginning to be seen as long-term, chronic diseases (Andrews 2001) and, although this is not always the case, systems of individual and organizational care need to take this into account. Within an individual practice there are many more people with disability resulting from long-term non-psychotic illnesses than there are those with psychosis. The burden is as a result of considerable comorbidity (Andrews *et al.* 1998) involving drug and alcohol problems and personality disorder as well as non-adherence to recommended treatment. The effects are profound on the individual, but also are significant when considering family members, particularly children, and the economy as a whole. This chapter will outline different ways of defining this complex group, consider deficits in care and propose ways in which individual care and the organization of care can be enhanced.

Defining the population

Ongoing mental illness is associated with social disadvantage, either as an aetiological factor or as a result of the mental health problem (Rogers and Pilgrim 2003). Only 26% of those disabled due to depression and other long-term neurotic conditions are in work, compared with a mean of 50% for all causes of disability (ONS 2005).

The three Ds is a useful way of defining the population with severe and long-term mental health problems for primary and community care (Slade *et al.* 1997). This requires a *diagnosis* of some kind, a *duration* of 2 or more years and ongoing *disability*, as defined in Table 19.1. It clearly moves the focus from the psychosis/common mental health problem dichotomy, and introduces duration and social functioning as a means of defining the problem. This opens up possibilities for outcome-based care with improvement in disability and social functioning and social inclusion as desired end-points.

Table 19.1. Three Ds model: inclusion criteria for long-term mental illness

Patients having:
Either:
One of the *psychoses*, including schizophrenia, paranoid psychosis, manic-depressive psychosis and psychotic depression (excluding those with no medication and no episode/care needs for 3 years)
Or:
One of the *chronic non-psychotic* disorders with a substantial *disability and a duration of 2 years or more*; for example: recurrent or continuing major depression, severe anxiety, panic and phobic disorders, obsessive-compulsive disorder and post-traumatic stress disorder
Duration: patient's disability must have been present for 2 years or more, including frequent recurrences or stable problems requiring ongoing medication or support)
Disability may be defined as being unable to fulfil any one of the following: • being able to hold down a job • maintaining self-care and personal hygiene • performing necessary domestic chores • participating in recreational activities
The disability must be due to any one or more of four types of impairment of social behaviour: • withdrawal and inactivity • avoidance behaviour • bizarre or embarrassing behaviour • violence towards others or self

In primary care long-term mental health problems are most likely to be due to depressive illness. People with long-term depression (LTD) lie along spectra of severity and recurrence. The spectra include those with recurrent brief episodes of moderate depression, through to those with severe and enduring depression and associated disability (Andrews 2001). Indeed the majority of those diagnosed with depression have a history of recurrent depression. There are a wide range of comorbidities associated with LTD, including chronic physical conditions, diagnoses such as general anxiety disorder, panic and post-traumatic stress disorder (PTSD), personality disorders and drug and alcohol problems. Only 12% of those with LTD have no comorbidity (Vuorilehto *et al.* 2005) and this adds further to the complexity of managing this condition. Although less common, those with ongoing problems such as chronic anxiety and other conditions such as PTSD, obsessive/compulsive disorder (OCD) and panic disorder may also be included in the three Ds definition (Slade *et al.* 1997).

Similarly those with chronic substance misuse problems often have recurrent or chronic depression and/or personality disorder, as do those with eating disorders. Many of these people can also be classified as having personality disorders, and many with significant personality disorders also have depressive symptoms or other diagnoses, although a significant proportion of those with borderline and histrionic personality disorders do not meet the criteria for depression illness. So in primary care depressive symptoms are part of many psychiatric conditions leading to chronic dysfunction and disability.

Socially excluded populations such as offenders, the homeless, the unemployed and asylum seekers have a particularly high proportion of people with long-term non-psychotic mental illness. 'Social' interventions and individualized treatment outcomes based on achievements towards social inclusion are therefore important.

Epidemiology

Prevalence of severe and enduring non-psychotic conditions varied from 1.3 to 8.3/1000 in recent studies (Kai *et al.* 2000; Kendrick *et al.* 1994). Long-term antidepressant prescribing is an additional and convenient marker in primary care; in one practice 36 per 1000 of the population were on long-term psychotropic medication, predominantly anxiolytics and antidepressants, and these patients were markedly more distressed than controls (Catalan *et al.* 1988). There are no recent UK studies examining prevalence and need, although we know that while anxiolytic prescription has dropped antidepressant prescribing has continued to rise. In the USA 75% of primary-care-treated patients with LTD reported persistent depression (Schwenk *et al.* 2004). So, while not all on long-term antidepressants would reach criteria for LTD, all would have care needs: those in remission from recurrence will merit preventive management; some will need support in overcoming fears to come off antidepressants; others will be in partial remission or an ongoing episode and will need assertive management to address depression and other physical and mental health conditions.

Improving care

Several components of care are necessary for managing chronic disease (Wagner *et al.* 1996). These include patient involvement (including self-help), collaboration with specialist services, an appropriate review function and service redesign to incorporate these features. Reviewing care in particular is associated with better outcomes for depression (Von Korff and Goldberg 2001). Medication combined with psychosocial modalities has been shown to improve outcomes (Arnow and Constantino 2003). Currently, primary care, with its mainly reactive response, and secondary care, with its emphasis on psychosis, are not fulfilling the needs of those with chronic and relapsing depression and other ongoing non-psychotic conditions. The use of recovery-based models, relapse recognition, self-help groups and facilitated self-help and new models for organizing care all require evaluation.

Individualized care

The lynchpin for this provision will often be the primary care practitioner, commonly a general practitioner, but perhaps an experienced nurse, and, in the future, we might see specialist mental health workers taking a lead. Having a named primary care worker addresses a major issue for many patients: i.e. continuity. This practitioner can then juggle, organize and coordinate various modalities, including the medical, the psychological and the social. These modalities will need to be introduced within an overall framework which is safe, involves an exchange of views, fully engages the individual concerned and offers choice and involvement in decision-making at all levels.

The medical perspective

The medical perspective is important in terms of managing an analysis of the problem with respect to diagnosis, assessing risk and providing medical treatments. Many people with long-term mental health problems feel stigmatized and may find it difficult to engage with practitioners in primary care. They may not recognize that they have mental health problems, being more concerned about ongoing comorbid physical health issues.

A trusting relationship between the doctor and patient is essential in order to address ongoing social problems. This should also involve an explicit discussion about psychological distress and, if possible, about diagnosis. Practitioners need to ensure that a range of specific psychiatric diagnoses are not missed, but care should be 'diagnosis-sensitive' rather than fixed according to diagnostic group. For example, those with long-term depression will need to have specific screening questions asked to ensure that they do not also have disorders that are obscured by depressive symptoms such as obsessive-compulsive disorder, post-traumatic stress disorder, generalized anxiety and panic, eating disorders or addictions. Bipolar affective disorder and other psychoses should also be excluded. Screening questions for personality problems are less well developed within the primary care setting but include enquiry about difficulties forming or maintaining close relationships, highly changeable mood, persistent self-hatred and episodes of self-harm such as overdosing or cutting. The aim of these questions is to identify specific problems or issues which may be amenable to particular medications or psychological treatment strategies as a part of the overall plan.

Medication is likely to continue to play a considerable role in the management of people with these long-term problems. Occasionally, in times of great distress benzodiazepines and other hypnotics or anxiolytics may be useful. While these have been shown to have effectiveness in the short term, their addictive potential may outweigh the benefits of introduction even for short-term treatment. They may also result in a sense of disempowerment and belief that only these particular medications will improve well-being.

Antidepressants will often have been used for those with chronic and recurrent depression as well as for those with diagnoses such as OCD, PTSD and chronic anxiety.

A number of important scenarios need to be considered for those with long-term mood disorders and the reader is referred to Chapter 7.

Chronic depression or failure to respond to antidepressants

In this situation it is worth trying further courses of a different antidepressant; switching after 6 weeks of each is reasonable practice. Increasing dosage is also possible with some medications. There are detailed protocols available for switching between antidepressants. Continued treatment failure suggests the need for lithium augmentation, combined treatments and other options requiring specialist support.

Partial recovery

This scenario is one of the most difficult for patients and practitioners to deal with. It is often unclear as to whether the antidepressant is working at all, or preventing decline into further, more severe depression. Decisions need to be made in the shared knowledge of this uncertainty and might include continuing, switching or increasing the dose.

Recovery

Standard treatment suggests that antidepressants should be continued for 6 months. A history of recurrence of three or more episodes raises the possibility of continuing treatment for 2 years or even for life in order to prevent further recurrences. This will not always be effective and many people find the idea unpalatable. Again, clear, explicit discussion about the risks and benefits is required with the practitioner supporting the decision of the individual patient, but revisiting this decision in future years. Recovery is a good point at which to consider several clinical matters relating to future progress. These include:

- strategies to prevent future recurrence
- documenting relapse signatures
- developing acute intervention/crisis plans.

Relapse and recurrence

Relapse is defined as symptom deterioration after a response to treatment but before full remission has occurred. Recurrence is defined as a new episode after remission. Both are disappointing for the patient, especially when the time period between treatment response/ remission and relapse/recurrence is short.

SSRIs such as citalopram and fluoxetine are now favoured as first-line treatment over tricyclic medications; although those who have responded well in the past to tricyclics or to another group may be re-started on the medication to which they responded initially.

Many will already be on maintenance antidepressants and difficult choices about switching medication, increasing dose or adding further antidepressants will have to be made, perhaps in conjunction with a psychiatrist.

Although not generally advocated, a pragmatic compromise for those who relapse during attempts to discontinue medication is to allow patients to restart or increase the dose of medication if they feel themselves slipping into a further episode of depression. Except for those who have considerable experience, this should normally be done in consultation with the prescriber, even if this is conducted over the telephone. For many patients additional social psychological strategies will be needed at this time. And accompanying a deterioration of mood there are likely to be recurrences of symptoms related to comorbid diagnosis and/or re-emergence of substance misuse.

Psychological treatment

Many people, both patients and practitioners, will want to know more about a range of other treatment options. Knowledge and understanding of these treatment modalities is restricted by lack of availability. Psychological therapy for this group of patients may be appropriate at the time of greatest distress during relapse or recurrence, but also may be relevant during periods of recovery as a buffer against further relapses. For example, cognitive behavioural therapy has now been shown to be as effective as antidepressants and additive to medication in the prevention of further episodes of depression for those with recurrence. A range of other psychological treatments, outlined more fully in Chapter 16, may well be relevant as part of a recovery and relapse prevention. The general practitioner's role will often be to discuss the possibility of various modalities, including whether it is one-to-one approach or group work, whether it is a short-term or long-term treatment package, or whether it involves interfacing with a computer or book, rather than a therapist. This discussion and triage function is important and if the generalist practitioner has insufficient knowledge then it may well be carried out by a specialist mental health practitioner based in primary care.

It is also important not to underestimate the psychological role of the generic practitioner. Some GPs and other PHCT (primary health care team) members will have undergone training to do more in-depth counselling or therapy within consultations. However, every practitioner has a role in listening, providing empathy and validating a patient's narrative (Launer 2002) and 'good medical care' includes basic psychological approaches within the consultation.

Intervening socially and promoting mental health

Mental health promotion is an important means of keeping people well. It is important for those with long-term mental health problems. Exercise has now been shown to be effective for those with depression. Advice and encouragement towards a more healthy lifestyle requires an understanding of the individual's preferences and social situation and a discussion about the balance between work and leisure, sleep, rest and activity, relaxation and stimulation and interaction with others, alongside time to reflect alone. Individuals may well have learnt what is best for them but might benefit from a structured discussion of the options.

An understanding of the individual's social context both contributes to defining the level of illness and also points the way towards recovery. This might include assessment of their work situation, their leisure activities, their housing, the number of social contacts they have, their family situation, their interest in exercise and sport and their involvement in religious or spiritual activities. People with long-standing mental health problems often participate less in these areas. Possibly the most critical of these is employment, which so defines our status. In some inner-city areas unemployment is not always a stigma but for most people lack of work or lack of engagement in productive or creative activity is a continuing source of demoralization. Whilst some people are genuinely caught in benefit traps and are unable to move easily into paid employment, most will be able to identify creative or learning experiences which they have enjoyed or would like to engage in. Practitioners can help facilitate involvement in opportunities within their locality.

Others are too unwell to return to work and many require support in obtaining benefits. Volunteering opportunities are also on offer and in a small way this can be both a step towards paid employment and a useful activity in itself. Limited hours of volunteering are allowable under the benefits system. It is likely that the Pathways to Work Initiative, available to all claiming incapacity benefits and the Employment and Support Allowance in Britain, will encourage volunteering as one of the paths back to paid employment. Currently, unfortunately, there are few organizations which combine advice on benefits, volunteering and employment. Time Banks are a particular form of volunteering where individuals join an organization and swap resources and favours. For example in south east London a Time Bank based in a practice was able to provide opportunities for individuals with a variety of mental health problems to gain confidence and feel empowered through doing rather than receiving (Byng and Smith 2001).

Continuity and integrated care

This range of possibilities for people with long-term mental health problems is the basis for ongoing commitment by primary care practitioners to support people with mental health problems in times of crisis and recovery. Each consultation requires empathy, real listening and shared decision-making about the next steps. The use of solution-focused approaches within consultations, building on positive achievements in times of recovery and what the individual is doing to help themselves in times of crisis can empower individuals by emphasizing strengths. This will help counter negative feelings about psychological dependence arising from the sole use of medications.

The 'inclusion web' is a useful tool which practitioners can use to identify and reflect on domains of life in terms of places frequented and contact with people. It can be used over a series of consultations to map out an individual's life and identify areas in which they would like to be more involved (Hacking and Bates 2008). This has an obvious role in those with long-term mental illness as it focuses on social support and social inclusion and can assist in guiding the patient in respect of these areas.

Continuity of care is crucial in managing those with long-term mental health problems. There are two aspects to this. Continuity may include ongoing contact with a named practitioner (longitudinal continuity) but it might be even more important for individuals to feel they are listened to and can trust practitioners (relational continuity). Holistic continuity involves making links between the medical processes of diagnosis and medication, and the wider social and psychological context. Continuity of information requires high-quality team-based records and transfer of appropriate information to others involved in the care of the patient. This can be challenging, especially as primary care teams are growing. Continuity can also be difficult when multidisciplinary input is required and for those such as offenders and the homeless who often move at short notice.

Developing systems for treatment and recovery

In the literature on collaborative care for depression coming from the United States, a system for regularly reviewing and monitoring the patient alongside specialist input has the best evidence base for improving outcomes (Von Korff and Goldberg 2001). Within the primary health care team there may be adjustments to roles and procedures and those involved with an individual patient must be fully au fait with the person's needs. This will require the development of comprehensive information systems.

Specialist input has been shown to improve outcomes and there are a number of ways in which this may occur; redesigning the organization of care and, in particular, systems to review care will be critical in improving primary-care-based services. Thus a designated case manager may be identified to regularly assess the person's symptoms, adherence to treatment, level of social activity and support systems while collaborating with the specialist community mental health teams as required.

'Collaborative care', developed out of the chronic disease model applied to depression, has now been recommended by NICE for people with comorbid depression and long-term physical conditions. It includes:

- patient-defined problems (as well as diagnosis)
- goals related to these problems
- self-management training to support achieving these goals
- assertive follow-up.

Involving individuals and providing information

Providing information and involving individuals in their own care are two facets identified as being crucial for chronic disease management (Wagner *et al.* 1996). When these are applied to people with long-term mental health problems a number of opportunities might be considered. These range from those focused on providing information to the patient to setting up systems for shared decision-making by doctor and patient and user-led care and will be examined in more detail.

Information is crucial to decision-making and the following systems are likely to be required within primary care settings:

- a full set of leaflets about a variety of conditions and treatments
- an up-to-date searchable website available to practitioners and users, detailing all of the local opportunities for care provision, across health, social care, and the voluntary sector
- a website with detailed information at a national level about conditions and treatments with links to other websites
- a full range of books and details of opportunities at local libraries and other public venues
- information about ways in which people can be involved in their own care and in developing systems of care (e.g. WRAP, inclusion web and patients as teachers, support organizations).

An important range of initiatives for which there is currently growing support is that of patient-led recovery tools. One particular example is the Wellness Recovery Action Plan (WRAP) (Copeland 2005). This is a system of care designed by users to identify ways to help themselves towards recovery and inclusion in social activities; it also details plans for dealing with relapses and crisis.

Some patients will move from becoming experts in their own care to taking wider roles:

- teaching students and professionals
- helping evaluate and plan services
- providing advocacy and signposting
- running patient support groups.

Assertive follow-up

Primary care in the UK is based mainly on reactive care and although the 1991 and 2004 contract revisions have 'incentivized' the use of systems of care for chronic disease management, these have been largely confined to physical conditions, and the small incentives for reviewing mental health care are now restricted to those with psychosis and bipolar affective disorder. The 2009 Quality and Outcomes Framework (QOF) now requires a review of depression symptom status for those recently diagnosed with a new episode of depression.

There is ongoing debate about whether the QOF should be extended to include an annual review for those with non-psychotic conditions. Such a review would need to include an assessment of patients' needs in terms of diagnosis, social inclusion, medication and the range of psychosocial interventions which may be appropriate. However, with the imperative to move towards a more user-centred care, there is a tension between the 'register and recall' system and ensuring that patients take responsibility for their ongoing management.

A minimum service might ensure that those flagged as having a long-term, disabling mental health condition should be called for a review once a year at a minimum. For those who are being followed up regularly this may involve just ensuring that areas not covered during the year are addressed; whilst for those who have not been seeking care during the year, it would provide an opportunity to systematically address a range of psychological, medication and social issues. For some people this might be carried out by the general practitioner or named primary care worker, whilst in some practices and for some patients it might be more appropriate for linked mental health workers to review psychosocial needs in more detail but in primary care.

Telephone recall has also been used to ensure that those with mental health problems adhere to treatment and maintain contact with services. It has been found to be particularly popular with patients and effective at improving outcomes in the treatment of acute episodes of common mental health problems and as part of a collaborative care arrangement for those with recurrent depression. This might be run by receptionists or counsellors, given additional training, but could also involve practice nurses or, indeed, GPs making calls.

Whatever the system chosen, there needs to be a named person responsible for contacting those who are not attending, and ensuring that no person is missed from the system. General practices have been particularly effective at ensuring that this process occurs for those patients whose follow-up is rewarded in the Quality and Outcomes Framework, and are in a position to offer a similar service for those with long-term depression and other conditions.

Summary

- The most common long-term emotional problem seen in general practice is 'depression'.

- A systematic approach to management in primary care is a vital ingredient.

- This involves engaging with the problems as defined by the patient, identifying the goals to achieving resolution, assisting in self-management to achieving these goals and assertive follow-up.

References

Andrews, G. (2001). Should depression be managed as a chronic disease? *BMJ*, **322** (7283), 419–421.

Andrews, G., Sanderson, K., and Beard, J. (1998). Burden of disease. Methods of calculating disability from mental disorder, *British Journal of Psychiatry*, **173**, 123–131.

Arnow, B. A., and Constantino, M. J. (2003). Effectiveness of psychotherapy and combination treatment for chronic depression. *Journal of Clinical Psychology*, **59**(8), 893–905.

Byng, R., and Smith K. (2001). Postcards from the 21st century: time heals! Using time as a currency. *British Journal of General Practice*, Nov, 950–951.

Catalan, J., Gath, D., Bond, A., *et al.* (1988). General practice patients on long-term psychotropic drugs. A controlled investigation. *The British Journal of Psychiatry*, **152**, 399–405.

Copeland, M. E. (2005). *Wellness Recovery Action Plan: A System for Monitoring, Reducing and Eliminating Uncomfortable or Dangerous Physical Symptoms*. Liverpool: Sefton Recovery Group.

Kai, J., Crosland, A., and Drinkwater, C. (2000). Prevalence of enduring and disabling mental illness in the inner city. *British Journal of General Practice*, **50**(461), 992–994.

Kendrick, T., Burns, T., Freeling, P., and Sibbald, B. (1994). Provision of care to general practice patients with disabling long-term mental illness: a survey in 16 practices. *British Journal of General Practice*, **44**(384), 301–305.

Launer, J. (2002). *Narrative-based Primary Care. A Practical Guide*. Oxford: Radcliffe Medical Press.

ONS. (2005). *Labour Force Survey*. London: ONS.

Rogers, A., and Pilgrim, D. (2003). *Mental Health and Inequality*. Basingstoke: Palgrave Macmillan.

Schwenk, T. L., Evans, D. L., Laden, S. K., and Lewis, L. (2004). Treatment outcome and physician-patient communication in primary care patients with chronic, recurrent depression. *American Journal of Psychiatry*, **161**(10), 1892–1901.

Slade, M., Powell, R., and Strathdee, G. (1997). Current approaches to identifying the severely mentally ill. *Social Psychiatry and Psychiatric Epidemiology*, **32**(4), 177–184.

Von Korff, M., and Goldberg, D. (2001), Improving outcomes in depression. *British Medical Journal*, **323**(7319), 948–949.

Vuorilehto, M., Melartin, T., and Isometsa, E. (2005). Depressive disorders in primary care: recurrent, chronic, and co-morbid. *Psychological Medicine*, **35**(5), 673–682.

Wagner, E. H., Austin, B. T., and Von Korff, M. (1996). Improving outcomes in chronic illness. *Managed Care Quarterly*, **4**(2), 12–25.

Chapter 20

Primary health care team and mental health care

Learning objectives

The magnitude of mental health problems in primary care issues
The role of the primary care team
Training needs of primary care physicians
The composition of primary care mental health teams
New models of primary care teams contributing to mental health

Primary care mental health is often characterized as the realm of common mental health problems. It lies at three critical interfaces:

- between the public and medical worlds
- between primary care and specialists
- between physical and mental health care.

Problems presenting a challenge to those who attend primary care services range in their severity, complexity, comorbidity and chronicity, and across the lifespan of patients. Most of the developments described below apply only in Britain. In other jurisdictions where different mental health care systems operate, similar developments have not been seen.

In Britain, a new policy, New Ways of Working for Primary Care Mental Health (Department of Health 2007), proposed that the workforce needs the skills, knowledge, attitudes and competencies to respond to the following range of clinical presentations:

(1) People with common mental health problems, consisting of short-lived distress related to life situation, low-grade ongoing mood and anxiety symptoms, through to diagnosable episodes of depression, anxiety or other psychiatric problems.

(2) People with mental health problems associated with physical health, including health anxiety, distress related to recent physical investigation or diagnosis, medically unexplained physical symptoms, and mental health problems resulting from long-term physical health problems.

(3) People with long-standing, complex, non-psychotic mental health problems, such as recurrent depression, chronic anxiety, post-traumatic stress disorder and obsessive compulsive disorder. There is often associated psychiatric and physical comorbidity, recurrent self-harm, substance misuse, homelessness and unemployment. This heterogeneous group has often fallen into the gap between primary care and specialist services.

323

(4) People with psychosis, consisting of new and recurrent episodes, often with ongoing disability, social exclusion and physical illness. They may or may not be looked after by a specialist mental health team. Primary care can be involved in early recognition and in ongoing physical and mental health care.

(5) People with cognitive impairment, including dementia, learning difficulties or developmental and organic disorders. These problems are also associated with physical and mental comorbidity and social exclusion.

The primary health care team

General practitioners are probably still at the fulcrum of primary care provision. As individuals they get to know patients over many years, and become experienced at dealing with undifferentiated, complex and long-term problems, as well as frequently providing immediate, short-term care.

Most GPs see mental health as core to their work but not all have had sufficient training at undergraduate or postgraduate levels. Furthermore there are some GPs who find working with people with mental health problems uncomfortable and, rarely, some who effectively deny their role – either by failing to recognize problems or by referring everybody with mental health problems to the specialist services. Professional bodies, such as the Royal Colleges in Britain, local commissioners and postgraduate deaneries, have a role in coordinating educational opportunities and assessing individual needs to ensure that whole populations, registered with particular practices or GPs, can obtain a minimum standard service.

Perhaps most important is the approach provided by all members of the practice staff, to ensure that people with mental health problems feel welcome and comfortable disclosing their problems without being disempowered.

Primary care teams are generally led in decision-making and in the process of care by GPs while practice nurses, district nurses, health visitors as well as practice-based mental health workers make up the extended primary health care team. Each of the three community-based nursing roles involves dealing with people with long-term mental health problems. District nurses often deal with the housebound elderly, who frequently have some type of mental health problem, often depression and anxiety, and experience bereavements and isolation. Health visitors have contact with young mothers, many of whom may have mental health problems, and also have responsibility for the mental health of children who may be psychologically affected by their parents' illnesses. Practice nurses come into contact with a wide range of the population whom they might screen for mental health problems but, perhaps more importantly, might also identify mental health problems in those with long-term physical health conditions. This role is now rewarded within the Quality and Outcomes Framework and will enhance the role of those working in primary care as promoters of both physical and mental well-being. Despite this contact with mental health problems, the training of these nurses in mental health, unless they have undergone registered mental nurse training, is often extremely limited. There are few requirements for ongoing postgraduate training and the nurses themselves are divided between those who want to take on a more psychosocial role and those who see their role as mainly concerned with physical health. Most nurses have excellent communication skills and are empathetic, but do not see themselves as having mental health care competencies. Education in the form of external training, in-house training, supervision and mentoring will be required as they are asked to formally take on mental health care roles and fit into new systems of review and assessment for those with mental health problems. Once community-based nurses gain experience of mental health problems they are enabled to take a lead role in the management of ongoing mental health care.

Receptionists, as the first point of contact within the primary health care team, are another under-used resource in respect of mental health and well-being. They have very little training in relation to mental health and understanding about how valuable their role could be. An initiative, as part of the Lewisham Depression Programme, involved the training of receptionists (South-east London Clinical Governance Resources Group 2004) in the recognition of mental health problems and understanding when they should consider informing a clinical member of staff about this possibility. It is also important that they work with practice managers to ensure that the job descriptions and team roles of receptionists facilitate this aspect of their work.

Previously counsellors and psychologists attached to practices were independent practitioners or employed by primary care or mental health trusts and occasionally by the general practitioners themselves. The relationship between general practitioners and counsellors, however, appears to be similar across organizations and consists of referral of individual patients, variable feedback from counsellors depending on their views about confidentiality and very little liaison work. Some practices have developed liaison models for counsellors and psychologists on a number of different levels. This liaison could consist of a discussion about individual cases when considering referral or regular reviews at practice meetings to discuss general issues or specific cases. Some practices have developed models where counsellors and psychologists provide consultancy and supervision to general practitioners and practice nurses who are seeing patients on an ongoing basis. As Improving Access to Psychological Therapy (IAPT) (Department of Health 2009b) services develop it is important that these positive advances are not lost.

The role of practice counsellors for care of people with longer-term serious mental illness is also debated. Some counsellors prefer not to become involved in supporting those with more severe disability and depression. However, some GPs' experience is that these rules, based on diagnosis, tend to be unhelpful and that it is more useful to examine the emotional, psychological and counselling support needs of the individual rather than their past psychiatric history when deciding whether a referral is appropriate. For example, someone with a long history of obsessive-compulsive disorder and depression may well benefit from a period of counselling to address an issue which is related but not central to these diagnoses. On the other hand some commissioners argue that the psychological needs of those with long-term mental illness should be provided for by the specialist teams. Many counsellors have been integrated into IAPT teams.

'Graduate mental health workers' were a new element of the primary care workforce in Britain over the past decade and primarily worked with those with mild to moderate conditions. They were often trained to provide psychological treatment in brief form and to link this to psychosocial interventions. Their lack of experience led to their roles being restricted to dealing mainly with those with new episodes and simple conditions. However, in some areas they have been specifically asked to provide reviews for those with more chronic conditions and apply similar approaches in making these assessments to those they employ with clients referred for time-limited common mental health problems. The graduate mental health worker role has now generally been merged with low-intensity (Psychological Wellbeing Practitioner) workers in the Improving Access to Psychological Therapies (IAPT) teams.

Table 20.1. Options for managing mental health problems which may be available in primary care

Direct access
Psychological approaches employed by generalist practitioners (watchful waiting)
Signposting advice about exercise and local opportunities
Volunteering, as a way of gaining confidence and a path back to employment
Local community groups with a role in promoting well-being: social groups, self-help groups, education and arts
Large group psycho-education courses are particularly useful for those who do not want to disclose their problems to others
Computerized CBT for those less comfortable with human contact
Bibliotherapy for those who prefer reading. There are now books available for those with poor literacy (libraries are increasingly stocking recommended books)
Referral from primary care clinicians and others
Facilitated self-help (signposting by specialists, eCBT or bibliotherapy)
Counselling
CBT
Solution-focused therapy, interpersonal therapy, couple therapy

In some areas the role of these new workers is being designed as an intermediate position between the community mental health team and counsellors. Their role will include reviewing those discharged from community mental health teams, but also assessing those with chronic problems referred from GPs whom the community mental health teams would not accept, based on the referral criteria.

Choice for general practitioners

With these developments in the availability and accessibility of therapists choice is now becoming a reality in mental health management in primary care. The service options available now for the treatment of the range of mental health problems enables patients to self-refer to therapists as well as following the more traditional routes. The options now available are listed in Table 20.1.

Specialist input is one of the pillars of severe and/or long-term illness management, and referral on to secondary care has been seen as an important function of the primary care consultation. Onward referral to outpatient psychiatry has largely been replaced by an array of mechanisms for achieving specialist support which include: referral on to assessment by community mental health teams; email or telephone consultation; consultation-liaison; primary-care-based counsellors and therapists; practice-based CPNs, OTs and social workers; and link workers. These models have often been developed by enthusiasts on both sides, but with the renewed emphasis on care closer to home, incentives may be in place to develop them further. The clinical functions of such specialist involvement include:

- assessing and sharing risk in crisis situations
- triage and onward referral
- sharing ongoing care
- consultation and advice about ongoing care or referral
- providing brief therapeutic input or facilitated self-help
- facilitation of discharge from intensive specialist input.

Common and new mental health roles for professionals in primary care

This section summarizes the differences between the traditional and the newly emerging roles for the different professional groups. These were developed by the New Ways of Working primary care group (Department of Health 2007).

GPs

Common roles

- Usually acting as the first point of contact for people accessing primary care
- Recognizing and engaging with patients who have mental health problems
- Treating with medication and referring for counselling or secondary care
- Providing ongoing support for people with common mental health problems
- Providing reactive physical care for people with mental health problems

New roles in primary care

- Developing more specific psychological skills such as cognitive behavioural and solution-focused approaches
- Directing people with common mental health problems to a wide range of social and psychological interventions, including IAPT services
- Proactively managing medically unexplained symptoms
- Providing proactive physical care of those with long-term mental health problems
- Leading and sharing care for those with long-term mental health problems
- Providing proactive mental health care for those with long-term physical health problems

Practice nurses

Although the role of the practice nurse has changed significantly over recent years, the focus has remained on physical conditions.

Common roles

- Informally supporting those experiencing emotional distress
- Managing the care of people with chronic diseases such as diabetes
- Providing physical health checks for individuals on the severe and enduring mental illness registers

New roles in primary care

- Screening and identifying depression and anxiety among those in at-risk groups
- Discussing therapeutic options
- Signposting and referring to interventions within the stepped care model
- Providing ongoing psychological support for those with long-term conditions as a part of collaborative care
- Providing follow-up and support in medication management

Practice receptionists and managers

Common roles

- Facilitating access to appointments with professionals
- Responding empathetically to those experiencing distress

New roles in primary care

- Noticing potential mental health problems and communicating concerns to clinicians
- Responding to distress and finding out how the practice can help
- Involving GPs in proactive reviews of services and primary care spending
- Organizing proactive reviews of progress to recovery for people with mental health problems
- Supporting the work of practice-based psychological therapists and other mental health specialists
- Distributing pre-appointment or post-appointment questionnaires including patient experience, some of which may have a mental health component
- Facilitating access to CBT

Health visitors

Health visitors are specially trained to assess the health needs of individuals, families and the wider community. Their work may include tackling the impact of social inequality on health or working closely with at-risk or deprived groups.

Common roles

- Using the Edinburgh Post Natal Depression Scale (EPNDS) to carry out postnatal depression screening at 6 weeks, 12 weeks and 8 months
- Supporting cases of postnatal depression with listening and increased contact
- Referring women with postnatal depression to GPs and/or a postnatal depression group

New roles in primary care

- Collaborating with midwives in the antenatal period to identify women with a pre-existing mental health disorder
- Working within an integrated care pathway for antenatal and postnatal, infant and family mental health

- Having a clear referral pathway into specialist perinatal services
- Assessing attachment difficulties
- Recognizing and managing a parent's mental distress in the postnatal period, identified with screening tools
- Managing the mental health and well-being of parents using a stepped care approach involving social prescribing, cognitive approaches, supported medication management and guided self-help
- Referring patients with mental health problems directly to specialist mental health services, including IAPT teams
- Working collaboratively with or within agencies involved with children's and families' mental health, e.g. Sure Start Children's Centres and nursery nurses
- Working to support extended families with multiple indicators of social exclusion

Midwives

Midwives have been identified as key professionals in predicting women at risk of perinatal mental health disorders.

Common roles

- Monitoring individuals in their care for previous or present history of mental ill health
- Running antenatal groups

New roles in primary care

- Supporting individuals within their care who have a previous or present history of mental ill health, through active listening and behavioural interventions
- Liaising with specialist mental health professionals or parental mental health teams to share care of the individual
- Incorporating basic psychosocial interventions into prenatal groups

District nurses

District nurses provide nursing at home and support to those with long-term physical health needs. Teams are linked to general practices.

Common roles

- Providing nursing care on discharge from hospital
- Providing palliative care
- Providing emotional support for those in distress

New roles in primary care

- Screening for and diagnosing mental health problems such as dementia and depression
- Integrating basic mental health care into care for physical health conditions
- Providing specific cognitive behavioural and solution-focused support for those with long-term conditions

Care assistants

Working in district nursing teams, home care teams and residential and nursing homes, care assistants provide essential help with personal care, mobility and supporting access to recreation.

Common roles

- Listening and providing support – but they are not seen as having a role in mental health care

New roles in primary care

- Identifying and referring those with suspected mental health problems to clinical staff or IAPT services
- Using behavioural techniques to help ensure social inclusion
- Supporting medication concordance

Occupational therapists

Occupational therapists work across the health and local authority divide, in acute trusts, community mental health teams (CMHTs) and community rehabilitation teams.

Common roles

- Assessing and treating physical and psychiatric conditions using specific, purposeful activity to prevent disability and promote independent functioning in all aspects of daily life
- Assessing need for aids to support independent living

New roles in primary care

- Working with general practice teams to support recovery and rehabilitation for those with physical and mental health problems
- Developing links between primary care and local mainstream resources (leisure, education, volunteering, self-help) to support recovery
- Delivering psycho-educational courses in stress management, focusing on the interaction between physical and psychological needs
- Working as part of the Conditions Management Programme attached to Jobcentre Plus, supporting Pathways to Work programmes and the Fit for Work programme

Community matrons

This is a new type of post, designed to enhance the health and social care of people with serious long-term or complex conditions. In their 'hands-on' case management role, these senior and experienced nurses will work in a community setting planning and organizing the care of this group. They will:

- work as members of the primary health care team to ensure a team approach to care, evaluating outcomes in partnership with GPs and hospital colleagues;
- collaborate with health professionals, social services, carers and relatives to understand all aspects of patients' physical, social and environmental condition; and

- assess and monitor the psychological well-being of clients and provide support or referral for mental health.

School nurses

School nurses can play a vital role in recognizing and assessing mental health problems, referring young people for help and managing children's mental health themselves.

Common roles

- Screening children and adolescents for physical health problems
- Signposting children with mental health problems for referral via their GP

New roles in primary care

- Working in an integrated school health team
- Screening for and recognizing mental health problems using validated instruments
- Utilizing self-help materials and problem-solving approaches to assist mental health problems
- Providing ongoing mental health care in liaison with general practice and specialist mental health teams
- Providing access and referral for advice from Child and Adolescent Mental Health Services (CAMHS)

Employment advisors and Conditions Management Programme workers

These posts are funded by the Department for Work and Pensions, which is also to pilot Employment Advice Workers within some new IAPT services; these workers will provide guidance on remaining in or returning to work for people who are experiencing common mental health problems but are not eligible for Incapacity Benefit.

Community pharmacists

The introduction of a new contract in 2004 encouraged pharmacists to expand their role in chronic disease management.

Common roles

- Offering advice on medication interaction
- Directing patients to their GP for further discussion on medication

New roles in primary care

- Supervising repeat prescriptions and medicines
- Reviewing the promotion of healthy lifestyles (including smoking cessation)
- Supporting patient involvement in medicine management via the delivery of medicines use reviews (MURs) in partnership with GP colleagues
- Supporting self-care

The Pharmacist Independent Prescriber (PIP) role allows qualified PIPs to prescribe any licensed medicine for any medical condition within their competence.

Future developments in primary care mental health services

These changing roles indicate significant training requirements. For primary care and general practice in particular, fulfilling these ambitions will require a shift towards (a) more mental health well-being work, (b) a new emphasis on recovery and social inclusion and (c) a requirement to increase collaboration with a number of other providers.

Likely service and pathway changes

While general practice will need to continue to provide a core NHS service recognizing and managing people with common mental health problems, with referral onto and collaboration with the IAPT teams, there are a number of other areas of primary mental health care which might also require significant development. These include:

- physical care for people with severe mental illness (see Chapter 8)
- mental health care for those with long-term physical conditions (see Chapter 12)
- care for those with medically unexplained physical symptoms (see Chapter 12)
- shared care and primary-care-based care for those with stable and less risky psychosis (see Chapter 8)
- integrated physical and mental health care for homebound people who are frail and have comorbid physical and mental health problems
- family-centred care for those families, particularly with young children, with multiple social and health problems
- care for those highly vulnerable people with common mental health problems who are often homeless or in and out of prison and have comorbid mental health, drug and alcohol and physical health problems.

Previous chapters have outlined the potential roles of primary care in the first three of these priorities. The skills and competency requirements are detailed below. This chapter closes with a view to the future, describing the potential formation of three other primary-care-based teams.

Developing knowledge and specific skills

Primary care practitioners will need to continue to adapt their basic and ongoing training. Improvements in knowledge and skills will be required. It is anticipated that new service models and supportive training as well as national policy directives will help to shift beliefs and culture about mental health with a new emphasis on:

- the importance of mental health well being
- the indivisibility of mental and physical health
- the importance of the social within the bio-psychosocial model (emphasizing not only social origins but perhaps more importantly social goals).

Knowledge

In a number of areas, knowledge will need to be updated. The following areas are particularly important:

- developing an understanding of new brain science (functions of the brain, the role of trauma and abandonment in producing psychopathology, interaction between genetics and environment)
- the pathophysiology of mind–body interactions
- understanding the mechanisms of psychological therapies and social interventions.

Skills

An improvement in key skills is probably the most important change for GPs in order to enhance primary care mental health services. This will require high-level political support from the key bodies representing primary-care-based professionals and joint working with a number of other key organizations to promote the role and develop the skills required of general practitioners and other front-line staff. Skills will be required in a number of areas:

1 Assessment and formulation

- Carrying out a comprehensive formulation over a series of consultations
- Integrating social and psychological with symptom and diagnosis based assessments
- Assessing and combining social goals and personal strengths into formulations and treatment plans.

2 Microtherapy

This is based on the premise that the consultation can contribute to health care not only by diagnosis and referral but through the act of communication within the consultation itself. A number of therapeutic modalities are likely to be useful and practitioners will gain from basic (and enhanced) training in the following areas:

- listening and counselling skills
- cognitive behavioural techniques
- other modalities such as solution-focused and problem-solving therapy
- understanding and awareness of transference.

3 Collaborative care

Key skills are required to provide ongoing collaborative care. These include:

- facilitation of self care
- liaison with other professionals
- taking on a part or a coordinating role of a 'package of care' for those with complex needs.

All of these changes will require a number of educational approaches which need to fit in with practitioners' workloads, learning styles, and previous experience and knowledge. They are likely to include e-learning, locality-based training (particularly when linked to role and service redesign) and team-based training.

Perhaps most importantly systems for providing ongoing support and mentorship for general practitioners need to be developed specifically to deal with new mental health functions. The development of peer supervision can contribute to this. However, it is likely when dealing with complex mental health problems that some form of support from an experienced mental health practitioner will be invaluable for individuals and teams.

Primary-care-based teams for specific groups – future possibilities

While general practice teams and the new IAPT teams will provide the core primary care mental health function in England, and in other parts of the UK and Ireland similar primary care psychological therapy teams are emerging, a number of other options for more specialized and integrated teams are possible. These include teams to support vulnerable and excluded adults and frail adults (who are often homebound) with mixed mental health and physical problems, and family-based teams focusing on multiply excluded families with children and adults.

Teams for frail elderly

For some people, especially those who are older, physical health problems can become the main focus of individuals' lives and the restriction of being housebound at home or in other settings, such as care homes, becomes the dominating feature of individuals' environments; depression in particular can supervene. In addition there are many individuals with long-term mental health problems such as depression and schizophrenia who with time develop a number of physical conditions. They were cared for by old-age mental health teams but with the new emphasis on providing care for people with dementia in specialized teams, this group of individuals are now considered a part of the remit of general adult mental health services, particularly in England. Meeting this group's physical health needs might not always be easy within adult mental health settings.

These two groups, therefore, have similar health and social care needs. One solution could be to develop integrated care for mentally and physically frail adults who may be housebound and have a combination of mental and physical health problems. Teams including general practitioners, district nurses, community psychiatric nurses, occupational therapists and physiotherapists and input from psychologists and psychiatrists could provide a valuable integrated service. The specific functions of such teams could include:

- ongoing mental and physical health care
- provision of social care needs
- delivery of social care
- delivery of medical care
- delivery of nursing care
- integrated assessment using a bio-psychosocial model
- assessment and delivery of carers' needs.

This team could be based at a locality level and work closely with a number of practices. Alternatively it could be a primary-care-based team with general practice records and with other professionals using general practice records in the same way as practice nurses. These could be seconded from other services, or employed by the general practices. The new PCT-level 'GP Health Centres' provide a mechanism for a mixed model with a core of patients who are permanently housebound being able to register with the practice specializing in this integrated care delivered at home. Others could receive shorter-term care for briefer periods from that same team. This model would mean an initial discontinuity from their original GP, but might provide more integrated ongoing care.

Care for excluded vulnerable adults

Every geographical area, whether rural or urban, has a group of individuals excluded from society in a number of (often multiple) ways. While for most the aim is to provide services from ordinary general practice and community-based teams (mainstreaming – and this would include the majority of those with long-term conditions, those from ethnic minority groups and most older people) there are a sub-population for whom specialized primary-care-based care may be the best way of delivering integrated services, for either a brief or an ongoing period of time. Such individuals include those who are homeless, those with significant alcohol and drug misuse problems and some individuals in contact with the criminal justice system (Department of Health 2010). Such a team could incorporate professionals with experience of dealing with mental health problems (in particular PTSD, complex trauma and personality disorder), practitioners with experience of dealing with drug and alcohol misuse and primary-care-based professionals with specific experience of integrating physical and mental health care, and the ability and willingness to work collaboratively with other workers and teams. The specific functions of such a team might include:

- full bio-psychosocial assessments
- specific diagnostic assessments (for learning difficulties, ADHD, anorexia, autistic spectrum and personality disorder) and integrated mental health and drug misuse care
- psychological therapies
- medication and physical health care.

Such a team would require some level of input from psychiatrists and a range of therapists (or pathways to) including, perhaps, CBT, cognitive analytic therapy (CAT) and psychodynamic therapy. Systemic therapy for working with families is also potentially important. Delivery of therapy would need to be re-engineered to reduce stigma, improve access and ensure a collaborative approach with other agencies. Therapists can also provide supervision to a variety of practitioners engaged in 'micro-therapy' or delivering community-based components of a therapy package, for example CBT.

Strong links would be required with a broad range of external agencies. These could include social services, for vulnerable adults and children, education and housing services and employment services. Links would also need to be established with a range of voluntary-sector providers such as those providing care for homeless people as a drop-in or in hostels, and specific services for resettlement of offenders. Key operational considerations include sharing information, co-location (possibly across a network of locations rather than fully centralized) and close liaison in order to develop coherent and consistent plans for achieving individual social goals.

These teams could in effect become the foundation for 'Bradley' style (Department of Health 2009a) criminal justice mental health services for offenders, tasked to provide integrated rehabilitation along with probation services, as well as court reports and forensic physician services to the police. Such a service could have a core general-practice-based registration system for medium/long-term ongoing primary care input, but also have the facility to provide briefer periods of integrated care and, if required, liaison with their client's own general practitioner. While there is a strong case for the setting up of 'one-stop shops' to provide integrated care alongside probation teams, social services and access to voluntary organizations, complete co-location for all teams is unlikely. Shared records for the core health teams using mobile laptops and a single record-keeping system across a range of locations in a network may be a more achievable objective. It might also provide more accessible services across a wider geographical area (by outreach) to a range of groups – offenders, the homeless and asylum seekers. By focusing on social inclusion, rather than population sub-groups, it might also reduce stigma.

As well as face-to-face or telephone-based liaison, information sharing of key pieces of data beyond health teams is also a requirement for integrated care. For example, while detailed medical records may not be shared, social inclusion goals regarding housing, relationships, education and training, as well as the main key teams involved and named workers, could be shared beyond health. Protocols for this exist and are being developed.

Family teams

The increasing emphasis on child mental health has resulted in new investment in child and adolescent mental health services. Systemic considerations are vital for these new services and it is increasingly recognized that children growing up in difficult family situations with problems related to trauma (witnessing violence or in receipt of abuse) and poor attachment are more likely to develop mental health problems. One way of addressing these in particularly vulnerable communities is to identify families with 'multiple vulnerability'. For example, in one family it is possible to often find someone with a major mental illness, someone with a learning difficulty, people with long-term physical conditions, such as strokes or multiple sclerosis, and ongoing involvement with drug and alcohol and contact with the criminal justice system. One approach to dealing with this is to set up teams focusing on family units including the extended family (and other key individuals) to ensure that families are in receipt of care and to help develop resilience and independence. While these teams are not yet in existence and there are no plans to commission them at national level pilot Family Intervention Projects (FIP) are now being reproduced. Their development might ultimately play a significant role in preventing the development of mental illness.

Summary

- Recent developments have led to expanded and new roles for many front-line workers in primary care.
- The development of mental health teams within primary care has been given impetus by the new policy aimed at improving access to psychological therapies.
- General practitioners will have to develop new skills and new knowledge so as to further develop the services offered in primary care to those with a range of mental health problems.
- For the future consideration should be given to developing specialist mental health teams in primary care with particular skills in meeting the mental and physical health needs of the frail elderly, those in the criminal justice system, the homeless and children in vulnerable families.
- At the heart of all these developments will be the requirement to break down barriers in terms of location, record-keeping and access to social care and to voluntary sector partners.

References

Department of Health. (2007). *New Ways of Working for Primary Care in Mental Health* in *New Ways of Working for Everyone*. London: Department of Health.

Department of Health. (2009a). *The Bradley Report*. London: Department of Health

Department of Health. (2009b). *Improving Access to Psychological Therapies (IAPT)*. Commissioning Toolkit. London: Department of Health.

Department of Health (2010). *High Quality Care for All. Primary Care and Community Services*. Inclusion health. Improving primary care for socially excluded people. London: Department of Health

South-east London Clinical Governance Resource Group. (2004). *Lewisham Mental Health Facilitation Project Progress Report*.

Mental health services and how they relate to primary care

Learning objectives

Historical background to the current services
Liaison between the voluntary sector and primary care
Traditional and new roles within community mental health teams
Traditional and new roles within primary care mental health teams
Managing interface responsibilities and shared care

Most countries have specialized mental health services and the United Kingdom and Ireland are no exceptions. Their separation from the general medical services is an embodiment of the Cartesian divide between mind and body which has dominated thinking in recent times. Specialized mental health services can be seen as originating with the 'Asylum' movement in the eighteenth century, initially with intentions related to the original meaning of asylum as a safe place. However, these initially small institutions with rehabilitation and outside life at their heart gave way to a period of mass incarceration for short, medium and long periods of individuals' lives. Not only were those with what we now call schizophrenia locked up but many others, exhibiting aggressive or anxious and agitated behaviour, were also admitted.

During the twentieth century various forms of psychotherapy were developed along with new antipsychotic and antidepressant medication in the middle half of that period. By the 1950s and 1960s it was clear that mental health institutions were too numerous, too large and often had a negative impact and prevented those who had been interned, either voluntarily or compulsorily, from being rehabilitated back into the community. This institutionalization was roundly criticized by the anti-psychiatrist movement and eventually a coalition between radical therapists and fiscal conservatives resulted in large-scale closure of asylums during the 1970s and 1980s.

Initially teams were set up in the community with the aim of rehabilitating those who had been institutionalized for many years. Alongside these teams a number of community psychiatric nurses and psychiatrists started working with general practices to provide care for those new cases of psychosis. This 'silent growth of a new service' (Strathdee and Williams 1984) came to a halt in the early nineties with the development of community mental health teams and the Care Programme Approach updated in 1999 (Department of Health 1999a). The elements of this included a multidisciplinary assessment of the health and social needs of those in contact with the mental health services by the community mental health team, a written care plan, a key worker (now called a care coordinator) and regular reviews with changes to the care plan as required. The Community Mental Health Teams (CMHTs) brought together psychiatrists, community psychiatric nurses, occupational therapists, social workers as well as other professions to deliver this service.

In the west midlands of Britain a number of pioneering approaches were developed with functional and structural splits between community-based teams delivering assertive outreach to patients who are hard to reach and hard to engage, home treatment teams providing care in people's homes as an alternative to hospitalization, and early intervention services (EIS) focusing on young people at risk of or experiencing new episodes of psychosis, with the aim of preventing institutionalization and promoting inclusion in terms of employment, housing and relationships. This multifaceted model became accepted as the template for mental health services in the National Service Framework for Mental Health (Department of Health 1999b) and was rigorously applied across all of England. Slightly different models appeared elsewhere in the UK.

In Ireland there were similar developments throughout the 1980s and 1990s culminating in A Vision for Change (2006), the Government's most recent blueprint for mental health services. The model is based on the delivery of multidisciplinary mental health services with care plans and service user and carer involvement where feasible. So far it has only been partially implemented.

Liaison between primary and the voluntary sector

Most areas have significant small and medium-sized voluntary-sector organizations in both Britain and Ireland. Branches of organizations such as MIND and Depression Alliance (AWARE in Ireland) exist in most major conurbations. In addition, there are small voluntary-sector organizations which have arisen as support groups, for carers or for individual patients and others which have arisen out of the principles of community development. They often offer patient-centred services which are based on principles of social inclusion but are frequently poorly funded. Funding is often renewed on an annual basis, making planning for expansion difficult. Relationships between primary care and these voluntary-sector organizations are normally patchy, with general practitioners often being unaware of their availability as local resources. In Britain graduate mental health workers (see Chapter 20) and some counsellors have had included in their role the identification and formation of links with these organizations to primary care settings. Voluntary-sector organizations can play a valuable role in assisting people with benefits advice, advice on voluntary work or perhaps the provision of this as well as assisting in pathways to employment. They operate in a number of ways, including increasing contact with other service users, increasing trusting relationships and networks, as well as promoting physical and mental activity. Links between general practices and these organizations can be enhanced by meeting face to face at local events or attendance at practice meetings. Systematic information about these resources should be available from local information systems. This should include clear information about referral criteria, work undertaken, locality, opening times and contact details.

Liaison between primary care and specialist mental health teams

Joint working between primary care and specialist mental health services has had a patchy history. Some patients, even in systems which are not designed to work together, will manage to access health care from both GPs and mental health specialists. However, some with significant mental health needs are discharged to practices with limited skills, or lost to follow-up. Others are seen regularly in secondary care, but miss out on physical care. Good liaison could resolve these problems but so far hopeful models have not received the research or policy attention required to refine and move mainstream.

During the 1970s and 1980s liaison between psychiatrists and general practitioners developed (Mitchell 1985). This varied regionally: by the mid 1980s 50% of Scottish GPs reported an attachment with a psychiatrist (Pullen and Yellowlees 1988) and in England almost 20% of consultant psychiatrists described spending time in general practice (Strathdee and Williams 1984). In a parallel development, community psychiatric nurses (CPNs) were being attached to practices so that by 1990 50% of practices had CPN attachments (Thomas and Corney 1992).

However, the form of this liaison was hotly debated. Mitchell (1985) suggested that four key elements were required: regular face-to-face contact, an acceptable meeting place, open communication and mutual understanding and trust. GPs wanted better communication, assessments by specialists in primary care, and to retain responsibility (Strathdee 1988). The shifted outpatient model, in which the general practitioner's surgery was in essence an outpatient clinic which the psychiatrist used as a convenience for the practice's patients, was the norm but liaison between the GP and the specialists, either after the consultation or during a shared consultation, was also common (Creed and Marks 1989). A more structured version of the liaison model ensured all possible referrals were seen and always discussed afterwards (Gask et al. 1997)

During this time there was increasing concern that the increased workload generated by this model left those with the most serious mental illnesses with reduced provision (Sayce et al. 1991). Large volumes of referrals from primary care to CMHTs were countered by the development of strict referral criteria for entry to specialist care. This led to deteriorating relationships between primary and secondary care. GPs recognized that patients with psychosis had better care in the reorganized services, but patients with non-psychotic illness were worse off (Harrison et al. 1997). GPs generally had low involvement and low satisfaction with the care responsibilities for patients under specialist services (Bindman et al. 1997).

A number of high-profile disasters catalysed a policy focus on specialist care for those with psychosis (Ritchie et al. 1994). The Care Programme Approach (CPA) and multi-disciplinary Community Mental Health Teams (CMHTs) were the mechanisms of implementation (Department of Health 1994). By the mid 1990s only fund-holding GPs retained linked CPNs and psychiatrists, mostly in the form of 'shifted outpatients' with little liaison. All of this developed in seeming contradiction of the guidance on shared care between primary and secondary care from the Joint Royal College Working Group (1993).

Since then government policy in Britain has continued to concentrate on patients with severe mental illness and the establishment of specialized functional teams. Guidance has been much less definitive about liaison between community mental health services and primary health care teams and in relation to the role of specialist mental health teams in supporting those with non-psychotic complex conditions.

Mental health liaison in primary care and the community mental health teams (CMHTs)

While the traditional roles of the members of community mental health team continue, new roles have been developed by the New Ways of Working policy for primary care mental health subgroup (Department of Health 2007). These changes have occurred in the context of a need to improve access to quality services for those with a range of mental health problems.

No such changes have been proposed in Ireland at the time of writing.

Community psychiatric nurses (CPNs)

These are key members of community-based mental health teams (CMHTs, primary care liaison teams, assertive outreach teams, crisis and home treatment teams and early intervention teams).

Common roles

- Carrying out full mental health assessments, using the Care Programme Approach (CPA), of people referred from primary care to CMHTs
- Liaising with GPs in relation to the continuing care for those with severe mental illness through CMHTs

New roles in primary care

- Providing assessments within primary care
- Providing psychological treatments and support to people within primary care settings
- Sharing care with primary health care team members
- Providing liaison functions for complex cases
- Utilizing primary care systems for record-keeping
- Providing independent/supplementary prescribing

Clinical and counselling psychologists

Most applied psychologists already working in primary care with CBT training can provide longer-term intensive psychological therapy to those with more complex problems; additionally they can be involved in the Improving Access to Psychological Therapies (DoH 2009) (see Chapter 20) either as high-intensity workers or supervising those delivering high- or low-intensity therapies.

Other roles will also be possible for other psychology grades:

- delivering psychological services and therapies directly to clients (graduate psychologists); and
- delivering group-based psycho-educational programmes for people with common mental health problems.

Community psychiatrists

Community psychiatrists are core members not only of CMHTs but also of assertive outreach, crisis and home treatment and early intervention teams.

Common roles

- Receiving referrals from primary care (normally via CMHT referral meetings) for work with individuals experiencing severe mental illness
- Delivering care according to the Care Programme Approach in outpatient settings
- Using expertise in prescribing psychotropic medication

- Undertaking the Responsible Medical Officer role for the current Mental Health Act
- Diagnosing complex and rare psychiatric conditions

New roles in primary care
- Providing liaison, consultation, advice and supervision for primary care and CMHTs via telephone, email and face-to-face contact
- Providing emergency appointments for brief reviews or assessments
- Considering co-location within general practices providing specialist liaison
- Providing sub-specialty advice and liaison for medically unexplained symptoms

Social workers
Social workers often work in local authority adult and children's teams and in 'mental health teams' under various partnership arrangements.

Common roles
- Acting as generic members of community-based mental health teams
- Assessing for 'social care packages', including housing and direct payments
- Carrying out Mental Health Act assessments as 'Approved' Social Workers – this will be changed under the new Mental Health Act to a role of Approved Mental Health Professional

New roles in primary care
- Taking on a link worker role (assessment and shared care)
- Developing a recovery and social inclusion function in primary care
- Supporting reviews of social care packages for those with primary-care-based mental health input, e.g. those with stable psychosis
- Supporting the implementation of personalization, individual budgets and direct payments

Support, time and recovery (STR) workers
An STR worker is part of a team that provides mental health services and this new role focuses directly on the needs of the people who use the service. They often work across traditional boundaries of care. Their role is to support, give time to and help the patient in their recovery. Many have previously been volunteers or people with lived experience of mental illness. Their training is focused on a supportive and listening role. Recovery values are based on the individual defining their recovery in their own terms and as far as possible self-managing their recovery process. The worker is there to help the individual define and achieve their recovery objectives. Roles include:

- sharing care with GPs for low-risk clients with psychosis who are in recovery and requiring support and short-term input
- supporting brief therapy on social interventions, e.g. to support cognitive behavioural work or attendance at mainstream vocational education or leisure activities.

Case study: the Mental Health Link project

The Mental Health Link project aimed to develop effective liaison between specialists and primary care and to develop shared care in response to the needs of patients, the practice and the associated specialist mental health team (Byng and Single 1999). The project also sought to establish processes for systematically reviewing patients in primary care. Facilitators met with a joint working group drawn from the CMHT and the practice in order to develop a shared care system from a selection of options contained in a toolkit. The two main focuses were, first, on the development of practice registers, minimum datasets for individual patients and recall systems, and second, on the development of the link workers' role when they were away from their base community team working within general practice.

Evaluation of the Mental Health Link project involved a cluster randomized trial (Byng *et al.* 2004) and an evaluation involving qualitative interviews in order to understand the process of service development and the influence of the project (Byng *et al.* 2005).

Practice CMHT vignettes have been composed from two or more of the original case studies (Byng 2004). This approach facilitates the representation of the findings in narrative form without making the practices and associated CMHTs recognizable. The following vignettes focus on the various roles of link workers.

Vignette 1

Integration of link worker achieved by helping solve crises and problems

A large practice with many GP partners in a relatively deprived inner-city area was allocated a link worker. They felt their case load warranted a practice-based CPN and, despite a strong interest in LTMI (long-term mental illness), they were suspicious that a link worker offering 2 hours a week would not contribute substantially. They found it difficult enough to meet as a team and so meeting regularly as a group with the link worker was not an option.

However, in collaboration with the link worker, they developed liaison arrangements to suit both sides. The link worker was introduced to the team in practice meetings and he attended the practice weekly, at a time when many of the team were in, and made himself available in the administrative hub of the practice as well as in quieter areas for in-depth consultations. He felt thoroughly welcomed by the practice and able to do a good and effective job. The practice on their part described him as a 'very special person' who would always take on their concerns and help solve a range of problems, including providing advice about complex patients with personality problems who were not in the trust's geographical area. He had experience of acute assessment as well as longer-term problems and knew the local services well. These attributes along with a willingness by the practice to collaborate resulted in effective reactive liaison in the absence of regular meetings.

Vignette 2

Undue focus on continuing care stymies effective liaison

A small practice in an inner-city area recognized its need to improve care for patients with LTMI and decided to join the Mental Health Link programme (see above). The GPs did not have particular interest or skills in primary care mental health but wanted collaboration with CMHTs. The patients were evenly divided between CMHTs from two different trusts. Initially both CMHTs engaged with the project but only one attended the first meeting. A link worker was appointed and it was agreed they would meet regularly with the practice.

Good relationships with the practice nurse and the GPs were maintained through informal contact with the continuing care team-based link worker. The joint meetings generated a trusting working relationship. There were a few patients with psychosis under the care of the continuing care team but discussions about them became repetitive and after six months the meetings died out. The GPs, lacking confidence in dealing with difficult new mental health cases, realized in retrospect that they would have preferred to improve their links with the assessment and brief treatment team, so they could gain specialist input to those patients without psychosis but presenting with complex needs.

Vignette 3

Liaison for proactive review

This medium-sized practice in an inner-city area, associated with a recently re-organized CMHT, had ambitions for developing practice-based shared care. However, when it came to planning the details of the liaison and the role of the link worker, the CMHT was reluctant to agree on a substantial role for the link worker other than as a channel for communication. In particular, the team voiced concerns that as the practice provided excellent mental health care, their priorities for liaison would lie elsewhere.

Meanwhile the practice itself underwent considerable disruption due to the loss of a partner. Over a year later the project was reviewed and a different link worker was appointed. The practice was more stable and, together, they worked out a system of joint review for all patients considered to have long-term mental illness. The practice manager organized one-to-one review meetings, with a list of patients, between the link worker and each of the GPs. The reviews were rapid with some patients who had been seen regularly and with few needs being discussed only briefly. The discussion of each patient ended with a decision about whether the patient:

- required any further immediate follow-up
- should be seen by the practice nurse for a physical health review
- should be seen by the GP for a mental health review
- or should be referred to the CMHT.

Each patient's care was reviewed once or twice a year and follow-up was targeted on those with most needs. The time allocated to these meetings was relatively limited and the GPs respected the link worker as a limited resource by making initial contact with the care coordinators of patients under the trust in times of crisis, and reserving more complicated cases for discussion with the link worker.

Lessons from the vignettes

The vignettes show that a variety of approaches to liaison can improve care, but that liaison is not easy and there are many inhibiting factors. There is no one model which will fit all contexts. The needs of particular organizations, the context in which they are operating and the needs of the patients all have to be taken into account when developing systems of shared care and liaison. Both sides need to be willing to engage with each other, links are needed to support decisions which GPs are most unsure about, and the discussion of real cases should lead to the development of trusting relations (Gilson 2003). The consultation–liaison approach, with all its theoretical advantages, has not been widely adopted within the UK. The low number of psychiatrists per head of population means that it is impractical for each practice to have a linked psychiatrist. The case studies above, however, have shown that the 'consultation–liaison' approach can be carried out by experienced non-medical mental health specialist workers in a variety of ways.

Sharing responsibility at the interface

This section provides a summary of the guidance to support the professionals in their new roles so as to enable them to carry out these in a high-quality, safe and defensible manner. It is adapted from the New Ways of Working (NWW) in Primary Care guidance (Department of Health 2007). The subgroup responsible for this piece of work included representation from different professions, unions, defence bodies, the Department of Health and Royal Colleges. As traditional boundaries between professionals and between primary and specialist care are broken down, the notion of medical responsibility is transformed into shared responsibilities between practitioners and the people who use services.

Providing advice about a patient or service user you have not seen

This occurs frequently when primary care clinicians ask for advice from specialists, and occasionally in reverse. The following principles should be adhered to:

- The person giving advice should ask for sufficient information about the clinical case, and record this.
- A record should be kept of the problem and the advice given, including the date and a patient identifier as an absolute minimum for good practice.
- Records should be secure and accessible but do not need to form part of the employing Trust's system.
- Best practice would indicate that for telephone contact, the advice should be subsequently provided in writing so that it can be incorporated into primary care or other records.
- Email advice provides a useful audit trail but needs to be incorporated into primary care records.

Advice for clinicians working within another team

Increasingly as part of NWW, team clinicians are asked to work alongside other teams in order to provide coordinated and multidisciplinary care. For example, CPNs, social workers and occupational therapists may be asked to take on the role of a link worker and provide advice and shared care for people with long-term problems. The following principles and guidance arose:

- It is good practice for clinicians working for other organizations to provide care within a primary care setting.
- Responsibilities for the roles should be documented in an agreement between the two teams.

- It is considered good practice for linked workers who are carrying out assessments or engaged in shared care to establish the principle of logging contact into the case notes of the team they are working with, rather than into those of their own team. Some may wish to keep supplementary records or copies of records for their own or for their organization's use. This is not considered essential practice.
- Agreements for the retrieval of records made by practitioners outside the organization they are working in should not cause a problem, as medical records are NHS property rather than belonging to primary care or the specialist trust.

Chronic disease management and shared care

The coordinating function for chronic disease management may well be located in primary care, and might be the joint responsibility of administrators and clinicians.

- It is essential to record the responsibilities for components of care in terms of which team and which professional is responsible for carrying out these. This is particularly critical for the various sub-components of care with respect to lithium, depot injections and clozapine treatment.
- Joint working within the Care Programme Approach (CPA) and other care navigator functions (e.g. the Quality Outcomes Framework 2009) should ensure proportionate engagement of all those involved in the care of individuals with complex needs.
- Invitations to attend lengthy CPA meetings or case conferences may not be the most appropriate way of engaging others. Alternative mechanisms, such as requesting that key information be sent to care coordinators or having verbal discussions prior to CPA meetings, are considered best practice when liaising with those unlikely to attend.

Medication risks at the interface

It is vitally important that anyone prescribing for patients with mental health problems has a complete record of any medication the patient is taking, the reason why drugs have been started, changed or stopped, plus details of future monitoring and planned reviews. It is therefore essential that:

- the name of the person responsible for prescribing, monitoring and reviewing any medication is recorded;
- in shared care, both primary and secondary care records should include records of all oral and parenteral medication (not just psychotropics) and significant diagnoses, in order to anticipate interactions and prevent prescribing against contraindications.

Information on changes in medication, along with related issues, should be forwarded to other teams involved, in a timely manner and usually before the patient is likely to be seen by them.

Other considerations

For children with mental health problems, health visitors (public health nurses) and school nurses are the very health workers who, along with early years practitioners (e.g. nursery nurses), need to work with the Child and Adolescent Mental Health Services. Many of the latter are now working in tiers according to complexity which should, in theory, make liaison easier.

Similarly, for older adults, liaison is often critical. Older people's mental health services are diverse and have not been subjected to rigorous performance management. Some have developed home treatment and crisis services in parallel with adult services. A recent initiative is the split into functional (depression/schizophrenia) and dementia services. This will have a profound impact on teams' structures. One potential gain is the possibility of the development of services for frail elderly in which teams have CPNs, OTs and district nurses caring for people at home with comorbid mental and physical health problems (See also Chapter 20 for the role of primary care teams).

Summary

- New Ways of Working has led to the development of new roles for mental health professionals working in CMHTs and in primary care.
- Outside the adult mental health services access to psychological therapies has improved.
- Collaborative care between primary and secondary is the ideal model.
- In this interface there must be a clear designation of responsibilities.
- Liaison and collaboration is also important for children's and older people's services.
- These developments pose considerable organizational challenges.

References

Bindman, J., Johnson, S., Wright, S., *et al.* (1997). Integration between primary and secondary services in the care of the severely mentally ill: Patients' and general practitioners' views. *British Journal of Psychiatry*, **171**, 169–174.

Byng, R. (2004). Link workers and liaison with primary care: lessons from case studies. *Mental Health Review*, **9**(4), 13–18.

Byng, R., and Single, H. (1999). *Developing Primary Care for Patients for Long Term Mental Illness – Your Guide to Improving Services.* London: King's Fund.

Byng, R., Jones, R., Leese, M., *et al.* (2004). Exploratory cluster randomised controlled trial of shared care development for long-term mental illness. *British Journal of General Practice*, **54**(501), 259–266.

Byng, R., Norman, I., and Redfern, S. (2005). Using realistic evaluation to evaluate a practice level intervention to improve primary health care for patients with long-term mental illness. *Evaluation*, **11**(1), 69–93.

Creed, F., and Marks, B. (1989). Liaison psychiatry in general practice: a comparison of the liaison-attachment scheme and shifted outpatient clinic models. *Journal of the Royal College of General Practitioners*, **39**(329), 514–517.

Department of Health. (1994). *Working in Partnership: The Review of Mental Health Nursing.* London: HMSO.

Department of Health. (1999a). *Effective Care Co-ordination in the Mental Health Services. Modernising the Care Programme Approach – A Policy Booklet.* London: Department of Health.

Department of Health. (1999b). *National Service Framework for Mental Health: Modern Standards and Service Models.* London: Department of Health.

Department of Health. (2003). *The Mental Health Policy Implementation Guide; Support, Time and Recovery (STR) Workers: Learning from the national implementation programme – Final Handbook (2008).* London: Department of Health.

Department of Health. (2007). New Ways of Working for primary care in mental health in New Ways of Working for Everyone. London: Department of Health.

Department of Health. (2009). *Improving Access to Psychological Therapies (IAPT).*

Commissioning Toolkit. London: Department of Health.

Department of Health and Children. (2006). *A Vision for Change. Report of Expert Group on Mental Health Policy*. Dublin: Department of Health and Children.

Gask, L., Sibbald, B., and Creed, F. (1997). Evaluating models of working at the interface between mental health services and primary care. *British Journal of Psychiatry*, **170**, 6–11.

Gilson, L. (2003). Trust and the development of health care as a social institution. *Social Science and Medicine*, **56**(7), 1453–1468.

Harrison, J., Kisely, S. R., Jones, J. A., Blake, I., and Creed, F. H. (1997). Access to psychiatric care; the results of the pathways to care study in Preston. *Journal of Public Health Medicine*, **19**(1), 69–75.

Joint Royal College Working Group. (1993). *Shared care of patients with mental health problems. Occasional Paper 60*. London: Royal College of General Practitioners.

Mitchell, A. R. (1985). Psychiatrists in primary health care settings. *British Journal of Psychiatry*, **147**, 371–379.

Pullen, I. M., and Yellowlees, A. J. (1988). Scottish psychiatrists in primary health-care settings. A silent majority. *British Journal of Psychiatry*, **153**, 663–666.

Quality Outcomes Framework. (2009). BMA and NHS Employers.

Ritchie, J. H., Dick, D., and Lingham, R. (1994). *Report of the Enquiry into the Care and Treatment of Christopher Clunis*. London: HMSO.

Slade, M., Powell, R., and Strathdee, G. (1997). Current approaches to identifying the severely mentally ill. *Social Psychiatry and Psychiatric Epidemiology*, **32**(4), 177–184.

Strathdee, G. (1988). Psychiatrists in primary care: the general practitioner viewpoint. *Family Practice*, **5**(2), 111–115.

Strathdee, G., and Williams, P. (1984). A survey of psychiatrists in primary care: the silent growth of a new service. *Journal of the Royal College of General Practitioners*, **34**(268), 615–618.

Thomas, R. V. R., and Corney, R. H. (1992). A survey of links between mental health professionals and general practice in six district health authorities. *British Journal of General Practice*, **42**(362), 358–361.

22

Providing primary care for people from diverse backgrounds

Chukumeka Maxwell and Maja Lelandais

Learning objectives

Disparities in access, experience and outcomes
Mental health in ethnic minorities – international and national picture
Asylum seekers, refugees and migrant workers
Improving access
Experience/outcome: assessment, formulation, intervention, peer support
Diversity in 10 minute consultations
Culture-bound syndromes

'The world in which you were born is just one model of reality. Other cultures are not failed attempts at being like you. They are unique manifestations of the human spirit'

Wade Davis

Health care in multicultural Britain

Twenty-first century Britain is more diverse than ever before. Our modern society is multi-cultural, multilingual and multilayered. According to the Office for National Statistics (ONS) UK Census, in 2001 nearly 8% of the UK population– over 4.6 million people – came from ethnic minority communities. And these communities are changing all the time. The growth of worldwide economies and the accession of European countries have provided a rapidly changing demographic landscape and there is no single service or area that has accurate data to deliver services. Health workers, however, are charged with providing high-quality care to meet every diverse need. Throughout this chapter a number of key questions lie behind the text.

- Is it best to be open to a wide range of different cultures and beliefs or ensure one knows all about the different ethnic groups in the locality?

- How do we acknowledge cultural differences and ensure everyone has equal rights?

- How to create a safe space to address potentially contentious issues such as racism and cultural differences?

- How do we make allowances for different beliefs and have consistent rules to ensure individuals are protected from abuse?

- Should services be designed to give the same access for everyone or be adapted for different cultural needs?

There are no easy answers to these questions. This chapter aims to help practitioners consider how they practise and design services by outlining and discussing some practical steps that can be taken.

BME defined

'Black Minority and Ethnic (BME) communities include people with different ethnic and/or national backgrounds living in the UK. This includes visible and non-visible minorities. Eastern Europeans, Gypsies and Travellers and the Irish Community. People of Mixed Heritage for example are also included under this term' (DoH 2005).

While attempting to be comprehensive this definition is still simplistic and does not take into account the complexity of interconnectedness or that people may not see themselves as 'BME'.

The BME population is not evenly distributed across the country, with members tending to live in the large urban areas. The different groups share some characteristics but there are often greater differences between the individual ethnic groups than between the minority ethnic population as a whole and the white British majority.

The national and international picture

Internationally, income inequality (see Figure 22.1) and being from a BME background has been found to be linked with poor mental well-being and health (Friedli 2009). It is likely that health differentials, whether derived from wealth or ethnicity, share common causative factors.

After the north east, the south west is considered to be the region with the lowest proportion of ethnic minority populations in the UK. According to the 2001 Census, individuals from BME background made up 1.25% of the total Devon population; however, more recent estimates suggest that the figure has substantially increased (Devon PCT 2007). People from BME backgrounds are much more likely to experience racism and discrimination in rural areas than in larger cities with a more established ethnic community presence. Asylum seekers are particularly vulnerable due to lack of legal services specializing in asylum, which impacts on all areas of their lives, including access to primary care health services.

It is widely recognized that BME people are over-represented within prisons and acute mental health services (DoH 2007), making up 20% of the prison population, despite making up only 8% of the general population (*National Body of Black Prisoners Support Groups SEED 4 BME Offenders Project*, 2007). Likewise, the Count Me in Census (2008) found that 23% of all mental health inpatients belonged to a BME group. African-Caribbean service users have reported a worse experience of care in mental hospitals compared with other ethnic groups and are more likely to be prescribed medication or ECT rather than psychotherapy or counselling (DoH 2005). These factors fuel the 'circle of fear' which can deter BME patients from seeking early treatment (Sainsbury Centre for Mental Health 2002; DoH 2003).

Part of the reason for this discrepancy is the assumptions and stereotypes which accumulate at various points within the public institutions, leading to a very high number of BME people in prison and acute mental health services (Fernando 2005).

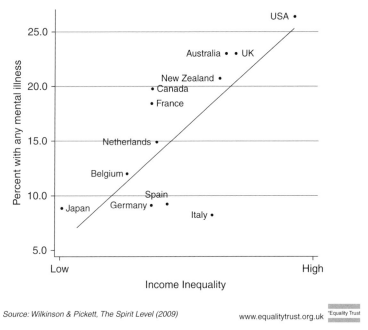

The Prevalence of Mental Illness is Higher in More Unequal Rich Countries

Source: Wilkinson & Pickett, The Spirit Level (2009)

www.equalitytrust.org.uk   "Equality Trust

Figure 22.1. International income inequality

As responsibility for care moves to general practitioners an understanding of local areas where the BME population reside, especially in areas where visibility is not so obvious, can contribute to locally sensitive redesign of services.

Ethnic minorities and access to services, experience and outcomes

'There does not appear to be a single area of mental health care in this country in which black and minority ethnic groups fare as well as, or better than, the majority white community. Both in terms of service experience and the outcome of service interventions, they fare much worse than people from the ethnic majority' (DoH 2003). The incidence of certain conditions appears higher, racism is believed to have an impact on stress and pathways to care are often complex or curtailed.

Transcultural psychiatry: the case of psychosis

Few areas are more controversial in transcultural psychiatry than ethnic differences in the incidence of psychosis. The whole debate and wealth of research generated are beyond the scope of this chapter, but here is a brief review of the main issues: African-Caribbean service users are more likely to be diagnosed with severe mental health problems such as 'bipolar disorder' and 'paranoid schizophrenia' than the majority population in the UK (Kirov and Murray 1999; Hemsi 1971). However, in Trinidad or Barbados the incidence of psychosis is lower than in the British Caribbean community (Bhugra *et al.* 1996, 1999). This makes a purely genetic predisposition unlikely. A higher incidence of psychosis has been found in the second generation of children of parents who migrated rather than in the migrants (Harrison *et al.* 1997). Interestingly the incidence is lower in south London, where there is a greater black population compared to other areas of inner London, which suggests the closeness of community or feeling less of a minority could be a protective factor. The explanations for these disparities continue to be debated (Singh and Burns 2006; Count Me In 2005).

Racism and its impact on mental health

Racial intimidation has been found to damage health, personal relationships and social functioning (Chahall and Julienne 1999). A qualitative study on mental health experiences confirmed that racism had a profound impact on respondents' mental and physical health (Nazroo and O'Connor 2002). Experiencing racism was reported to require an enormous amount of energy to cope with the situation itself and its 'internal' consequences. Racist incidents ranged from bullying at school, verbal abuse and physical attacks to more hidden, institutional racism (collective failures, unwitting behaviours, poorer outcomes) such as job loss and lack of promotion. This does not mean that individuals in organizations are powerless to intervene. On the contrary, we believe that practitioners can be part of a solution to overcoming inequalities in health using their whistle-blowing policies if needed. Practitioners can work alongside colleagues, challenging them if needed, to help them practise in a non-racist manner.

Pathways to services

Black and Asian people are less likely to be registered and have lower attendance rates with their general practitioner. Even when they attend with psychological symptoms, they are less likely to be diagnosed with a psychiatric disorder; but having been diagnosed are less likely to be referred for psychological treatment than white people. Ethnic minorities have more complex pathways to specialist services than do white people and this route is not due to lack of help-seeking behaviour: almost half the black patients seen for initial assessment with psychiatric services had contacted a helping agency in the previous week. The police are also more likely to be involved in the admissions of both black and Asian patients and this is more likely to be done under the Mental Health Act than with white patients. One possible explanation may be that as general practitioners are less involved with these patients they present in crises, often with the emergency departments as the initial point of contact (Bhui *et al.* 2003). However, since being single and lacking a close friend or relative are even more important determinants of compulsory admission it may be that the pattern among ethnic minorities is primarily a reflection of social isolation.

There is a clinical impression that those from ethnic minorities lose contact with the specialist services as time passes. However, studies vary in their findings, with some services maintaining similar contact with white as with ethnic minority patients whilst others seem to have less follow-up. It is possible that service quality rather than ethnicity may be the factor that determines continuity of care.

Gender differences in mental health needs

It has been suggested that the convergence of immigration, changing gender roles and race-related issues create a unique set of risk factors for mental health problems among women from BME backgrounds (Bryce-Laporte and Delores 1981; Sellers *et al.* 2006); one of the reasons for this discrepancy for women migrants in particular may be linked with having to renegotiate family expectations and responsibilities, which may have consequences for their health and well-being.

There is clear evidence of the adverse effects of domestic violence on women's mental health (Golding 1999). However, survivors of domestic violence from black and other minority ethnic communities are less likely to access statutory services, because of racism, culture, religion, immigration status, knowledge of English, safety and gendered decision-making. For example, Asian women could have great difficulty leaving their partners in these circumstances and could be blamed for 'letting down the family's "izzat" (honour)' (Rai and Thiara 1997). Practitioners need to be clear that violent or illegal behaviour is not excused by ethnic or cultural factors.

Mixed-heritage experience

Mixed-heritage families make up a significant percentage of the ethnic minority populations. Mixed-heritage individuals' experience of racism can be more complex due to uncertainty of how they may be perceived. Some mixed-heritage individuals may be accepted by both white and non-white extended families, others may feel that they do not easily find cultural under-standing and solidarity in either community. Children from a mixed heritage have been found to experience exclusion by both black and white peers (Department for Education and Skills 2004). Teachers tended to have low expectations due to perception of 'confused' identity in children of mixed heritage, leading to what is perceived to be challenging forms of behaviour.

System-wide changes

In addressing the inequalities in access and experience, the Delivering Race Equality (DRE) programme (2005) took the following steps:

- improving information (monitoring, dissemination, effectiveness)
- developing responsive services (general services and specifying groups)
- appointing community development workers (CDWs) in every Primary Care Trust.

The core of the CDW's role is to work with and support communities, including the BME voluntary sector, to help build capacity within them, and ensure that the views of the minority communities are taken into account by the statutory and other sectors in the planning and delivery of services.

Working with refugees and asylum seekers

The term 'asylum seeker' refers to those in the process of claiming asylum, while 'refugee' refers to those at all stages of the asylum process including those who have been given a positive decision on their claim. The term 'migrant worker' refers to those who come to a new country for the purpose of seeking employment. Although all of those groups are entitled to free health care (in Britain), asylum seekers and migrant workers have restricted access to welfare benefits and social care services which may have significant impact on their health and well-being.

Common mental health issues among asylum seekers, refugees and migrant workers

For many asylum seekers fear of persecution and trauma in the home country can be compounded by issues in the country of seeking asylum. These may include: adjustment or cultural shock, uncertainty, traumatic life events, racism and stereotyping by host community, language barriers, immigration status and fear of negative decision (Franks *et al.* 2007).

In addition to loss of home, family, language and culture, refugees and asylum seekers need to cope with isolation, lack of employment and poor living conditions in the host country (Harris and Maxwell 2000). Extreme sadness and distress, poor sleep patterns, grief, shame and bereavement are among common psychological responses, as well as experiences we understand as 'anxiety' and 'depression' (Burnett and Fassil 2002). In addition, practical issues such as the uncertainty of the asylum process, difficulty obtaining or lack of legal representation, relocation and destitution all pose further difficulties. Mistrust of authority and fears about confidentiality may also be a barrier to engagement.

Post-traumatic stress disorder is a particularly common result of torture, warfare and other violence (Ashton and Moore 2009; Burnett and Gebremikael 2008). However, there are a range of barriers to accessing secondary mental health care, including a failure to use translation services to enable identification of mental health problems by health care professionals.

Migration is also a source of stress, which may involve difficulties with communication, limited educational and employment opportunities, as well as risk of social isolation and depression. Pickett and Wilkinson (2008) found that the material advantages that accompany higher socio-economic status do not provide an adequate protection against stigma, segregation and discrimination.

'Spiritual well-being' has been found to be linked with lower stress levels, greater resilience and higher self-esteem among a sample of African migrants (Kamya 1997), suggesting that practitioners need to be aware of a range of processes linking socio-cultural factors with well-being when working with immigrant populations (Sellers *et al.* 2006)

Therapeutic and social group work has been found to be highly supportive in reducing isolation, sharing experiences and inspiring hope and resilience (Burnett and Gebremikael 2008). Psychological interventions have been found to be more effective when the help is extended beyond the therapy room into political alliance, advocacy, campaigning and helping with practical problems such as housing and access to social services and coordinating services with other agencies.

Some research suggests that traumatic life events can challenge spiritual beliefs and search for meaning (Carli 1987; Gorst-Unsworth *et al.* 1993); however, for many trauma survivors spiritual life can remain intact.

Creating a culturally capable service

Understanding your own biases

Despite an increasing awareness of culture and a call for reform, it has been suggested that the issues of race have tended to be overlooked in clinical work (Erskine 2002). Sewell (2009) explained how practitioners may feel anxious about broaching the subject of race due to fear of getting it wrong, worry about being perceived as over-compensating for racist feelings, and fear of backlash if it leads to tailored or 'special' provision for BME service users. Peer support, external mentors or community development workers can be used to reflect on and overcome your own fears and anxieties.

Using interpreters

Failure to use interpreters in consultations can reduce identification of mental health issues in service users who do not speak English. This in turn can reduce timely and proactive referrals. Both one-to-one and language line services are available in most practices, and the staff can familiarize themselves with the relevant procedures.

Suggestions for making services more accessible and welcoming of those from BME backgrounds are listed below.

Developing more accessible services

Issues to consider:

- Are BME service users over/under-represented (Count me In Census 2008)?
- Who are the local BME contacts, e.g. CDWs?
- Who are the local BME groups and resources?
- What are the staffing ratios – do they reflect the local population?
- Is there a policy on equal opportunities or discrimination?
- Are interpreters easily available?
- What are the best contexts in which to deliver services?

Suggestions:

- Promote services in different languages
- Consider non-traditional psychology (i.e. community) and healing approaches
- Evidence-base based on the majority culture, may not be culturally appropriate

Check whether there have been any complaints in the past year from BME service users or their families. Also check whether there is language support available for using the complaints procedure.

Mapping out cultural issues

Transparency, collaboration and consideration of power relationships are some of the pertinent features of a culturally sensitive assessment (Patel 2000; Tizard and Phoenix 2002). Practitioners might want to consider and reflect upon the significance of their gender, ethnicity and their role as a health professional in gathering background information (Patel 2004).

Showing a genuine interest in a service user's culture is a useful aid to engagement and building of trust. Sensitizing to the service user's and their family's culture and identifying strengths and the culture clashes is also desirable, as is being mindful of the ethnic cultural factors in relation to current services and local culture (Canino and Spurlock 2000).

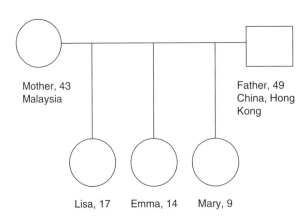

Figure 22.2. A cultural genogram

Mother, 43
Malaysia

Father, 49
China, Hong
Kong

Lisa, 17   Emma, 14   Mary, 9

Cultural genograms can be used to explore cultural and identity issues (Erskine 2002) in a very accessible way. They are helpful in mapping both the family structure and cultural factors.

E.g. Lisa is the eldest in a family of three children. Her mother is Malaysian and her father Chinese, born in Hong Kong. Both parents migrated to the UK as young adults. Lisa lives with her parents and two younger sisters (Figure 22.2).

The next steps include adding: the (==) symbol to identify intercultural marriages, colours to illustrate the cultural composition of each person's cultural identity, and the symbols denoting pride/shame issues. Cultural differences in marriage often have a significant influence on the nature of the relationship and on children. Additional issues to explore may be how different cultural issues were negotiated and the intergenerational consequences of the intercultural union.

The experience of using cultural genograms can be highly emotional and clinicians should remain supportive throughout the process. Rather than using the information as the basis for perpetuating stereotypes, it allows practitioners to generate culturally *and* individually based hypotheses that can help shape the course of treatment.

While it can be too time-consuming to do cultural genograms as a part of everyday general practice clinics it is possible to ask individuals to come back for an additional appointment. Doing genograms – which appear part of the technical/medical realm – can be a useful way of starting to talk about difficult areas of family conflict.

The interview – general principles

The principles of openness and empathy apply in the context of evaluating those from other cultures as they do to the indigenous culture. However, there are also likely to be differences and specific aspects that require special consideration.

- The speed of the interview may be slower than usual if an interpreter is used. While it may be tempting to use a family member for this, it would be inappropriate. If the person is speaking in English comprehension of language may vary and more time may be required. Some cultures are also uncomfortable 'getting to the point' early in the interview.

- Non-verbal communication (use of gestures, body language, eye contact and gaze can be different across cultures). For example, direct eye contact may be regarded as a sign of disrespect among some South American, African and South and East Asian service users (Hollins 2009).
- Verbal communication (accent pronunciation, jargon, tone of voice and intonation differ across cultures). In Somali culture, praise and adulation may be considered to bring about an 'evil eye', causing harm or illness, either purposely or accidentally (Hollins 2009).
- The doctor should speak simply and clearly, avoiding jargon.
- The patient is likely to feel comfortable if issues relating to extended family and culture generally (e.g. diet, customs) are inquired about.

The interview should evaluate the possible range of traumas that a person may experience. Thus sexual orientation, gender, disability, domestic violence, faith, religion and spiritual needs can also be taken into consideration in arriving at a holistic formulation as people can be and often are marginalized along multiple dimensions.

Assessment of trauma in torture survivors

Disclosing traumatic and personal experiences can be assisted by building trust, offering a choice of gender of health worker and an interpreter and working at their own pace. This is possible in general practice but will normally involve a couple of double appointments with an interpreter. Common psychological responses following trauma among refugees and asylum seekers need to be understood in a context of their occurrence and not just as medical diagnoses. Distressing dreams, poor sleep patterns, recurrent vivid memories, headaches, palpitations, sweating, trembling, choking, chest or abdominal discomfort, muscle pains, tiredness, loss of concentration, jumpiness or exaggerated startle reflex, low mood, frequent crying and irritability are all common responses to traumatic events. According to the Medical Foundation for the Care for Victims of Torture (1996) the diagnosis of post-traumatic stress disorder (PTSD) is of limited value and does not reflect the complexity of how historical, political and social factors interact and impact on refugee communities. This relates to the concept of 'complex trauma', which is useful for people with long histories of abuse, abandonment and ongoing traumas which require a different psychological approach from PTSD related to single traumatic episodes.

Torture survivors may be suspicious of the health care workers if they have had experiences of torture in their home countries in which professional agencies including health staff may have been complicit. Survivors of torture may avoid or feel anxious about being touched and examined and it may take time to earn and build trust.

Sexual violation is used by perpetrators as a means of degrading not only individuals and their families but whole communities. Deep shame is the dominant emotional response, and survivors may find disclosure difficult for fear of being ostracized from their own community. Sexual violation may also have resulted in unwanted pregnancy and birth and/or HIV.

Symptoms which may cause concern and warrant referral for more specialist services include: consistent failure to function properly with daily tasks; active suicidal ideation, precipitated by the refusal of asylum claim; detention and threat of deportation; social withdrawal and self-neglect; behaviour or talk not acceptable within the service user's own culture; and aggression (Burnett and Gebremikael 2008).

Formulating the problem

It is important to bear in mind that different cultures have different ways of defining health and illness, and that Western models of mental illness may be interpreted differently as spirit possession, a sign of divine punishment, or normal behaviour. Whilst basic familiarity with the service user's culture is helpful, the most important issue is to ask the service user for explanation and resist making assumptions.

Pointers for formulation – issues to be mindful of

- Never assume that 'BME' people can be viewed as a homogeneous group of people.
- Understand issues that may be faced by people from BME backgrounds, e.g. discrimination, racism, stigma, culture conflict, housing, employment, isolation, culture shock, socio-economic factors, trauma, impact of negative media, concerns over immigration status.
- For asylum seekers and refugees, awareness of how practical issues such as the uncertainty of the asylum process, difficulty obtaining or lack of legal representation, relocation and destitution, may undermine emotional well-being (Ashton and Moore 2009).

Some of the issues relating to the formulation will be illustrated in the case study below.

Case study: F's story

Dear colleague,

Re: FC

Thank you for accepting this referral for an assessment of my patient, F.

F has a diagnosis of schizophrenia and is prescribed antipsychotic medication. Although he had some initial side effects he was and remains compliant. F claims that he has always had 'special powers' since he was very young and converses with voices that he hears.

He has been a mental health service user for nearly three years and during that time there have been significant concerns about risk: two years ago he was sectioned following threatening behaviour to a member of the public and assaulted a police officer and a nurse on admission (following a Section 136). It was during this admission that he received the diagnosis.

He has been keeping quite well although over the last couple of years he has become more withdrawn, no longer working or seeing his friends at The Africa Centre. There may be some cultural issues that I confess I haven't got to grips with but I'm sure the Centre can help you out with this.

I haven't seen much of him over the last 9 months but recently he has been getting more agitated again and I am concerned about increasing risk both to himself and others.

F has episodes of low mood when he suggests he may kill himself when his mother dies (although my understanding is that although HIV positive his mother is healthy and successfully maintained on medication). His low mood seems to exacerbate his psychotic symptoms, strengthening his belief that somehow his father's death puts him and his remaining family in danger. He feels compelled to return to Africa at these times.

He currently lives with his mother, his dad having killed himself. They are in receipt of some home support but there have been some difficulties between F and the home care agency.

I'd be grateful for your perspective of what might be behind his deterioration and whether or not you could give advice on his management. I have looked at the NICE guidelines and wonder if CBT for psychosis might be indicated?

Best wishes
GP

Comment on the case study of FC

This relatively full and empathic letter is nevertheless written primarily from a medical perspective. A culturally sensitive formulation in response would involve understanding F's difficulties from a cultural perspective, such as that his spiritual beliefs are understandable within his culture and not misperceived by the mental health system. F has a status of a 'svikiro', a spiritual leader revered by the community in his home country. He emigrated from Africa to care for his mother, who is HIV-positive, following his father's suicide, and by doing so lost his support networks and spiritual and social status. The diagnosis of schizophrenia may be inappropriate and misleading, masking the wider family, social and political issues causing distress and this would need to be discussed with the MDT.

Risk to self and to others needs to be acknowledged within a recovery-model framework which may involve an honest dialogue with F to develop a collaborative 'crisis' plan. Intervention should involve acknowledging the importance of his mother's well-being and an integrated care package should include respite, housing, financial support and professional development. Community development workers could provide useful information on community groups and resources such as African AIDS helpline. F may need support to get in touch with his spiritual resources and go back to Zimbabwe to 'complete' and perform a ritual on his father's grave and options and possibilities to support him should be considered. CDWs may also advise on community mental health interventions, such as the 'tree of life' narrative approach. The 'tree of life' is used internationally to explore cultural identity and emotional wellness in a way which is not retraumatizing. It also allows us to explore peoples' strengths and abilities and hopes for the future.

Management

The most important advice is to manage the person as an individual not a 'BME group'. It is important not to jump to conclusions about the service user's culture based on what can be read in the literature. Rather, it is helpful to attend to the themes, beliefs and explanations of service users (Vetere and Dowling 2005) and responding accordingly. The contextual perspective of family therapy offers possibilities to understand the interaction of psychological difficulties and social arrangements. It considers social and political issues in personal dilemmas without pathologizing the individual. Likewise, narrative therapy has been identified as a particularly promising critical approach to therapy (Prilleltensky and Nelson 2002).

Although a recent study has found a culturally adapted CBT to yield some positive outcomes in the treatment of psychosis (Rathood *et al.* 2009) its application would be of limited value to F in the case example provided above as his spiritual beliefs were misperceived by the professionals.

The link between social support and mental health has been widely investigated, and evidence suggests that social support is an important protective factor for mental health (Orford 1992). By expanding social networks, community psychology interventions such as the 'tree of life' can greatly improve the emotional well-being of individuals, families and communities.

Pointers for intervention and evaluation

- Critical stance toward cultural appropriateness of existing interventions.
- Applying standard interventions in culturally sensitive ways
- Integration of social and psychological interventions, e.g. community groups and resources.
- Using a 'recovery model' to move beyond symptom-based measures to consideration of what is subjectively meaningful (Care Services Improvement Partnership 2007).

Peer support for practitioners

Self-awareness and reflection are some of the prerequisites for cultural sensitivity in those working with ethnically diverse groups (Patel 2004). Practitioners may construct their own cultural genograms individually or with other colleagues to help understanding of their cultural backgrounds and the influence of their own values and beliefs on practice. Here are some pointers for peer support and questions to be considered.

- Exploring own identities, assumptions and prejudice and development of worldview.
- How may it impact on others who are culturally different from ourselves?
- How safe is it to ask open and direct questions about cultural identity?
- How safe is it to explore our own prejudice? Is 'political correctness' likely to lead to change and reduce stereotyping and discrimination?
- Acknowledge power imbalances between supervisors, trainees and service users, on the basis of 'difference', especially when perceived as 'less able' e.g. expert/service user.

Specific culture-bound emotional experiences

The dominant discussion in transcultural psychiatry is that Asian women present their mental distress as physical symptoms, the 'somatization thesis'. This thesis has masked the complexity of Asian women's mental health issues. Rogers and Pilgrim (2005) point out how the phenomenon could reflect weaknesses of Western psychiatric constructs which assume a neat division of mental and physical illness, a split which is not evident in all cultures. Krause (1989) and Fenton and Sadiq-Sangster (1996) found that in South Asian culture sadness may be articulated as a heart 'sinking' or 'falling', and that this can be understood from the point of view of the centrality of the heart in this culture. In other words Asian women have been found to express their emotional distress in a culturally specific way which in many ways corresponds to a Western psychiatric category of depression.

General practitioners need to consider how they interpret symptoms and avoid both extremes of:

(1) labelling all BME as somatizers and

(2) failing to consider mental health because presentations differ from text book descriptions.

The wealth of experiences from diverse cultures cannot always be fitted into the Western models of mental health and definitions of psychosis.

There is debate about whether the commonly described culture-bound syndromes are best regarded as illness or not and this is reflected in the fact that neither DSM-IV nor ICD-10 includes them in the main body of the text but in the appendix and annex respectively. Moreover some cross-cultural psychiatrists argue that these are false categories arising from misunderstandings of the behaviours and emotional reactions in different cultural settings.

Although hundreds of these culture-bound phenomena are described in the literature, ICD-10 1has condensed them into 13 as follows.

Amok – an unprovoked episode of aggressive behaviour culminating in multiple homicide or suicide. Described in Malaysian culture.

Brain fag syndrome – found in West Africa and attributed to the pressure put on young people to be successful. Tightness in the chest, blurring of vision, pain around the head, anxiety, depression.

Dhat – a type of anxiety in young South Asian men associated with a white discharge in the urine and muscle pains, distortion of penis shape, anxiety, depression and fatigue.

Frigophobia – fear of wind and cold leading to excess clothing. This rare condition is found in China and among Chinese immigrants.

Koro – occurs in Chinese men and is associated with a fear of impending death due to a belief that his penis is shrinking into his abdomen.

Latah – an exaggerated startle response among Indonesians, the Lapps of Scandinavia and some communities in South America. It is associated with an exaggerated flight and fright response followed by echolalia, echopraxia, automatic obedience and a trance-like state.

Nervois – this occurs in women in South and Central America and consists of episodes of sadness or anxiety, distress and somatic complaints.

Piboloktoq – also called Arctic hysteria, it consists of acutely disruptive behaviour preceded by irritability or withdrawal. The person may tear off his clothes and develop echolalia, echopraxia, coprophagia and violence. It ends with either a fit or sleep after which the person has amnesia.

Susto – diverse symptoms including apathy, anxiety, nightmares, depression, anorexia. Seen in Central and South America and in Latino immigrants in the USA.

Taijin kyofusho – found in Japan, it is characterized by fear of offending others and manifests itself as stuttering, making improper facial expressions, flatulence and very high anxiety levels in public places. Hypersensitivity to certain body parts is also prominent such as the eyes or bodily blemishes.

Ufufyane (or Saka) – a trance-like state described in southern Africa in which the person falls under the spell of magic potions administered by rejected lovers or spirit possession. Emotional lability and conversion symptoms are present.

Uqamairineq – described in the Inuit of the Arctic, this presents with sudden paralysis, hallucinations and agitation, which after a few minutes are followed by complete remission.

Windigo (or Witiko) – found in those living in north-eastern Canada, it resembles amok. Homicidal and cannibalistic impulses are directed usually at members of the individual's family. It is accompanied by delusions of transformation into the Windigo monster, a mythical man-eating beast.

Many of these conditions bear a resemblance to either conversion or anxiety disorders and none resembles psychotic illness. Even when a culture-bound condition is identified it should not be the end-point in itself but should take account of the context stressors and be fully assessed within the person's social framework.

Summary

- People from ethnic minorities are at increased risk of mental health problems stemming from a number of social and personal factors.

- Those who are asylum seekers or refugees also have particular vulnerabilities stemming from trauma, uncertainty of status, grief and unemployment.

- Psychological and social interventions are required.

- General practitioners have a key role in providing culturally accessible and sensitive services.

- The symptoms of mental health disorders may differ in those from BME groups and GPs should be aware of this.

- A number of culture-bound disorders have been described and there is debate as to whether these represent psychiatric disorders in themselves or transient distress.

References

Ashton, L., and Moore, J. (2009). *Guide to Providing Mental Health Care Support to Asylum Seekers in Primary Care*. Royal College of General Practitioners.

Bhugra, D., Hilwig, M., Hossein, B., *et al.* (1996). First-contact incidence rate of schizophrenia on Barbados. *British Journal of Psychiatry*, **169**, 587–592.

Bhugra, D., Leff, J., Mallett, R., and Mahy, G. E. (1999). First-contact incidence rate of schizophrenia on Barbados. *British Journal of Psychiatry*, **175**, 28–33.

Bhui, K., Stansfeld, S., Hull, S., *et al.* (2003). Ethnic variations in pathways to and use of specialist mental health services in the UK. Systematic Review. *British Journal of Psychiatry*, **182**, 105–116.

Bryce-Laporte, R. S., and Delores, M. M. (eds.). (1981) *Female Immigrants to the United States: Caribbean, Latin American, and African Experiences*. Washington DC: Research Institute on Immigration and Ethnic Studies, Smithsonian Institution.

Burnett, A. and Fassil (2002) *Meeting the health needs of refugee and asylum seekers in the UK: an information and resource pack for health workers*. NHS/ Department of Health publication.

Burnett, A., and Gebremikael, L. (2008). The psychological wellbeing of refugees and asylum seekers. *Delivering Mental Health in Primary Care*. RCGP Publishers.

Canino, I. A., and Spurlock, J. (2000). *Culturally Diverse Children and Adolescents: Assessment, Diagnosis and Treatment*, 2nd edn. New York: Guilford Press.

Care Services Improvement Partnership (CSIP). (2007). *A Common Purpose: Recovery in Future Mental Health Services*. Royal College of Psychiatrists (RCPsych) and Social Care Institute for Excellence (SCIE).

Carli, A. (1987). Psychological consequences of political persecution. The effects on children of the imprisonment of their parents. *Tiddsskrift for Norsk Psykoloforening*, **24**, 82–93.

Chahall, K., and Julienne, L. (1999). *We Can't All Be White! Racist Victimisation in the UK*. York: Joseph Rowntree Foundation.

Count Me in Census. (2005). Healthcare Commission.

Count Me in Census. (2008). Healthcare Commission.

Department for Education and Skills. (2004). *Understanding the educational needs of mixed heritage pupils*. Retrieved on 17 May 2007 from www. dfes.gov.uk/ research.

Department of Health. (2003). *Department of Health Equality Framework: Priorities for Action*. London: HMSO.

Department of Health. (2005). *Delivering Race Equality: A Framework for Action*. London: HMSO.

Department of Health. (2007). *Positive Steps: Supporting Race Equality in Mental Healthcare*. London: HMSO.

Devon Partnership NHS Trust. (2007/8) *Monitoring Equality Performance Report*. 01/12/08. Available from: http://www.devonpartnership. nhs.uk/uploads/tx_mocarticles/ Trust_Equality_Monitoring_Report_0708. doc.

Equality in Later Life. (2009). A National Study of Older People's Mental Health Services. www.cqc.org.uk/_db/% 20_documents/Equality_in_later_life.pdf.

Erskine, R. (2002). Exposing racism, exploring race. *Journal of Family Therapy*, **24**, 282–297.

Fenton, S., and Sadiq-Sangster, A. (1996). Culture, relativism and mental distress. *Sociology of Health and Illness*, **18**(1), 66–85.

Fernando, S. (2005). 'Ethnic issues' in the mental health field: Is psychiatry racist? 28/11/08: http://www.narrativepractice.com/Articles.

Franks, W., Gawn, N. and Bowden, G. (2007). Barriers to access to mental health services for migrant workers, refugees and asylum seekers. *Journal of Public Mental Health*, **6** (1), 33–41.

Friedli, L. (2009). *Mental Health, Resilience and Inequalities*. Mental Health Foundation and World Health Organization (WHO) Europe: www.euro.who.int/document/e92227.pdf.

Golding, J. M. (1999). Intimate partner violence as a risk factor for mental disorders: a meta-analysis. *Journal of Family Violence*, **14**(2), 99–132.

Gorst-Unsworth, C., Van Velsen, C., and Turner, S. (1993). Prospective pilot study of survivors of torture and organised violence: examining the existential dilemma. *Journal of Nervous and Mental Disease*, **181**, 263–264.

Hardy, K., and Laszloffy, T. (1995) The cultural genogram: Key to training culturally competent family therapists. *Journal of Marital and Family Therapy*.

Harris K., and Maxwell, C. (2000). A needs assessment in a refugee mental health project in North-East London: extending the counselling model to community support. *Medicine, Conflict and Survival*, **16**, 201–215.

Harrison, G., Glazebrook, C., Brewin, J., *et al.* (1997). Increased incidence of psychotic disorders in migrants from the Caribbean to the United Kingdom. *Psychological Medicine*, **4**, 799–806.

Hemsi, L. (1971). Psychiatric morbidity in West Indian Immigrants. *Social Psychiatry*, **2**, 95–100.

Hollins, S. (2009). *Religions, Culture and Healthcare: a practical handbook for use in healthcare environments*, 2nd edn. Oxford: Radcliffe Publishing.

Hutchinson, G., Takei, N., Fahy, T. A., *et al.* (1996). Morbid risk of schizophrenia in first-degree relatives of white and Afro-Caribbean patients with psychosis. *British Journal of Psychiatry*, **171**, 776–780.

Kamya, (1997) In Sellers, S. L, Ward, E. C and Pate, D (2006). Dimensions of depression: a qualitative study of wellbeing among black African immigrant women. *Qualitative Social Work 2006*. **5**, 45

Kirov, G., and Murray, R. M. (1999). Ethnic differences in the presentation of bipolar affective disorder. *European Psychiatry*, **14**, 199–204.

Krause, L. B. (1989). Sinking heart: a Punjabi communication of distress. *Social Science and Medicine*, **29**(4), 563–567

Nazroo, J., and O'Connor, W. (2002). *Ethnic Differences in the Context and Experience of Psychiatric Illness: A Qualitative Study*. London: National Centre for Social Research Healthcare Commission.

Orford, J. (1992). *Community Psychology Theory and Practice*. Chichester: Wiley.

Patel, N. (2000). *Clinical Psychology, 'Race' And Culture: A Resource Pack for Trainers*. Leicester: British Psychological Society.

Patel, N. (2004). Difference and power in supervision: the case of culture and racism. In Fleming, I., and Steen, L. (eds.), *Supervision and Clinical Psychology: Theory, Practice and Perspectives*. Bruner: Routledge.

Pickett, K., and Wilkinson, R. G. (2008). People like us: ethnic group density effects on health. *Ethnicity and Health*, **13**(4), 321–334.

Prilleltensky, I., and Nelson, G. (2002). *Doing Psychology Critically: Making a Difference in Diverse Settings*. New York: Palgrave Macmillan.

Rai, D. K., and Thiara, R. K. (1997) In A. Parmar and A. Sampson, University of East London and A. Diamond, Home Office Domestic Violence: providing advocacy and support to survivors from Black and other minority ethnic communities: Home Office Development and Practice Report.

Rathood, S., Kingdon, D., Phiri, P., *et al.* (2009). *Developing culturally sensitive cognitive behaviour therapy for psychosis for ethnic minority patients*. In 10th Annual International CBT For Psychosis Conference Program, Philadelphia, USAm 21–23 May 2009.

Rogers, A., and Pilgrim, D. (2005). *A Sociology of Mental Health and Illness*, 3rd edn. Maidenhead: Open University Press.

Sainsbury Centre for Mental Health. (2002). *Breaking the Circles of Fear*.

Sellers, S. L., Ward, E. C., and Pate, D. (2006). Dimensions of depression: a qualitative study of wellbeing among black African immigrant women. *Qualitative Social Work*, **5**, 45.

Sewell, H. (2009). *Working with Ethnicity, Race and Culture in Mental Health*. London: Jessica Kingsley.

Singh, S. P., and Burns, T. (2006). Race and mental health: there's more to race than racism. *British Medical Journal*, **333**, 648.

Tizard, B., and Phoenix, P. (2002) *Black, White or Mixed Race: Race and Racism in the Lives of Young People of Mixed Parentage*. London: Routledge.

Vetere, A., and Dowling, E. (2005). *Narrative Therapies with Children and their Families: A Practitioner's Guide to Concepts and Approaches*. London: Routledge.

Further reading

Papadopoulos, I. (2008). *Transcultural Health and Social Care: Development of Culturally Competent Practitioners*. London: Churchill Livingstone Elsevier.

Sewell, H. (2009). *Working with Ethnicity, Race and Culture in Mental Health*. London: Jessica Kingsley.

Shulman, L. (1999). *The Skills of Helping: Individuals and Groups*. Itasca, IL: F.E Peacock.

Useful websites for practitioners and service users

National Mental Health Development Unit: http://www.nmhdu.org.uk/nmhdu/en/our-work/mhep/delivering-race-equality/.

Ferns Associates: http://www.fernsassociates.co.uk/.

Suman Fernando: http://www.sumanfernando.com

Chapter

23

Capacity, compulsory admission and treatment

Cornelis de Wet and James de Pury

Learning objectives

How to assess mental capacity
The role of the general practitioner in compulsory admission
Differences and similarities between the legislation in England and Wales, Scotland, Northern Ireland and Ireland

When a person's disordered mind renders them vulnerable to risk, and they are unable (or unwilling) to accept the necessary help, the decision to intervene may need to be made by others, in some cases their general practitioner. Under such circumstances, one of two legal frameworks may apply, and then depending on the cause of the mental disorder and the nature of the intervention required, the action that is taken could be:

(1) If an adult person *lacks mental capacity for any reason whatsoever*, then medical, welfare and financial decisions can be made on their behalf under the Mental Capacity Act 2005 (in England and Wales) or the Adults with Incapacity (Scotland) Act 2000. Such 'best interest decisions' can be made by anyone involved with the person's care (and include a range of medical, social or financial decisions), but can only be justified when made exclusively in the best interest of the person lacking capacity. General practitioners may be expected to decide on medical treatment or investigations for incapacitated patients who are unable to fully understand its purpose and give consent. The Mental Capacity Act 2005 provides a legal definition of capacity, the process for arriving at a decision that is in the person's best interest, and mechanisms for the incapacitated person's wishes to be considered in the decision making process.

The Mental Capacity Act (and Mental Incapacity Act in Scotland) was introduced to provide the first statutory framework to existing common law, and to ensure consistency with European Human Rights legislation.

In the Republic of Ireland and Northern Ireland there is no specific mental capacity legislation, and common law still prevails, but professionals are well advised to be guided by the principles that underpin the Mental Capacity Act.

(2) If a person *suffers a mental disorder and presents a risk to themselves or others*, and they refuse intervention (due to lacking capacity or not), then they can be compelled to accept admission and treatment for their mental disorder under the relevant Mental Health Act. General practitioners play an important role in deciding when and whether to admit patients to hospital for compulsory treatment for their mental

illness. The Mental Health Act does not apply to people lacking capacity for any reason other than a mental disorder and so cannot be used in situations involving intoxication, delirium or unconsciousness. Neither can the Mental Health Act be used to enforce any interventions other than the treatment of the individual's mental disorder. In practice, the use of the Mental Health Act applies to a relatively small number of people and circumstances compared with the Mental Capacity Act. The decisions to detain and treat are made only by appropriately clinically trained and approved professionals along clearly formalized procedures which include a number of statutory safeguards, such as second opinions, tribunals and appeal proceedings to protect the person's rights. In contrast to the Mental Capacity Act, the rationale for decisions made under the Mental Health Act can be in the detained person's best interests, for their own health and safety *or* be intended to protect others.

The Mental Capacity Act

The England and Wales Mental Capacity Act 2005 (MCA) and Adults with Incapacity (Scotland) Act 2000 are relevant to everyone who may care for a person who lacks capacity, whether in a professional role (e.g. nurses, doctors, social workers, etc.) or informally (e.g. family, friends, carers). Every day, millions of decisions are made on behalf of incapacitated people, ranging from seemingly small everyday care and welfare decisions, to more formal and important financial, legal or medical decisions. The Act will apply in all areas of medical and social care for people who are unable to make decisions for themselves, and the MCA is particularly relevant to doctors working in general practice, emergency medicine, care of the elderly and palliative care. The principles of the Act apply equally to informal caring acts in the community, e.g. helping a forgetful neighbour with her groceries, assisting a stranger collapsing in the street. Before the MCA, these decisions were made and could be justified under common law, but now this relatively new Act provides a clear statutory responsibility decisions of this kind, in order to provide legal protection not only to incapacitated people, but also to those who have to care and make decisions for them. The Act provides guidance for everyone on how to assess a person's capacity and how to ensure that decisions are made in the intersts of that individual.

The Act is underpinned by the following five core principles:

- Every adult is assumed to have capacity to make his or her own decisions unless proven otherwise.
- People retain the right to make their own decisions even if their decisions seem unwise or eccentric.
- All people must be given the appropriate help and support in making their own decisions before it is decided that they are unable to do so themselves.
- If a decision has to be made on behalf of a person who lacks capacity, the decision must only be made in that person's best interest. By definition, a best interest decision cannot include bringing about the person's death.
- Decisions made on behalf of people who lack capacity should be made with the least amount of restriction of their freedom and human rights.

Types of actions health staff commonly perform on, or on behalf of, incapacitated people may include administering treatment or medication or taking them to clinic or hospital, often without their explicit consent. Doctors may often have to perform medical or dental examinations, diagnostic tests, medical procedures, surgery or emergency resuscitation, by necessity, without the patient's consent.

General practitioners may also be asked to become involved with decisions about people's personal care and household management, e.g. help with washing, feeding, self-care, cleaning, mobility, shopping or paying for rent or services. Bigger decisions, such as making someone move home permanently, may require an application to the Court of Protection.

In England and Wales the Act is supplemented with a Code of Practice, which offers case examples and guidance on the practical application of the legislation. The Scottish Act does not have a separately published Code of Practice.

Certain kinds of decision are specifically excluded under the Mental Capacity Act. These include decisions made on behalf of an incapacitated person may *not* include consent to marriage, civil partnership, consent to sexual relations or divorce, or decisions relating to adoption, parental responsibilities or fertilization treatment, even if these decisions are thought to be in the person's best interest. Other decisions need to be referred to the courts for decision, for example withholding nutrition from people in a vegetative state, bone marrow or organ donation by an incapacitated person, or treatments that are untested, or not indisputably in the person's interest (such as may be used in clinical research trials). Decisions to detain and treat people who suffer with mental illness are also excluded from the MCA. These decisions are made under the Mental Health Act (below), and in these cases the Mental Health Act 'trumps' the Mental Capacity Act. The Mental Capacity Act governs all other decisions made for people who cannot decide for themselves.

The Mental Capacity Act 2005 in England and Wales introduced a number of specific new provisions:

- The Act clarifies the law in connection with care and treatment of incapacitated people provided for people who are unable to consent to this care. In doing so it provides legal protection (i.e. indemnity from liability) for people who give treatment for (or make decisions on behalf of) people who cannot consent, provided they act in good faith and in accordance with the principles of the Act. By the same token, the Act makes it a criminal offence to ill-treat or wilfully neglect an incapacitated person.

- The Act makes the first provision for people to make legally binding Advance Decisions about the medical treatment they would want to receive in the event of their becoming incapacitated at a future time, including 'Living Wills'. Advance Decisions may include *refusal* of life-saving or other specific treatments (i.e. advance refusals), but cannot include a demand for any specific treatment or any form of assisted suicide (Department of Health 2010). To be valid, an Advance Decision has to be signed, dated and witnessed, and be readily available to the person's treating clinical team. In addition, the clinician should ensure that they are absolutely certain of the current validity of a written Advance Directive before considering departure from any procedures necessary to prolong life.

- The Act provides for the appointment of certain people to assist in making decisions on behalf of people who lack capacity. The Act enables any adult to give other people (partner, friends, relatives or anyone of their choice) power of attorney to make legal, financial and/or welfare decisions on their behalf in the event of their becoming incapacitated at a future time. Before the MCA, powers of attorney were limited to financial decisions only, but since 2007 a person can donate powers to make different decisions (e.g. health, legal, financial) to different people. Where an incapacitated person is unable to formally give power of attorney to someone themselves, then the Court of Protection can appoint a deputy to act on the person's behalf (Age Concern 2009). The Act created a special Court and Public Guardian to oversee these deputies and attorneys, and to investigate any allegations of abuse. Finally, for people who have no friends or family to speak on their behalf, and for whom potentially life-changing decisions have to be made (e.g. serious medical treatment, changing residential placement) the Act provides for the appointment of an Independent Mental Capacity Advocate (IMCA) to support and represent them in the decision.

When can someone be said to lack capacity?

Capacity is decision-specific and time-specific, i.e. capacity has to be assessed *in relation to a particular decision, at a particular time*. A person who suffers a medical condition (e.g. head injury, shock, intoxication, stroke, delirium, confusion, psychosis, learning disability, etc.) may still have capacity to make certain decisions, and should not be assumed to lack capacity on the basis of their medical diagnosis alone. The judgement of someone's capacity should also not be influenced by any other unjustified assumptions about their age, appearance, intellect, religious beliefs or culture, etc. Every adult should be assumed to have capacity until an assessment indicates specific reasons to doubt their capacity. In certain cases a person's capacity may *fluctuate over time* (e.g. bipolar disorder, confusional states), or their incapacity may be only *temporary* (e.g. acute illness, intoxication). Wherever possible decisions should be delayed until a time when the person has recovered or regained sufficient capacity to make the decision for themselves, or at least participate in the decision more.

A person can be deemed to be incapable of making a particular decision, at a particular time, if they are *unable to do any one of the following*:

- *understand* the information relevant to their decision, despite all reasonable efforts to enhance their comprehension of the facts (e.g. simple language, using visual aids, etc.)
- *retain* (or remember) the information for long enough to make a decision
- *weigh* the information and consider the consequences of deciding one way or another, or the consequences of not making a decision at all
- *communicate* their decision verbally, in writing, or with other physical indications (for example: writing, blinking, pointing).

The assessment of capacity must be about a particular decision at a particular time and not about a range of decisions or decisions in general. If someone cannot make complex decisions this does not mean that they are incapable of making simple decisions. All reasonable efforts should be made to enhance decision-making, including allowing the person to talk things over with someone they know or trust, giving them adequate time and support, and making numerous attempts to help them reach a final decision. Capacity to make a particular decision requires full understanding of all the relevant information. This information must be shared with the person assessing capacity, but confidentiality and consent to disclosure must be respected as far as possible.

Who decides whether someone lacks capacity?

Before a person (e.g. professional or carer) can make a decision or act on behalf of another person, they have to have reasonable grounds for believing that the person lacks capacity to make the decision at that particular time. It is the responsibility of the person intending to act or decide on the person's behalf (i.e. the decision-maker) to judge whether the person has capacity or not. Although clinical teams may collaborate in providing care for incapacitated people, it is up to the individual making the best interest decision for the person to satisfy themselves that the person they are making a decision for indeed lacks capacity.

A medical or other expert opinion on capacity might be indicated where the decision to be made (or its consequences) is very important (e.g. serious medical treatment, re-housing), or the person suffers a condition that is best understood by someone with expertise in that area. A specialist opinion may also be advised when a person repeatedly makes decisions that put them at risk, or when a person expresses different views to different people, or their capacity is disputed or might be contested at a later stage (e.g. contesting a will). An expert assessment of capacity (by a psychologist or psychiatrist) will always be required where a certification of capacity is required to sign a legal document, or where the courts require a formal decision on someone's capacity, as in fitness to plead, for example.

How is it decided what is in a person's best interests?

The Act provides protection from liability to people who make decisions and perform acts on behalf of incapacitated people. It gives legal protection to someone who, say, needs to touch a person or enter their property without their permission to help them, from later accusations of assault or trespassing. This is similar to actions previously performed 'under common law', and the legal protection is valid without the need for legal formalities. Care can proceed as if the incapacitated person had given their consent, without fear of liability, provided that the person lacks capacity, and the action is the least restrictive and in their best interest (i.e. that the principles of the Act have been applied).

To ensure that a decision made on behalf of a person who lacks capacity is in their best intersts, it is the clear responsibility of the person making the specific decision to ensure that:

- the decision is not influenced by preconceived assumptions or prejudices based on the person's age, appearance, culture, language, etc.
- all relevant circumstances have been considered – at least all circumstances of which the decision-maker is aware and reasonably regards as relevant
- the incapacitated person has been allowed and encouraged to express their views, and to participate in the decision as far as is reasonably practical (maybe assisted by an advocate)
- the person's past and present wishes, feelings, beliefs and values have been taken into account as far as possible.

Where practicable and appropriate, the decision-maker should take into account the views of others engaged in caring for the person, anyone named by the person to be consulted on particular matters (e.g. relative or advocate) or anyone legally appointed to act on their behalf (e.g. a deputy of the Court of Protection, donee of lasting power of attorney). Blood relatives do not necessarily have to be involved if they are not involved in their care. When important decisions about serious medical treatment, long hospital admissions or changes in accommodation are considered, and the person is entirely unbefriended, an Independent Mental Capacity Advocate (IMCA) should be appointed.

Quite reasonably, the more important the action or decision, or the greater its consequences, the greater is the burden of proof that these principles have been considered. For example, a carer helping someone get dressed does not stringently have to go through the procedure above on a daily basis, while a doctor performing an amputation will be expected to apply (and record) professional steps at assessing capacity, and to demonstrate that attempts have been made to include the person and their close ones in the decision, that the decision was made in the person's best interest and that less serious interventions were considered. The law is also 'reasonable' and in England and Wales the Code of Practice specifically acknowledges that such rigour will not always be possible in emergency situations.

In summary, when making a decision (or acting) on behalf of a person who lacks capacity, always ensure that all the following steps have been followed (and where appropriate, recorded in case notes):

- First, assume capacity. Explain the relevant information and ask their opinion. If in doubt, *assess the person's capacity to make the particular decision, at the particular time, i.e. assess whether they can* understand *all the information relevant to the decision,* retain *the information for long enough to make a decision,* weigh *the information, and consider the consequences of their decision, and* communicate *their decision.*

- If the person lacks capacity, consider whether anything can be done to *enhance their capacity* (e.g. given better explanation or more time), whether the person is likely to regain capacity at a future time (e.g. fluctuations or recovery), and whether the decision can safely be postponed until a time when their capacity has improved. Consider seeking a second opinion on the person's capacity (from a psychiatrist or psychologist) if the person repeatedly makes decisions that put them at risk, if there is dispute over their capacity (or might be in the future), or if the decision to be made is a very important one or has legal implications.

- Before making a decision (or taking an action) on behalf of an incapacitated person, *encourage them to participate in the decision as far as practicable.* Consider their past and present wishes and appropriate information that may be relevant to the decision, including any previously held instructions (or Advance Statements).

- *Consult the views of others interested in the person's welfare, for example, family, carers, advocates, IMCA (where appropriate), donee of power of attorney, deputy of the Court, or any other named person.*

- Finally, when making the decision (or acting) on behalf of the incapacitated person, remember to consider other, less restrictive options that can achieve the desired outcome, and ensure that the decision is *in the person's best interests only.*

- *Record* the assessment of capacity, consultations with others, and rationale for decisions made in the person's case records, in free text. There are no statutory forms required by the Mental Capacity Act, but case records should be appropriately clear, detailed, signed and dated, as usual.

The Mental Health Act

The purpose of the Mental Health Act is intended to protect and regulate the care of people who require assessment or treatment for their mental disorder, but who are unable or unwilling to consent. The Scottish Parliament has its own powers over mental health legislation and passed its own Mental Health (Care and Treatment) (Scotland) Act in 2003 (Office of Public Sector Information 2003). Although the Scottish legislation has the same broad aims as the England and Wales Mental Health Act 1983 (as amended 2007; Department of Health Code of Practice

2008), there are some differences between the two, likewise in respect of the Irish Mental Health Act (2001) and the Mental Health (Northern Ireland) Order 1986.

At its core, the Mental Health Act in all the above jurisdictions has one purpose. This is to provide the legal framework to justify and authorize the use of compulsory detention, assessment and treatment (whether in hospital or in the community), without the consent of a person with a serious mental disorder where it is considered that they are a risk to their own health and/or safety or to protect others. Such detention can only take place where the person has been clinically assessed by professionals with the appropriate training. Furthermore, in their pursuance of this decision, there must be no other way to prevent their health deteriorating or prevent them from causing harm to themselves or others.

Underpinning the approach in England and Wales, it is important to understand the Guiding Principles in the Code of Practice. In essence, these principles aim to provide those responsible for making decisions under the Act the means to inform their practice based on a series of values in order to help support their deliberations when it comes to considering the use of compulsory powers. These values are also in place to ensure compliance with the Human Rights Act as far as is possible when detaining someone against their wishes. While there has been a recent decline in general practitioner involvement in compulsory detention, new policies promoting GP-led commissioning and the forthcoming Mental Health Strategy may lead to more involvement in both detention and treatment orders.

Guiding principles

These are derived from the principles enshrined in the Mental Health Act England and Wales (as amended 2007).

Purpose: any decisions taken under the Act must be taken with a view to minimizing the undesirable effects of mental disorder, by maximizing the safety and well-being (mental and physical) of the patients, promoting their recovery and protecting other people from harm.

Respect: those responsible for making decisions under the Act must recognize and respect the diverse needs, values and circumstances of each patient, including their race, religion, culture, gender, age, sexual orientation and any disability. They must also consider the patient's views, wishes and feelings (whether at the time or expressed in advance) so far as they are reasonably ascertainable, and follow those wishes wherever practicable and consistent with the purpose of the decision. There should be no unlawful discrimination.

Participation: all patients must be given the opportunity to be involved, as far as is practicable in the circumstances, in planning, developing and reviewing their own treatment and care to ensure that this is delivered in a way that it is as appropriate and effective for them as possible. The involvement of carers, family members and other people who have an interest in the patient's welfare should be encouraged (unless there are particular reasons to the contrary) and their views taken seriously.

Least restriction: those taking action without a patient's consent must attempt to keep to a minimum the restriction they place on the patient's liberty, having regard for the purpose for which the restrictions are imposed.

Effectiveness, efficiency and equity: people taking decisions under the Act must seek to use the resources available to them and to patients in the most effective, efficient and equitable way to meet the needs of patients and achieve the purpose for which the decision was taken.

No one principle is more important than the others and in individual situations, the responsibility rests with the decision-makers who are considering the use of compulsory

Table 23.1. Inclusion and exclusion under the Mental Health Acts

Mental Health Act	Includes	Excludes
England and Wales Mental Health Act (amended 2007)	Dangerous and severe personality disorder (DSPD) and learning disability associated with grossly irresponsible or abnormally aggressive behaviour; dementia; paedophilia	Dependence on alcohol or drugs
Mental Health (Care and Treatment) (Scotland) Act (2003)	Any mental illness, personality disorder, mental impairment (dementia) or learning disability	Sexual deviance, dependence on drugs or alcohol, behaviour causing alarm, distress or harassment or acting imprudently
Mental Health (Northern Ireland) Order (1986)	Learning disability; dementia	Personality disorder; substance misuse or dependence
Mental Health Act Ireland (2001)	'Severe' dementia or 'significant' intellectual disability	Personality disorder, substance misuse and 'social deviancy'

powers to weigh each of these in order to support best practice when applying the provisions of the Act.

The Scottish Act has its own ten, very similar guiding principles but also includes *reciprocity*, whereby the individual's obligation to comply imposes a parallel obligation on authorities to provide care for the person beyond the period of compulsion.

Who can be detained under the MHA?

Any person who appears to be suffering a mental disorder, the nature or degree of which may threaten their health and safety or the safety of those around them, may be considered liable to be detained under the Mental Health Act if they refuse to accept informal intervention. The definitions of mental disorder are broadly similar in the various jurisdictions and the Acts refer to 'any disorder or disability of the mind' (England and Wales), 'a state of mind which affects a person's thinking, perceiving, emotion or judgement to the extent that he requires care or medical treatment in his own interests or the interests of other persons' (Northern Ireland and Ireland). Thus conditions such as bipolar disorder, schizophrenia, eating disorders, depression and so on are included in all. Learning disability and dementia are contained within the definition but only if there are associated features that require compulsory treatment such as aggression or psychosis. There are, however, differences with regard to the exclusions. All exclude substance misuse or dependence but there are differences in relation to personality disorder, learning disability and paraphilias (see Table 23.1). While these distinctions may seem of theoretical interest, it is crucial that GPs are aware of the inclusions and exclusions in their own jurisdictions when deciding on the appropriateness of compulsory admission.

The 2007 amendment of the England and Wales Mental Health Act 1983 repealed a previous exclusion of 'immoral conduct or sexual deviancy' so as to bring paedophilia (and other 'clinically significant' paraphilias) into the definition of a mental disorder.

Table 23.2. Duration of general practitioner's recommendation/request

England and Wales	14 days
Scotland	72 hours
Northern Ireland	2 days (up to 14 in exceptional circumstances on application to the Commission)
Ireland	7 days

How can someone be detained under the MHA?

In England and Wales a person who is liable to be detained is compulsorily admitted to hospital by the decision of the professionals who conduct a Mental Health Act Assessment, or by an order of a Court.

A Mental Health Act Assessment under the English and Welsh Act comprises two independent doctors (at least one of whom must be approved as having specific expertise in mental disorder under Section 12) and an Approved Mental Health Professional (AMHP, who is usually a social worker, but could be a mental health nurse, psychologist or occupational therapist, who has received appropriate training). There are many general practitioners with an interest in mental health who undergo training to gain Section 12 approval in order to undertake additional Mental Health Act Assessments, who work as part of their surgery, or often, on out-of-hours duties. Where there is concern for a person's mental health and risks, any professional (or the patient's nearest relative) can request for the person to undergo a Mental Health Act Assessment to consider the need for compulsory admission. Ordinarily Mental Health Act assessments are coordinated and convened by the AMHP. These can assess a person anywhere, but most commonly this occurs in hospitals, clinics or sometimes in a person's own home. The person's own general practitioner is usually asked to assess the person with the AMHP (with or without the second doctor present, depending on the circumstances). These assessments may also be convened in so-called 'places of safety', which can include police stations if the person came to their attention first.

The police have powers to convey a person *in public* (Section 136) to a 'place of safety' such as hospital or police station for up to 72 hours in order for consideration to be given to further intervention or a MHA Assessment. In other circumstances, warrants can be obtained via the Courts under Section 135 to allow mental health professionals the authority to convey a person without their consent from a specified location in the community, to be taken to a 'place of safety' and for them to undergo a full Mental Health Act assessment there.

In all jurisdictions the relevant professionals must complete specific statutory MHA forms (stating the reasons for and place of admission), before a person can be legally detained. The slightest omission or error in completing these forms may render them invalid, and the person's detention would not be legal. It is also important to be aware that, once a general practitioner has assessed a person who potentially might be admitted compulsorily to hospital, the assessment is only valid for a certain time within which the individual must be seen in an approved centre – the time periods are shown in Table 23.2.

It is not unusual for a Mental Health Act assessment to conclude with no intervention, or with the person agreeing to informal admission or treatment. If the person refuses and the professionals undertaking the Mental Health Act assessment unanimously agree that the criteria are met then the person can be immediately detained and conveyed to hospital, with the support of the police if necessary. The main powers under the civil Sections are as follows:

Emergency detention (Section 4)

If required in an emergency a person can be detained for up to 72 hours if recommended by only one doctor and another professional, usually a specially trained social worker, i.e. an Approved Mental Health Professional (AMHP) in England and Wales. Similar provisions apply under the Scottish Act and any medical practitioners, including general practitioners, can issue the certificate and where practicable must have consulted with and obtained the consent of a Mental Health Officer (MHO) in Scotland. This is only used where there would be significant delay in obtaining a second doctor to attend an assessment and is therefore rarely used.

Short-term detention

A person can be detained in hospital for up to 28 days, i.e. Section 2 in England and Wales. This requires two medical recommendations (one with special approval) and an application by an AMHP.

In Scotland detention under Section 44 requires a recommendation by one specially trained doctor (a psychiatrist) and agreement by a Mental Health Officer (MHO) and the detention period is for 28 days. In Ireland an admission order can detain a person for up to 21 days under Section 15. In Northern Ireland admission for assessment can be for up to 7 days and for treatment for up to 6 months in the first instance.

In Northern Ireland an application for detention is made by the patient's nearest relative or an approved social worker and recommended by a registered medical practitioner. The medical recommendation along with the reasons for the recommendation are then conveyed to the admitting hospital managers and an examination is carried out normally by the responsible medical officer but failing this by any medical practitioners in the hospital or by a medical practitioner appointed by the Mental Health Commission. If approved compulsory admission for assessment is not to exceed 7 days. Detention for treatment can be for up to 6 months.

In Ireland an application is made by a relative, police officer, member of the public or an 'authorized officer' to a registered medical practitioner (RMP), who then examines the person within 24 hours of receipt of this. The RMP then makes a recommendation to the clinical director of the approved centre. If the consultant psychiatrist is satisfied that the person has a mental disorder within the meaning of the Act the admission order is completed (Section 15).

All the Acts require that once in hospital the person should have their rights explained, including their right of appeal to an independent panel with the support of a free and independent legal representative and an independent advocate.

Long-term detention

In Ireland an admission order may be followed by a renewal which extends the person's detention for another 3 months, which may be extended by a further 6 months, and then extended to further periods of 12 months' detention, subject to appeal.

In England, Wales and Scotland a person may be detained, from the outset, for a compulsory treatment period of up to 6 months. Such a detention in England and Wales under Section 3 of the Mental Health Act 1983 requires a person to be admitted to hospital for treatment but, as with Section 2, patients subject to Section 3 may be granted periods of leave from hospital to assist with their gradual rehabilitation back into the community. In Scotland detention under a Compulsory Treatment Order or CTO (not to be confused with a Community Treatment Order as applies in England and Wales; see below) does not inevitably lead to hospital admission and a person may receive the entirety of their treatment in the community, consistent with the principle of least restriction. In England, Wales and Scotland these longer-term provisions include an additional safeguard, which allows a person's nearest relative (in England and Wales, which since 2007 includes civil partners) or named person and primary carer (in Scotland) to have their objection to the detention heard. After the first six months clinicians may apply for the renewal of the order as long as the legal criteria still apply and pass the challenge of rigorous appeals proceedings.

Detaining a patient who is voluntary

In a hospital, where there is concern for the mental well-being of a patient wanting to take their own discharge, or where it may be that informal or voluntary admission of the patient is no longer appropriate, in certain circumstances they can be detained by a registered mental health or learning disabilities nurse under Section 5(4), for up to 6 hours; or by an approved clinician or a nominated approved clinician or registered medical practitioner in charge of the patient's care, under Section 5(2), for up to 72 hours in order for their mental state to be assessed by appropriately qualified staff, or for a full Mental Health Act assessment to be carried out.

In Northern Ireland Section 5 of the Act allows for the emergency detention of a person already in hospital for up to 72 hours, as in Scotland. In Ireland the emergency detention period must not exceed 24 hours. Thereafter, all jurisdictions require that a decision must be made to allow the patient to self-discharge or apply another section of the relevant Act.

Supervised Community Treatment (in England, Wales and Scotland only)

A person may be well enough to remain in the community, but be required to comply with conditions to ensure that they accept. Under a Community Treatment Order (or Section 17A) in England and Wales, the responsible clinician is able to set conditions on a person's discharge from Section 3, such as adherence, but not compulsion to enforce, to medication without the patient's consent, identify a specified place of residence, their attendance for appointments or any other conditions agreed with an AMHP. The responsible clinician has the power to recall the person back to hospital at any time to reassess the person, or to reinstate treatment, if necessary, under another term of Section 3. Under the Scottish Act a Compulsory Treatment Order can compel a person to accept treatment in the community from the outset, and it is not required that a person must first be detained under long-term provisions in hospital. The introduction of supervised community treatment in England, Wales and Scotland reflects the shift in mental health service delivery away from hospital-based care and toward more community and home-based treatments. In Scotland, where compulsory community treatment was first introduced (in 2005), the total number of people subject to long-term compulsion remained stable, but with about a third of people being treated in the community. Although not yet strictly supported by clinical outcome studies, similar legal mechanisms for compelling mentally disordered people to agree to community treatment on an outpatient basis had previously been introduced in North America, Australia, New Zealand and Israel (Institute of Psychiatry 2007). Community treatment orders are not included in the Irish Mental Health Act 2001 or under the Northern Ireland Order (1986).

From time to time courts can order a mentally disordered offender's transfer to hospital for assessment or treatment of their mental illness. Rather than sentencing a mentally disordered person to prison, courts often sentence offenders to hospital for treatment of their mental illness in forensic units with appropriate levels of security. Once in hospital they can appeal against their detention or be discharged by their doctor, unless their crime was particularly serious, in which case they are likely to remain subject to supervision and restrictions by the Ministry of Justice for very many years.

What treatment can be given against a person's will?

In considering the use of compulsory powers, the professionals making the decision to recommend admission under the amended Act are required to justify not only that the grounds for admission are met, but that the hospital where this is planned has the appropriate medical treatment to meet the patient's needs.

The definition of medical treatment can include nursing, psychological therapies, specialist mental health 'habilitation' (meaning equipping someone with skills and abilities they have never had), rehabilitation and care.

For the person who has been formally admitted and detained under Section 2 and Section 3, the Mental Health Act allows their compulsory treatment for their mental disorder even if this is without their consent. This is also the case for the majority of patients who are admitted via the courts to receive treatment for their mental disorder. Exclusions apply to those patients who are admitted and placed under some of the shorter-term powers (under Sections 4, 5(2), 5(4) or 136) and certain Court Orders (Section 35) who cannot be compelled to receive any medication, without their consent, and, if so required, it is only to be given based on the justification for its use under common law (or equivalent of the Mental Capacity Act)

A person can be prescribed any treatment for their mental disorder without their consent for a period of up to 3 months (or 2 months in Scotland). In England and Wales, beyond 3 months of detention, it is the statutory responsibility of the responsible clinician to determine the individual's capacity and consent to treatment, and, if they refuse treatment or lack the capacity to understand the nature, likely effects and purpose of medication, then a Second Opinion Approved Doctor (SOAD, appointed by the Care Quality Commission) is required to visit the patient and consult with professionals involved with their care. The result of their discussion will then determine the agreed medication to be given to the detained patient and will also specify the method of administration, the route and the maximum dosage and, often, the length of time any specific medication is authorized. Consent to treatment for the patient who is detained under the Mental Health Act relates only to psychotropic medication authorized for the treatment of the mental disorder. It does not permit the authorization of medication to be given for any physical disorder. This is covered by the provisions of the Mental Capacity Act.

There are specific rules governing electroconvulsive therapy (ECT). Under the Mental Health Act 2007 ECT cannot be given to a person who refuses, and has the mental capacity to refuse, at any stage of their detention, nor can it be given to a person who has a valid advance decision in relation to not receiving ECT. In Ireland ECT can be given to a detained patient against their will but this requires a second independent psychiatric opinion.

Summary

- To demonstrate the capacity to make a decision, a person must be able to understand and retain the relevant information, weigh the consequences of each of their options, and be able to communicate their decision.

- Judging a person's capacity should be considered in relation to a particular decision at a particular time.
- In England and Wales the Mental Capacity Act 2005 provides a framework for making medical, welfare and financial decisions on behalf of people who lack capacity. In Scotland, the Incapacity (Scotland) Act 2000 is the relevant legislation.
- The Mental Health Act can be used to compel a person to accept treatment for their mental disorder, but not to accept any other medical or social interventions.
- The general practitioner has a key role in initiating compulsory admission.
- The legislation, while differing in detail, is broadly similar in the various jurisdictions.

References

Age Concern: Factsheet 22 September 2009. Available at: http://www.ageuk.org.uk/publications/health-and-wellbeing-publications/.

Department of Health (2008).*Code of Practice to Mental Health Act 1983* (2008 revised). London: TSO (England and Wales).

Department of Health. (2010). *NHS Choices*. Available at: http://www.nhs.uk/livewell/endoflifecare/pages/rightsandchoices.aspx.

Institute of Psychiatry. (2007). *International Experiences of Using Community Treatment Orders*. Available at: http://www.iop.kcl.ac.uk/news/downloads/final2ctoreport8march07.pdf

Mental Health Act 2001. Available at: http://www.mhcirl.ie/Mental_Health_Act_2001/Mental_Health_Act_2001.pdf (Ireland).

The Mental Health (Northern Ireland) Order 1986. Available at: www.legislation.gov.uk/nisi/1986/595.

Office of Public Sector Information. (2000). Adults with Incapacity (Scotland) Act. Available at: http://www.opsi.gov.uk/legislation/scotland/acts2000/20000004.htm

Office of Public Sector. (2003). Mental Health (Care and Treatment) (Scotland) Act 2003 Information. Available at: http://www.opsi.gov.uk/legislation/scotland/acts2003/asp_20030013 (Scotland)

Fennell. P. (2007) *Mental Health: The New Law*. Bristol: Jordans.

Jones, R. (2009). *Mental Health Act Manual*, 12th edn. London: Sweet and Maxwell.

Useful websites

Mental Capacity Act 2005 (England and Wales): http://www.opsi.gov.uk/acts/acts2005/20050009.htm.

Mental Capacity Act 2005 Code of Practice, Chapter 11 (England and Wales): http://www.dca.gov.uk/menincap/legis.htm#codeofpractice.

Adults with Incapacity (Scotland) Act, 2000: http://www.opsi.gov.uk/legislation/scotland/acts2000/20000004.htm.

Care Quality Commission (England and Wales): www.cqc.org.uk.

Mental Welfare Commission for Scotland: www.mwcsof.org.uk.

Mental Health Commission (Ireland): www.mhcirl.ie.

National Mental Health Development Unit (within Department of Health, England and Wales): www.nmhdu.org.uk.

Office of Public Guardian (England and Wales) Mental Capacity Act 2005 matters (England and Wales): www.publicguardian.gov.uk.

Further reading

Barber P., Brown R., and Martin, D. (2009). *Mental Health Law in England and Wales: A Guide for Mental Health Professionals*. Exeter: Learning Matters.

Useful information for patients and carers

http://www.patient.co.uk/doctor/Consent-To-Treatment-(Mental-Capacity-and-Mental-

Health-Legislation).htm (England and Wales).

http://www.carersscotland.org/
Policyandpractice/Keylegislationandpolicy/
MentalHealthAct2003 (Scotland).

http://ec.europa.eu/health/ph_determinants/
life_style/mental/green_paper/
mental_gp_co062.pdf (Northern Ireland).

http://www.mhcirl.ie/ (Ireland).

Useful telephone numbers

Mental Health Commission, Ireland: 01 6362400.

Mental Welfare Commission for Scotland: 0131 3138777 or 08003896809.

The Care Quality Commission (England and Wales): 0300616161.

Regulation and Quality Improvement Authority (Northern Ireland): 02890517501.

Appendix: Alternative and complementary therapies

Learning objectives

Familiarity with the common herbal and complementary therapies in current use
To become familiar with the evidence base for their use

Complementary and alternative therapies mean different things to different people. They might refer to herbal and vitamin supplements, acupuncture, meditation or traditional healing methods. Alternative therapies replace medical or conventional interventions while complementary therapies are used in addition to these.

The general public is increasingly interested in alternatives to conventional medicines in the treatment of all illnesses, including psychiatric disorders. Indeed psychiatric disorders are the most common reasons for individuals resorting to these remedies. In Britain 14–30% of the population use these therapies and acupuncture is the most popular. A US study by Kessler et al. (2001) found that 56% of those with severe depression in a US population chose alternative therapies in the year before the study. In light of the popularity of these products general practitioners need to be aware of the evidence base for their effectiveness and also of their likely side effects and interactions with conventional medicines. GPs will need to come to their own conclusions about both the actual efficacy of the substance, the potential value of the likely placebo response and how much they are willing to condone or recommend the wide range of approaches used by alternative practitioners.

A number of these have been examined scientifically and are described below.

Saint John's wort

Also known as hypericum, this is perhaps the most commonly used herbal remedy for psychological disorders. A number of placebo-controlled trials have been studied in a Cochrane systematic review (Linde et al. 2008). It has demonstrated superiority when compared to placebo, and when compared to established antidepressants, i.e. SSRIs and tricyclic antidepressants, it is equally effective. However, this study found that those studies from Germany, where is has been well established for many years, tended to be more positive. The authors suggest that this may be due to the inclusion of different types of depression in small studies reporting over-optimistic results. Side effects were fewer with St John's wort. The authors point out that the content of St John's wort differs with different preparations on the market. Of note also, this study only examined those with mild and moderately severe depression. For depressive and anxiety symptoms associated with the menopause there is some suggestion of benefit.

St John's wort suffers from a lag period of 2–4 weeks before the onset of symptom relief and a full therapeutic response can take up to 12 weeks. Side effects are much less common than with standard antidepressants, the main ones being gastrointestinal, allergic reaction and either tiredness or restlessness. There is a case report of sub-acute polyneuropathy and a photosensitivity rash co-occurring.

As St John's wort can increase the activity of cytochrome P450 the possibility of interactions with drugs metabolized using this system exists. It is recommended that concomitant use with warfarin, other antidepressants, digoxin, anticonvulsants, oral contraceptives and anti-migraine drugs be avoided where possible. An oral dose of 900 mg per day is suggested. However, use of St Johns wort is not recommended by NICE guidelines and we are not therefore recommending that UK practitioners prescribe it.

Omega-3 oil

Fish oils contain the fatty acids eicosapentaeonic acid (EPA) and docosahexaenoic acid (DHA) and these act by maintaining the neuronal membrane structure. They are also involved in the production of prostaglandins and leukotrienes. It has been suggested that EPA might help in the treatment of depression in those who do not respond to standard antidepressants. Theories on the benefits of these fatty acids stem from findings that there are abnormalities in CNS omega-3 fatty acids in those with depression and some studies have found that low blood levels have been found in those with Alzheimer's disease, schizophrenia, attention deficit hyperactivity disorder and depression. A placebo-controlled study in those with depression already receiving antidepressant treatment found a significant reduction in symptoms compared with the control group (Peet and Horrobin 2002) when prescribed with 1 g daily. Case reports and prospective studies suggest that it might be helpful in residual schizophrenia, particularly in patients responding poorly to clozapine, but further studies are required (Taylor *et al.* 2003). A Cochrane systematic review of omega-3 oils in bipolar disorder identified five studies meeting inclusion criteria, of which one showed benefits as an adjunctive treatment in those with depressive symptoms (Montgomery and Richardson 2008), leading them to caution in recommending this treatment. At this point the evidence for benefits from fish oils in depression, schizophrenia or bipolar disorder is limited.

Kava

This is the extract of a Polynesian plant, *Piper methysticum*, and is used in religious ceremonies and recreationally in the South Pacific. It is ingested in beverage form or by chewing. Early double-blind studies suggest that it may be superior to placebo and equivalent to benzodiazepines in the treatment of anxiety. In addition the incidence of side effects is reported to be very low with probably little risk of dependence. However, these studies are limited in number, the diagnostic criteria for anxiety were non-specific and there is no clear information on optimal dosage. In addition the duration of treatment was no longer than a few months and so firm information on the dependence potential is lacking.

A Cochrane review (Pittler and Ernst 2004) examining six studies found that patients receiving kava extract did improve significantly more than those on placebo. The report concluded that kava was effective and safe but for no longer than six months as further studies into its long-term efficacy and safety are required. As well as being used as an anxiolytic it also has muscle relaxant and hypnotic properties. It is mildly intoxicating and there have also been reports of its abuse, the latter causing scaly skin lesions, known as kavaism. It interacts with alcohol, antidepressants and analgesics and should not be used in pregnancy or when breastfeeding. A further problem is its potential for hepatotoxicity (Ernst 2007), making it unsuitable for clinical use. This has led to its banning in several European countries, while in the UK the importation or sale of most of its derivatives is prohibited.

Valepotriates (valerian extract)

This substance has been suggested as being a potential anxiolytic and has recently been examined in a pilot study comparing placebo, diazepam and valerian extract (Andreatini *et al.* 2002). Using a random allocation following a placebo wash-out period, 36 outpatients meeting DSM criteria for generalized anxiety disorder were randomized to one of the three treatments for 4 weeks. Diazepam and valerian extract showed a significant reduction in the cognitive aspects of anxiety but valerian did not impact on other features such as physical symptoms. This small study, while preliminary, does suggest that valerian extract might have an effect on the psychic component of anxiety. Clearly larger studies are required. A Cochrane systematic review (Miyasaka *et al.* 2006) identified this study also as the only one suitable for inclusion of a total of eight that were identified. The conclusion was that, based on this single study, no conclusions could be drawn about the efficacy of valerian in comparison with placebo or diazepam. Thus there is little to support the use of these derivatives in those with anxiety.

Ginseng

A herbal remedy that is widely recommended for treatment of fatigue and to ward off adverse reactions to stress is Siberian ginseng. Used for several millennia in China, it only became popular in the West in the 1950s. It has been used by Russian athletes to improve stamina and it is often prescribed by Russian doctors to improve general health, much as doctors prescribe tonics in Britain and Ireland. A recent study from the University of Iowa (Hartz *et al.* 2004) compared Siberian ginseng against placebo in a group of patients with chronic fatigue and found that only those with less severe fatigue showed a positive response. As this was the first trial to examine ginseng the authors recommend further studies.

Acupuncture

Acupuncture has not been as widely investigated as other alternative remedies. In anxiety disorders it may have a role in those with hyperventilation and in those with PTSD although there have been few studies and these have methodological problems.

A Cochrane systematic review of acupuncture in the treatment of depression (Smith *et al.* 2010) identified 30 studies that met the inclusion criteria involving over 2800 subjects. The authors concluded that there was insufficient evidence of benefit compared to waiting-list control or sham acupuncture. Two found that it may have an additive benefit in combination with medication. There was a high risk of bias in the inclusion criteria. The authors found that there was insufficient evidence to recommend acupuncture for the treatment of depression. Similar conclusions were reached in another systematic review (Leo and Ligot 2007), albeit with smaller numbers.

Acupuncture is also used in the treatment of generalized anxiety and while some benefit has been demonstrated in acute anxiety its role in generalized anxiety disorder is less clear. Moreover, the studies vary in quality and sample sizes are small. An excellent review of the effect of acupuncture on depression and anxiety is provided by Pilkington (2010). Thus, based on the totality of the information to hand, the use of acupuncture for either depressive illness or generalized anxiety has a questionable evidence base and clearly further studies are required.

Other

Aromatherapy has been the subject of some investigation but the studies have major methodological flaws and more robust studies are required to justify its use (Perry and Perry 2006). It may help reduce anxiety and depressive symptoms in women who are experiencing menopausal symptoms. Massage has been used as an adjunctive therapy in those with cancer to reduce anxiety and physical symptoms due to chemotherapy. However, in those with primary psychiatric disorder there is little evidence supporting its use although it may reduce symptoms of anxiety in the short term. However, the few studies that are available in this group are non-randomized and have small sample sizes.

Meditation in the treatment of anxiety disorders has also been the subject of a Cochrane review but only two studies were identified and while the effects were similar to other interventions the dropout rate was high (Krisanaprakornkit *et al.* 2006).

Summary

- The evidence for the efficacy of herbal remedies is patchy.
- There are also indicators that some are worthy of further scientific examination.
- St John's wort has the strongest evidence but only in mild to moderate depression.

References

Andreatini, R., Sartori, V. A., Seabra, M. L., and Leite, J. R. (2002). Effects of valepotriates (valerian extract) in generalised anxiety disorder: a randomised placebo-controlled pilot study. *Phytotherapy Research*, **16**, 650–654.

Ernst, E. (2007). Herbal remedies for depression and anxiety. *Advances in Psychiatric Treatment*, **13**, 312–316.

Hartz, A. J., Bentler, S., Noyes, R., *et al.* (2004). Randomised controlled trial of Siberian ginseng for chronic fatigue. *Psychological Medicine*, **34**(1), 51–61.

Kessler, R., Soukup, J., Davis, R. B., *et al.* (2001). The use of complementary and alternative therapies to treat anxiety and depression in the United States. *America Journal of Psychiatry*, **158**, 289–294.

Krisanaprakornkit, T., Sriraj, N., Piyavhatkul, N., *et al.* (2006). Meditation therapy for anxiety disorders. *Cochrane Database of Systematic Reviews*, **1**, CD004998.

Leo, R. J., and Ligot, A. (2007). A systematic review of randomised controlled trials of acupuncture in the treatment of depression. *Journal of Affective Disorders*, **97**, 13–22.

Linde, K., Berner, M. M., and Kriston, L. S. (2008). St. Johns Wort for major depression. *Cochrane Database of Systematic Reviews*, **4**, CD000448.

Miyasaka, L. S., Atallah, A. N., and Soares, B. (2006). Valerian for anxiety disorders. *Cochrane Database of Systematic Reviews*, **4**, CD004515.

Montgomery, P., and Richardson, A. J. (2008). Omega-3 fatty acids for bipolar disorder. *Cochrane Database of Systematic Reviews*, **2**, CD005169.

Peet, M., and Horrobin, D. F. (2002). A dose ranging study of the effects of ethyl-eicosapentaenoate in patients with ongoing depression despite adequate treatment with standard drugs. *Archives of General Psychiatry*, **59**, 913–919.

Perry, N., and Perry E. (2006). Aromatherapy in the management of psychiatric disorders: clinical and neuro-pharmacological perspectives. *CNS Drugs*, **20**, 257–280.

Pilkington, K. (2010). Anxiety, depression and acupuncture: a review of the clinical research. *Autonomic Neuroscience*. Epub ahead of print. DOI.10.1016j. autneu.2010.04.002.

Pittler, M. H. and Ernst, E. (2004). Kava extract for treating anxiety (Cochrane Review). *The Cochrane Library*, Issue 1. Chichester: Wiley.

Smith, C. A., Hay, P. P. J., and MacPherson, H. (2010). Acupuncture for depression. *Cochrane Database of Systematic Reviews*, **1**, CD004046.

Taylor, D., Paton, C., and Kerwin, R. (2003). Fish oils in schizophrenia. In *The Maudsley 2003 Prescribing Guidelines*, 7th edn. London: Martin Dunitz.

Further reading

Ernst, E., Pittler, M. H., Stevinson, C., *et al.* (2001). *The Desktop Guide to Complementary and Alternative Medicine.* London: Harcourt.

Index

TERMS AND CONDITIONS OF USE

1. Licence

(a) Cambridge University Press grants the customer a non-exclusive licence to use this CD-ROM **either** (i) on a single computer for use by one or more people at different times **or** (ii) by a single user on one or more computers (provided the CD-ROM is used only on one computer at one time and is always used by the same user).

(b) The customer must not: (i) copy or authorise the copying of the CD-ROM, except that library customers may make one copy for archiving purposes only, (ii) translate the CD-ROM, (iii) reverse-engineer, disassemble or decompile the CD-ROM, (iv) transfer, sell, assign or otherwise convey any portion of the CD-ROM from a network or mainframe system.

(c) The customer may use the CD-ROM for educational and research purposes as follows: material contained on a simple screen may be printed out and used within a fair use/fair dealing context; the images may be downloaded for bona fide teaching purposes but may not be further distributed in any form or made available for sale. An archive copy of the product may be made where libraries have this facility, on condition that the copy is for archiving purposes only and is not used or circulated within or beyond the library where the copy is made.

2. Copyright

All material within the CD-ROM is protected by copyright. All rights are reserved except those expressly licensed.

3. Liability

To the extent permitted by applicable law, Cambridge University Press accepts no liability for consequential loss or damage of any kind resulting from use of the CD-ROM or from errors or faults contained in it.